Mapping AIDS

In this innovative study, Lukas Engelmann examines visual traditions in modern medical history through debates about the causes, impact and spread of AIDS. Utilizing medical AIDS atlases produced between 1986 and 2008 for a global audience, Engelmann argues that these visual textbooks played a significant part in the establishment of AIDS as a medical phenomenon. However, the visualizations risked obscuring the social, cultural and political complexity of AIDS history. Photographs of patients were among the earliest responses to the mysterious syndrome, cropped and framed to deliver a visible characterization of AIDS to a medical audience. Maps then offered an abstracted image of the regions invaded by the epidemic, while the icon of the virus aspired to capture the essence of AIDS. The epidemic's history is retold through clinical photographs, epidemiological maps and icons of HIV, asking how this devastating epidemic has come to be seen as a controllable chronic condition.

Lukas Engelmann is a Chancellor's Fellow at the University of Edinburgh.

Global Health Histories

Series editor

Sanjoy Bhattacharya, *University of York*

Global Health Histories aims to publish outstanding and innovative scholarship on the history of public health, medicine and science worldwide. By studying the many ways in which the impact of ideas of health and well-being on society were measured and described in different global, international, regional, national and local contexts, books in the series reconceptualise the nature of empire, the nation state, extra-state actors and different forms of globalization. The series showcases new approaches to writing about the connected histories of health and medicine, humanitarianism, and global economic and social development.

Mapping AIDS

Visual Histories of an Enduring Epidemic

Lukas Engelmann

University of Edinburgh

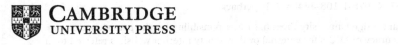

CAMBRIDGE
UNIVERSITY PRESS

CAMBRIDGE
UNIVERSITY PRESS

University Printing House, Cambridge CB2 8BS, United Kingdom

One Liberty Plaza, 20th Floor, New York, NY 10006, USA

477 Williamstown Road, Port Melbourne, VIC 3207, Australia

314-321, 3rd Floor, Plot 3, Splendor Forum, Jasola District Centre, New Delhi - 110025, India

79 Anson Road, #06-04/06, Singapore 079906

Cambridge University Press is part of the University of Cambridge.

It furthers the University's mission by disseminating knowledge in the pursuit of education, learning and research at the highest international levels of excellence.

www.cambridge.org
Information on this title: www.cambridge.org/9781108444057
DOI: 10.1017/9781108348959

First published 2018
First paperback edition 2020

A catalogue record for this publication is available from the British Library

Library of Congress Cataloging in Publication data
Names: Engelmann, Lukas, 1981- author.
Title: Mapping AIDS : visual histories of an enduring epidemic /
    Lukas Engelmann.
Other titles: Global health histories (Series)
Description: Cambridge, United Kingdom ; New York, NY : Cambridge
    University Press, 2018. | Series: Global health histories | Includes
    bibliographical references and index.
Identifiers: LCCN 2018023525| ISBN 9781108425773 (hardback : alk. paper) |
    ISBN 9781108444057 (pbk. : alk. paper)
Subjects: | MESH: Acquired Immunodeficiency Syndrome–history |
·   HIV Infections–epidemiology | History, 20th Century | History,
    21st Century | Atlases
Classification: LCC RA643.83 | NLM WC 17 | DDC 614.5/99392–dc23
    LC record available at https://lccn.loc.gov/2018023525

ISBN   978-1-108-42577-3   Hardback
ISBN   978-1-108-44405-7   Paperback

To Kate

Contents

Figures

Acknowledgments

Writing about the history of AIDS would not be possible without the tireless efforts of those who have struggled and fought to save lives and to change the course of AIDS. This book pays tribute to the memory of the lives lost in the epidemic and is dedicated to the remembrance of the past of a devastating disease that continues to disrupt our present.

Pointing out beginnings is difficult. But I would like to start with a series of undergraduate seminars organized by Isabell Lorey and Linda Hentschel, which introduced me, first, to the adventures of thinking visually about history and, second, to thinking politically about disease and immunity. From developing my master's thesis to the completion of my dissertation, which forms the basis of this book, I am profoundly grateful to my advisers: the historian of medicine Volker Hess and the feminist sociologist of knowledge Sabine Hark. Volker Hess provided persistent and patient guidance into the historical worlds of medicine; his extensive expertise on the production of medical knowledge was an essential and tenacious foundation for this project. Sabine Hark has shown me how to conduct a history of the present and has been a brilliant guide in learning to negotiate the complex political waters of HIV/AIDS with zeal, integrity and political compassion.

The colloquium at the Center for Interdisciplinary Women's and Gender Studies (ZIFG) at Technical University–Berlin allowed me to unpack intricate and difficult questions in an inspiring forum, characterized by a shared commitment and rare intellectual friendship. The colloquium at my graduate school "Gender as Category of Knowledge" boasted an abundant wealth of expertise, experience and knowledge that I have come to miss ever since. I would like to thank all who have contributed to the lively and productive discussions in these thought-incubators. Among the peers and colleagues, of which many have become friends, I would like to warmly thank Nana Adusei-Poku for knitting together visual frameworks in search of our academic milieu; Mike Laufenberg for the pleasure of reading and teaching Canguilhem and Foucault together; Sarah Speck for balancing intellectual collaboration with political comradery in fundamentalist times; Lisa Malich for together uncovering new ways of doing medical history; and Gabriele Dietze for resolute questions about my project's stakes. I would like to thank Gregg Bordowitz, who came to Berlin to share his impressive work. And I am indebted to Brigitte Weingart, whose book on infectious words has been my key reference for many, many years and whose commentary on my project was generous, insightful and productively challenging.

Without the support of Ilana Löwy, I would have not taken up a visiting PhD student fellowship at the Department for the History of Science at Harvard University. Thanks largely to the fantastic mentorship from Jeremy Greene, my term at the department has been an enriching and inspiring experience. My gratitude to the graduate students and especially to Lisa Haushofer for a warm welcome, David Jones for taking me on his course, Peter Galison for advice on atlases, Charles Rosenberg for his thoughtful comments on the normalization of AIDS and Allan Brandt for his generosity in sharing deep insights into the history of AIDS. It was a most remarkable experience to witness the premiere of "United in Anger" in New York's MoMA in 2012, and I am deeply indebted to Jim Hubbard for the generous invitation and for sharing thoughts about his life and work.

Finishing the PhD, supported by a helpful write-up retreat at the Fondation Brocher in Geneva, would have not been possible without the critical and careful reading that Mike Laufenberg dedicated to my manuscript. My gratitude goes also to Sarah-May Dang, whose feedback and patience carried it through to the printer. The transition into this book began at the Institute for the History of Medicine, now the Center for Medical Humanities at the University of Zurich. I would like to extend my warm thanks to Flurin Condrau for supporting my work all the way through and giving me the pleasure of collaborating with the brilliant Janina Kehr on the blurred lines between anthropology and history and between tuberculosis and HIV/AIDS. Many thanks to Mark Honigsbaum, Sandra Eder and Niklaus Ingold. In Zurich, I was also fortunate to be able to consolidate collaboration with Beate Schappach and Sophie Junge along the lines of our shared commitment to AIDS history.

In Cambridge, working on the visual history of bubonic plague since 2014, I would like to thank Christos Lynteris, who showed compassion and inspiring encouragement towards this book. Warm thanks to Branwyn Poleykett, Nick Evans, Emma Hacking, Catherine Hurley,

Simon Goldhill, Tim Lewens and all members of CRASSH for their inputs, questions and helpful critiques. Also, closer to the end, many thanks to Richard McKay, Karen Jent and Lisa Haushofer for their feedback on the final manuscript. Furthermore, this book became real through the encouragement of Sanjoy Bhattacharya, the series' editor, and Lucy Rhymer, who I am thrilled to call my editor at Cambridge University Press. And finally, my thanks to the anonymous reviewers for their attentive and productive feedback.

But beyond all these inputs, friendly and fierce critiques, one outstanding person deserves my utmost gratitude. Kate Womersley has single-handedly given me the courage to translate my German thesis; she has shared her incredibly sharp intellect, her brilliant eye and her impeccable writing skills to teach me invaluable insights into my work and into the finesse of style and tone in English, and she has lent an unsurmountable amount of dedication and commitment to the book. Thank you, this book would not be here without you. I am lucky to call you my partner, and I am sure our shared and deeply intermingled future will allow me to give back. Here's to many more books you and I will write together.

I owe my parents a great deal, but also this book. Without their enduring support and their unshakable belief in my work, I would have struggled to maintain focus and my economic independence. Also, Emanuel Kann has contributed more to this book than he would believe. Friends are essential, and without them this book would have remained an impenetrable mental obstacle. My warmest thank you and big hugs for engaging discussions, caring commitment and brilliant distractions to Anne Lenz and Lotte Lenz, Michi Brosig, Resa Haeckel, Magali Mander, Sonja Neuweiler, Mathias Boehm, Paul Buntzel, Vojin Saša Vukadinović, Tatjana Kononenko, Vanessa De Vries, Lena Kahle and my siblings Julez and Jonas.

What is left is to express thanks to all the participants in workshops, conferences, seminars and meetings who, over the years, generously engaged with my presentations. Financial support has been given to this book through a fellowship of the DFG in Germany and through a fellowship from the Fondation Brocher in Switzerland. My thanks also to the staff of the Staatsbibliothek zu Berlin and the Widener Library as well as the Countway Library in Harvard for their invaluable support in writing this book.

Introduction

Looking back on his medical practice during the mid-1980s – a time when the acronym AIDS was widely known but little understood – the dermatologist Alvin E. Friedman-Kien recalled that at the New York Hospital where he worked, not all doctors would see the immuno-compromised patients. Selective physicians who turned these cases away knew that Friedman-Kien had a different attitude. These doctors would "walk [the patients] over to my office," he remembers, "and say, 'This doctor will take care of you. I don't see this disease.'"[1] Their resistance toward "seeing the disease" may have been the result of widespread prejudice, anxiety about how this new syndrome threatened medical authority or simply fear of infection. Even though AIDS was certainly not invisible, it could be left unseen.

Friedman-Kien's account reminds us how difficult it was to see, recognize and diagnose AIDS more than 30 years ago. Very few doctors – most by circumstance rather than intent – had cared for patients affected by the emerging epidemic. The medical profession struggled to recognize the blurred pattern of this new disease and showed hesitation toward its patients. A lack of biomedical information, speculation about the syn-drome's association with sexual identities and bodily practices, and public response structured by a toxic combination of fear, bigotry and blame all obstructed AIDS from being seen within the confines of a straightforward clinic consultation.

Today, it is once again difficult to see AIDS. In the West, full-blown cases are rare. Even if they appear, clinicians are encouraged not to speak of AIDS. They refer to consequences from an unmanaged Human Immunodeficiency Virus (HIV) infection, perhaps even call it *HIV disease*. Three centuries of activism, reforming public and global healthcare and tireless advocacy against stigma, rejection and isolation have all shifted the image of the AIDS epidemic away from many of its original

---

[1] Ronald Bayer and Gerald M. Oppenheimer, *AIDS Doctors: Voices from the Epidemic* (Oxford: Oxford University Press, 2000), 102.

1

associations and anxieties. The introduction of HAART (highly active anti-retroviral treatment) in 1995 shifted the experience of AIDS for patients and turned the threat of impending death into a manageable infection with HIV; that is, if life-saving medication is accessible.[2] Our contemporary difficulty in seeing AIDS is very different in kind to that of the 1980s. This book asks how the challenges of seeing the epidemic have changed, and what we can learn about the normalization of a disease from the perspective of its visible and invisible histories.

AIDS is not a disease. It is not a condition composed of an exclusive set of unique symptoms. Rather it is understood as an underlying disposition, an immunodeficiency, that lays the body vulnerable to a series of opportunistic infections that appear in unusually severe and lethal patterns. The syndrome is caused by an HIV infection, as was hypothesized in 1983 and confirmed in 1986. HIV is best described as a retrovirus that slowly depletes the body's defenses against common and normally trivial infections like herpes. In the host, HIV remains mostly invisible within human cells, leading to an asymptomatic stage that is often called clinical latency. An unrecognized and untreated HIV infection will – after eight years, on average, though there is wide variation – leave the patient vulnerable to critical illness. Only then do the emerging patterns of disease suggestive of the underlying syndrome enable a doctor to "see the disease."

To this end, a small, medically trained minority repurposed one of the nineteenth century's most powerful empirical instruments of medical classification to assert the profession's authority. Their collaborative clinical response to the crisis was to create an atlas and reinvent this historical pinnacle of medical taxonomy in the context of an unknown disease. They adapted traditions of medical visualization, including clinical photography to portray AIDS as a disease, geographical mapping of AIDS as epidemic and modeling viruses to picture the infection. The AIDS atlas, first published in 1986, was set up to map out the contours of the syndrome. It promised to establish order where there was little.

This is a book about seeing AIDS in the atlas: It is a book about the challenges of mapping AIDS as a disease through photographs, seeing the syndrome as an epidemic in maps and its identification with the HIV infection in models of the pathogen. AIDS may have been one of the most formidable challenges in history to the medical perspective of

---

[2] HAART is a combination therapy whose last element, the protease inhibitor Saquinavir, was approved by the Food and Drug Administration (FDA) in 1995. HAART succeeded in suppressing the replication of the virus, leading to a dramatic and at times indefinite extension of the clinical latency of HIV.

definition and diagnosis, as it seemed so deeply entrenched in social, cultural and political conflict. But endeavors to see AIDS as an object of medical knowledge were informed by long-standing routines of visualization in medicine. These practices and procedures were mobilized in the atlas to continuously separate signs of medical significance from the manifold ways of seeing AIDS as anything other than a medical subject.

What does it mean to see a disease? Scholarship in the history of medicine has developed two modes to address the visibility of diseases, epidemics and infections. The first approach considers seeing disease as a metaphor for representation. Seeing neglected diseases, previously unknown conditions and symptoms whose definition lacked specificity, promises recognition of patients' suffering. "Making visible" is an ethical process of accepting the social structure of sickle-cell anemia, for example, seeing lung cancer as an outcome of smoking, recognizing the mental and physical strain imposed by office buildings or illuminating the backgrounds of rare genetic conditions.[3] AIDS, with its venerable history of stigmatization, neglect, identity politics and social struggle is to historians a recurrent case to demonstrate how deeply seeing enabled the syndrome's representation as a political, social and cultural subject.[4]

A second approach to seeing disease is associated with visualization of a disease as an object of medical knowledge. Visualization here should be understood as the pursuit to identify a disease's cause, classify its appearance and refine its scientific definition. Focus falls on the technical and scientific challenges of visualization, concern for how pictures contributed historically to knowing a disease medically, how pictures have enabled identification and diagnosis and how they have structured biomedical practices.[5] These questions can never be fully disconnected from

[3] Keith Wailoo, *Dying in the City of the Blues: Sickle Cell Anemia and the Politics of Race and Health* (Chapel Hill: University of North Carolina Press, 2014); Allan M. Brandt, *The Cigarette Century: The Rise, Fall, and Deadly Persistence of the Product That Defined America* (New York: Basic Books, 2007); Michelle Murphy, *Sick Building Syndrome and the Problem of Uncertainty: Environmental Politics, Technoscience, and Women Workers* (Durham, NC: Duke University Press, 2006); Diane B. Paul and Jeffrey P. Brosco, *The PKU Paradox: A Short History of a Genetic Disease* (Baltimore: Johns Hopkins University Press, 2013).

[4] See, e.g., Sander L. Gilman, *Disease and Representation: Images of Illness from Madness to AIDS* (Ithaca, NY: Cornell University Press, 1988); Roger Cooter and Claudia Stein, "Visual Imagery and Epidemics in the Twentieth Century," in *Imagining Illness: Public Health and Visual Culture*, ed. David Harley Serlin (Minneapolis: University of Minnesota Press, 2010), 169–92; Tara Burk, "Radical Distribution: AIDS Cultural Activism in New York City, 1986–1992," *Space and Culture* 18, no. 4 (2015), 436–49, doi:10.1177/1206331215616095.

[5] The obvious case here is, of course, the history of mental illnesses and their reflection in visualization practices. See, e.g., Georges Didi-Huberman, *Invention of Hysteria: Charcot and the Photographic Iconography of the Salpetriere* (Cambridge, MA: MIT Press, 2003).

the politics of a disease's representation, but coaxing this separation is useful to emphasize different modes in the historical analysis of disease visualizations. The first – the metaphorical approach to visualization – tends to presuppose an ethical imperative of radical and indefinite illumination, while the second approach is one of selection, focusing and curation. As I show here, the challenge of seeing AIDS as a disease is inevitably a process structured by principles of stringency, decisiveness and accuracy.

Such a medical visualization was encouraged, organized and subsequently archived in the AIDS atlas. It rests on three modes of seeing and thinking through its subject: clinical photographs, geographical disease maps and models of viruses. They combine a practice of mapping AIDS; a practice of visualization that measures, gauges, appraises, calibrates and informs understanding of AIDS. Pictures were cropped, framed, assembled and annotated to produce meanings for a professional audience; this process made the pictures medically legible and tamed the abundant implications associated with immunodeficiency at the time. A medical vision was separated from and cleansed of popular perception, and constantly actualized to keep track of the rapid transformation of AIDS. With each renewal and revision of the atlas from 1986 to 2008, as it transformed into new editions and subsequent series, under changing editorships and in different publishing houses, the consecutive adaptation and refinement of the atlas have left us with a precious set of sources. This series provides us today with the archive of many consecutive medical visions of AIDS.

This study offers a medical visual history of AIDS that looks beyond the strategies of making AIDS merely visible. It unfolds a series of visualizations in which the shifting social appearance of AIDS, the emerging geographical diversity of the epidemic and the microbiological depth of the HIV infection was depicted and presented, curated, arranged, focused and mapped. In this story, AIDS does not become increasingly visible, more brightly lit until we are able to see every facet

---

Reflections on the productive forces of pictures in medicine is usually scattered among rather general approaches to visual history and "image science." A German collection has reflected on the relationship between pictures and *Gestalt* in medicine, which is perhaps most closely associated with the argument made in this book. W. J. T. Mitchell, *What Do Pictures Want? The Lives and Loves of Images* (Chicago: University of Chicago Press, 2005); Bernd Hüppauf and Peter Weingart, eds., *Science Images and Popular Images of Sciences* (New York: Routledge, 2008); Frank Stahnisch and Heiko Bauer, *Bild und Gestalt. Wie formen Medienpraktiken das Wissen in Medizin und Humanwissenschaft?* (Hamburg: Lit Verlag, 2007); Hans-Jörg Rheinberger, "Experimental Systems: Historiality, Narration, and Deconstruction," in *The Science Studies Reader*, ed. Mario Biagioli (New York: Routledge, 1999), 417–29.

of its enormously complex social, cultural and medical appearance. A moving focus from the patient's body to the geographical distribution to the hidden workings of a virus might suggest increasing the field of sight, extending the depth of focus and revealing unseen truths. But the analysis of the historical layers of pictures of AIDS does not contribute to an increased transparency, and neither has medical sobriety ever achieved to overcome the subject's many faces.[6] Rather, this book pursues the conviction that AIDS has never been liberated from the shadows of doubt, uncertainty and confusion that were associated with the epidemic from its earliest days. Instead, we witness a process of unseeing AIDS. With each new frame, with each new perspective offered by doctors, epidemiologists and scientists, other visions, older versions and past representations move out of focus and into history.

Each time a claim was made about what counted as a real representation of the epidemic, other perspectives were condemned to the archive. In the changing arrangements of useful medical representation, wider questions arise for the history of medicine, such as how visual sources inform and shape the appearance and perception of diseases, epidemics and infections. Furthermore, I ask how the medical visualizations of AIDS engaged with the epidemic's broad social, political issues and cultural implications. How is a medical picture separated from other ways of seeing? Can we ever speak of a medical visualization that is a cleansed picture of the disease, or do we rather see the reassertion of medical authority through successive integration of the political and social questions that emerged with the arrival of AIDS? This leads to the historical outline of this book, which questions how practices of medical visualization that long predate the emergence of AIDS became part of the destigmatization, scientification and, most notably, normalization of AIDS.

The AIDS atlas proposes its own order; the political, epistemological and social implications of this medical order constitute the subject of this book. But such order has been – and remains – under continual strain: There was the emergence of an epidemic that did not fit with established classifications and frameworks in the once supposedly dying field of infectious diseases in the 1980s. There was the sociology of risk associated with the epidemic, which resisted calls for medical rationality and attached notions of infection to sexual identity and the supposed pathology of certain homosexual and urban lifestyles. And there was a rapidly

---

[6] On the often-misunderstood political risks of transparency, see: Stefanos Geroulanos, *Transparency in Postwar France: A Critical History of the Present* (Stanford, CA: Stanford University Press, 2017).

changing geography, deeply tied to the longer natural history of the epidemic, its globalization and its devastating future. And finally, the intricacies of HIV catalyzed the development of a rapidly mounting research industry that reshaped the epidemic into a techno-scientific stream of interventions and innovations.

Looking at the history of AIDS through its configurations in the atlas is an opportunity to reconstruct the normative character of the syndrome at different points over the past 30 years. Visual traditions have shaped the process of normalizing AIDS by supporting the transformation of an old AIDS into a new AIDS. Traditions of medical photography encouraged the historical shift of seeing AIDS beyond symptoms of opportunistic infections and the persons affected by the syndrome. Conventions of medical geography shaped new perspectives on the epidemic's societal impact and its emerging global shape. Routines of visualizing a pathogen iconized the countless abstract and artificial instantiations of HIV. Stripped of obvious pathological connection, the models and technical diagrams of the virus as an inconspicuous submicroscopic entity signal the arrival of a manageable and normalized time of the epidemic.

Since Georges Canguilhem's seminal thesis, we have routinely worked under the assumption that the normal is not the necessary and certainly not always the logical opposite of the pathological. Canguilhem encouraged appreciation of norms associated with the pathological to move beyond an impoverished positivist framework in which health and normality were thought of as one and the same.[7] The healthy, he writes, are not only those without clinical signs and lacking experience of symptoms, but health needed to be understood as more than normal, as "an exuberance that is not limited to and by norms, but indeed constructs them."[8] Diseases, however, present themselves as situations in which humans are constricted by norms, governed by the failure of organs, for example. They are also directed through regimens of treatment, coaxed to adopt therapeutic behaviors, manuals of visitation and routines of living with a disease. Visualizing the disease, and especially portraits of pathogens as images of a disease's most reliable nature, were to Canguilhem vital instruments through which to devise the norms and routines of dealing with a disease. "To see an entity is already to foresee an action," he suggests.[9] Accordingly, as the AIDS atlas offers different norms of seeing

---

[7] Georges Canguilhem, *On the Normal and the Pathological* (Dordrecht, the Netherlands: Reidel, 1978).

[8] Stefanos Geroulanos and Todd Meyers, "Introduction: Canguilhem's Critique of Medical Reason," in *Writings on Medicine*, ed. Georges Canguilhem (New York: Fordham University Press, 2011), 3.

[9] Canguilhem, *On the Normal and the Pathological*, 40.

and thus proposing the shape of the entity of AIDS through time, it predisposes different kinds of actions.

For Canguilhem, the norms of seeing a disease were grounded in the transition from thinking of diseases as poorly differentiated situations of life, to an entity of scientific inquiry that has a qualitative difference to health. "A vulgar hierarchy of diseases still exists today," Canguilhem wrote in the 1950s, "based on the extent to which symptoms can – or cannot – be readily localized."[10] This division continues to structure contemporary ways of seeing diseases and its analytical capacity is decisive to the history of AIDS visualization in the atlas. Canguilhem recognized that some diseases were associated with dispositions, malignant excesses of life's forces, and mutation and monstrous deformation of health and normal physiology. Examples include cancers, endocrine dysfunctions or chronic conditions of deteriorating physiology, such as diabetes. For Canguilhem these conditions, often given the prefix *dys*, can be only incrementally differentiated from the normal condition to which they are seen in quantitative difference: as an excess or deficiency of an otherwise healthy body. Diseases that are defined through constitutive difference are by contrast usually attributed to the presence of an infective organism, or seen in localized causes that exist and persist relatively independently from human physiology. Such an ontology of diseases assists thinking a fully disclosed nature of a disease, which is seen in qualitative difference to human life. The disease agent, from a bacterium to a virus, Canguilhem suggests, appears as a picture that claims to be evil, an entity whose entire figuration is constituted as an antithesis to human life.[11]

The history of AIDS normalization resonates between the two edges of this framework. It exposes how a poorly defined, underlying condition of immune deficiency was deeply implicated in the lifestyle of a subpopulation, before the disease became separated from patient identities and societal mores, and instead was confined to the complex but discrete mechanics of a microbiological agent. Within this history, we find the differentiation of the morphology of a Kaposi's sarcoma (KS) lesion from the patients' identity; the diffusion of AIDS as an ecological condition of communities, cities and nations; and the successful separation of a virus from the ways in which it travels, infects and multiplies. This is the history of the sequential mapping of AIDS through clinical photographs,

---

[10] Ibid., 39.

[11] Canguilhem argues that a rational optimism would need to reject any notion of the reality of evil and rather consider the kind of values that are placed in absolute opposition to what is considered to be health. Ibid., 103.

geographical maps and virus models. In the atlas, we trace how the medical perception of AIDS went from questioning *who* got the disease, to *where* the epidemic was moving, to a fixation about *what* AIDS is.

*

Inevitably, this is a book about pictures, or rather an AIDS history presented as a visual triptych of photography, mapping and modeling. My inquiry begins when pictures addressed pressing issues about AIDS but follows them as they disappeared or moved to the edge of the frame as new challenges in the epidemic's history demanded new ways of picturing, seeing and thinking about AIDS. Pictures move across history as much as they cross boundaries of knowledge and fields of thinking about AIDS. Photographs linked the clinical imaging laboratory to the politics of activism and AIDS art; maps merged epidemiology with governments' public health communications; virus models bridged the submicroscopic worlds of molecular biology and the human experiences of millions across the globe. These three pictures – photographs, maps and models – do not exclusively belong to one practice, one way of thinking or seeing, but rather embody the relations and connections of an object across boundaries of disciplines and fields.

AIDS provoked the most substantial and extensive crisis to biomedicine in the late twentieth century. The emerging epidemic buried the 1970s utopia of a world without infectious diseases, and submerged medicine into an open-ended stream of politically and culturally charged interpretations of the unfolding crisis, sentencing medical professions to helplessness and passive observation as otherwise healthy, young men died in great distress. With infectious disease doctors unable to define a stable entity causing this suffering, or a discrete disease to fight, the shapes, meanings and dooming prospects of AIDS seemed to develop at an unrelenting pace. Many scholars have argued, that in the early years of the epidemic, medicine was effectively sidelined by other voices.[12] Where pharmaceutical and conservative treatment failed, practices of prevention were devised behind activist picket lines, fortified by a growing corpus of social studies. Assessment of the epidemic's societal impact seemed better articulated through cultural critiques then by public health departments, which were struggling on both sides of the Atlantic with the highly sexualized crisis at hand.

---

[12] See, e.g., the contribution to this excellent collection of poignant cultural analysis of the epidemic: Douglas Crimp, ed., *AIDS: Cultural Analysis, Cultural Activism* (Cambridge, MA: MIT Press, 1988).

Despite previous signs to the contrary, medicine seems to have prevailed. Looking back to a time when those beyond medical profession – patient advocates, activists, historians and social scientists – seemed to have a firmer grip on the questions that mattered (both to persons with AIDS as well as to society's fears about AIDS), the weakness of medicine has been largely forgotten and today seems unthinkable. In an unforeseen twist, the medical profession – from clinicians to lab scientists – not only regained authority, but also AIDS today appears as a crisis more easily attributed to failures of national or international politics and inhumane patent regulations than any failure of medical knowledge or proficiency.

This book searches for an answer to the question about how medicine regained this control over the epidemic, in terms of administering care as well as managing the disease's social and cultural repercussions. Was medical authority reinstalled after an initial period of shock and despair by finding systematic and rigorous treatment regimens to deal first with opportunistic infections, then with social attitudes and false conceptions, to arrive finally at a techno-scientific pharmaceutical solution? Or should we take a step back and ask if medicine after the AIDS crisis was still the same compared to what it had been before. In other words, is this a history of medically guided integrating, adapting, appropriating and sustaining criticism that were posed to the medical professions by patient-cum-activists, social scientists, historians and policy advocates?

The answers lie in the larger history of visualizing disease, far beyond the history of AIDS after 1981. Photographs of patients were in circulation almost immediately after the invention of photography in the mid-nineteenth century, geographical mapping had a decisive impact on perceptions of epidemics as measurable and manageable entities, while the visualization of pathogens was not just a result of laboratory medicine but essential to the transformation of microbes into agents of infectious disease. The long nineteenth century and its characteristic push for modernization, the introduction of scientific practice and mounting political regulation of medicine shaped visualization practices into powerful and spectacular instruments of medical classification.[13] To make sense of AIDS, to stake the importance of a medical vision, the tradition of these practices mattered. Clinical photography, medical

---

[13] See, e.g., John Harley Warner, "The History of Science and the Sciences of Medicine," *Osiris* 10 (1995), 164–93; Steven Sturdy and Roger Cooter, "Science, Scientific Management, and the Transformation of Medicine in Britain c. 1870-1950," *History of Science* 36, no. 114 (1998), 421–66; Michael Worboys, *Spreading Germs: Disease Theories and Medical Practice in Britain, 1865-1900* (Cambridge: Cambridge University Press, 2000).

geography and pathogen visualization had become routinized practices with agreed-upon conventions. They each had unique and extensive capacities to render signs and patterns into objects of medical significance. The atlas of AIDS harnessed this history of visualization and the abundant visual culture of AIDS to distill and present a stringent and accurate medical form.

My analysis encourages a perception of AIDS pictures as moving objects claimed by different protagonists at different times to articulate various ways of seeing and understanding the epidemic.[14] The book reaches from opinions about what is significant within a photograph or map, to the associations that are expected when one sees a suffering person, a moving geographic distribution or the outline of the virus. Motives, shapes and figures have no inherent medical nature, but can be made medically meaningful. To look at pictures as objects characterized by an interpretative flexibility, we can point beyond the historical analysis of the political and rhetorical oppositions that structured so much of AIDS history. Instead, the pictures provide a historical archive of the obstacles and complexities that were referenced across activism, medicine and politics. A source and a starting point of problematization practices, pictures lead us to an archive of strategies and tactics employed to make sense of AIDS.[15] They encourage us to reflect on the three central embodiments of a disease that modern medicine has made available: the individual body in the clinic, the diseased space in epidemiology and the pathogen in microbiology.[16]

Histories of AIDS

Photographs were the earliest images of AIDS. Since 1981, cameras – on the streets and in the clinics – captured the mysterious appearances of unusually severe infections on what the Center for Disease Control

---

[14] For the original discussion on boundary objects, see John R. Griesemer and Susan Leigh Star, "Institutional Ecology, 'Translations' and Boundary Objects: Amateurs and Professionals in Berkeley's Museum of Vertebrate Zoology, 1907–39," *Social Studies of Science* 19, no. 3 (1989), 387–420. For a recent discussion of the continued relevance of the concept and beyond, see Geoffrey C. Bowker et al., *Boundary Objects and Beyond: Working with Leigh Star* (Cambridge, MA: MIT Press, 2016).

[15] This only hints at the extensive discussion of problematization as a method of historical research, which Foucault repeatedly compared to a kind of diagnostic perspective onto the archive, comparable to the clinician's gaze. See, e.g., Michel Foucault, "Polemics, Politics and Problematizations," in *Ethics: Subjectivity and Truth*, ed. Paul Rabinow and Robert Hurley (New York: New Press, 1997), 111–19.

[16] Michel Foucault, *The Birth of the Clinic: An Archaeology of Medical Perception* (New York: Pantheon Books, 1973), 9.

(CDC) referred to as otherwise healthy young men. Artists like Nan Goldin took haunting stills of infected friends in despair, while journalistic photographers tried to communicate the fear of the disease in portraits of people with AIDS.[17] In hospitals, the camera was often the only way to arrive at a medical representation of the severe infections and shocking symptoms in entirely unfamiliar demographics. Photography enabled a perception of AIDS as a series of discrete diseases, played out on individual patient bodies, to support clinical theories and approaches regarding the new syndrome. Before the close of the 1980s, the photograph had become a contested mode of visualization, criticized by cultural scholars and activists for being too "medical," for being "phobic images,"[18] while in clinical settings, criticized for lacking diagnostic value.

To see disease impact and visualize the actual epidemic, the geographer Peter Gould co-wrote a paper in 1991 that sought to predict the "next map" of AIDS. With three colleagues, he tagged incidence rates of infection to terrain coordinates and geographical features "to find those linkages, those invisible connections on an invisible, but tragically real, human landscape."[19] Gould, like many geographers at that time, wanted to draw global attention to the moving localities of AIDS, and dismantle the misconception that social categories and sexual identities were particularly susceptible. AIDS's forceful first appearance in its infamous and intimate relation to the male homosexual community of American urban centers had contributed to making invisible the epidemic's effects in the hinterland of the United States, its impact on IV drug users, prevalence among women and its catastrophic extension across the African continent.[20] Crucially, maps supported the development of an epidemiological approach to AIDS, a figuration of a spatial metaphor beyond the individual body. But with geographic clarification of the epidemic's

---

[17] Sophie Junge, *Art about AIDS, Nan Goldin's Exhibition Witnesses: Against Our Vanishing* (Berlin: De Gruyter, 2016), doi:10.1515/9783110453072; Lukas Engelmann, "Photographing AIDS: Capturing AIDS in Pictures of People with AIDS," *Bulletin of the History of Medicine* 90, no. 2 (2016), 250–78; David Campbell, *The Visual Economy of HIV/AIDS*, 2008, www.visual-hivaids.org; J. Currie, S. Trejo, and C. Goldin, *Gran Fury: Read My Lips* (New York: NYU Steinhardt, 2011).

[18] Douglas Crimp, "Portraits of People with AIDS," in *Melancholia and Moralism: Essays on AIDS and Queer Politics*, ed. Douglas Crimp (Cambridge, MA: MIT Press, 2002), 83–107.

[19] Peter Gould et al., "AIDS: Predicting the Next Map," *Interfaces* 21, no. 3 (1991), 89.

[20] Abraham Verghese, Steven L. Berk, and Felix Sarubbi, "Urbs in Rure: Human Immunodeficiency Virus Infection in Rural Tennessee," *Journal of Infectious Diseases* 160, no. 6 (1989), 1051–5; Gena Corea, *The Invisible Epidemic: The Story of Women and AIDS* (New York: HarperCollins, 1992); Helen Epstein, *The Invisible Cure: Why We Are Losing the Fight against AIDS in Africa* (New York: Picador, 2008).

breadth came bewildering spatial diversity. The many different epidemics of AIDS that emerged through this geographic revision complicated a unified perception of what AIDS was and what it continues to be.

By the mid-1990s the idea of "seeing HIV itself" remained a trusted signifier of the disease. It is an old trope to think of a virus such as HIV as an invisible enemy. Pictures of the virus – whether an electron micrograph, or a stylized model of its viral component parts – provide us with a singular entity of HIV, in which scientists, public health campaigners, affected communities, activists, pharmaceutical companies and patients could locate a common adversary. Fundamentally, seeing HIV as a pathogen allowed a sighting of a new disease beyond AIDS's bodily representation or geographic burden. Visualizing HIV empowered a techno-scientific perspective on AIDS, governed by the disciplines of virology and microbiology, and it symbolized the pathway to the end of AIDS, to its control and one day its eradication.

All three genres of visualization – photographs, maps and models – carry indices of the social and cultural struggle that dominated much of the epidemic's past. Paula Treichler has brilliantly shown that AIDS can never just be defined as a disease, secure in the hands of medical institutions. Rather it appeared as an "epidemic of signification."[21] From the plethora of conspiracy theories to religious declarations of guilt and divine punishment, the early discourses of AIDS revolved almost entirely around the trope of the homosexual male body. Questions of *who* would get AIDS, were at risk and posed risk to others were short-circuited by a renewed merging of homosexuality and pathology.[22] Gayle Rubin has described the depth of the predicament of these dangerous stereotypes and stigmatizations:

Just when homosexuals have had some success in throwing off the taint of mental disease, gay people find themselves metaphorically welded to an image of lethal physical deterioration. The syndrome, its peculiar qualities, and its transmissibility are being used to reinforce old fears that sexual activity, homosexuality, and promiscuity led to disease and death.[23]

---

[21] Treichler used this phrase to characterize the open-ended stream of meanings, interpretations and theories that had been attached to AIDS in science, medicine and media, which claimed to signify the true nature or to represent the true picture of the epidemic. Paula A. Treichler, "AIDS, Homophobia, and Biomedical Discourse: An Epidemic of Signification," in *AIDS, Cultural Analysis, Cultural Activism*, ed. Douglas Crimp (Cambridge, MA: MIT Press, 1988), 31–70.

[22] For a summary of the debate see: Vernon A. Rosario, *Homosexuality and Science: A Guide to the Debates*, Controversies in Science (Santa Barbara, CA: ABC-CLIO, 2002).

[23] Gayle S. Rubin, "Thinking Sex: Notes for a Radical Theory of the Politics of Sexuality," in *The Lesbian and Gay Studies Reader*, ed. Henry Abelove et al. (New York: Routledge, 1993), 164.

Where medicine failed to provide a stable explanation or a unanimous definition of the disease, the excess of its meanings fell out of proportion, leaving us with the impression of an "epistemic anomaly," as Brigitte Weingart wrote.[24] Medical authority, discussed by Alex Preda in his study on AIDS rhetoric, lacked the "rules of seeing" that were necessary to establish clear guidelines for clinical practice and for the syndrome's interpretation.[25] Susan Sontag, in her groundbreaking essay on the metaphors of AIDS, declared that AIDS was a crisis of medical categories and classification systems. The "medical inference"[26] did not integrate smoothly into then-existing textbooks and atlases of medicine. Furthermore, the crisis of AIDS was emphatically seen as a crisis of the social fabric, sexual identity and racial categories. A model of epidemic uncertainty and a crisis of medical authority, AIDS reorganized the relationship between medicine and society.[27] "The brief history of AIDS," Charles Rosenberg had already written by 1986, "illustrates both our continuing dependence on medicine – for better or worse – and the way in which disease necessarily reflects and lays bare every aspect of the culture in which it occurs."[28] An early lesson of AIDS, as Allan Brandt has described in detail, was that a medical perception of the epidemic could not possibly emancipate itself from social struggles, cultural values and economic problems that constituted the "epidemiological nature" of the syndrome, even if that might have been desirable.[29] The same, of course, accounts for the epidemic's visualization in an AIDS atlas.

---

[24] Brigitte Weingart, *Ansteckende Wörter, Repräsentationen von AIDS* (Frankfurt am Main: Suhrkamp, 2002), 79.

[25] Alex Preda, *AIDS, Rhetoric, and Medical Knowledge* (Cambridge: Cambridge University Press, 2005), 48.

[26] Susan Sontag, *AIDS and Its Metaphors* (New York: Farrar, Straus and Giroux, 1989), 20.

[27] Allan M. Brandt, "AIDS in Historical Perspective: Four Lessons from the History of Sexually Transmitted Diseases," *American Journal of Public Health* 78 (1988), 367–71; Allan M. Brandt, *No Magic Bullet: A Social History of Venereal Disease in the United States since 1880*, Oxford Paperbacks (New York: Oxford University Press, 1987); Allan M. Brandt, "How AIDS Invented Global Health," *New England Journal of Medicine* 368, no. 23 (June 6, 2013), 2149–52, doi:10.1056/NEJMp1305297; Gerald M. Oppenheimer, "In the Eye of the Storm: The Epidemiological Construction of AIDS," in *AIDS: The Burdens of History*, ed. Elizabeth Fee and Daniel M. Fox (Berkeley: University of California Press, 1988), 267–300.

[28] Charles E. Rosenberg, "Disease and Social Order in America: Perceptions and Expectations," *The Milbank Quarterly* 64, no. 1 (1986), 53. See also his well-known consideration of epidemics as sampling device for underlying social and cultural questions: Charles E. Rosenberg, "What Is an Epidemic? AIDS in Historical Perspective," in *Living with AIDS*, ed. Stephen R. Graubard (Cambridge, MA: MIT Press, 1989), 1–17.

[29] Brandt, *No Magic Bullet*, 5.

The atlas was embedded within, not just affected by, cultural conventions and social structures.

The impurity of scientific accounts of AIDS that were intended as immune to homophobia, politics of neglect and outright ignorance have been analyzed and exposed by Steven Epstein. His study points to the genesis of ill-defined categories, such as the prototype term for AIDS, "Gay-Related Immunodeficiency Syndrome" (GRIDS). His work encourages consideration of how lesbian, gay, bisexual, and transsexual (LGBT) activism, lay experts and political movements penetrated the closed ranks of committees and professions and how community-based research projects turned into large-scale campaigns to get "drugs into bodies."[30] Winning access to the committees that devised national research direction was essential to the activists, who finally in 1990 conquered the meeting rooms of the National Institutes of Health (NIH) in Bethesda through direct action.[31] Not only were the gay communities of the early 1980s most affected by AIDS, they battled against stigmatization in their bid to find strategies to overcome, or at least contain, the crisis. "AIDS became a 'gay disease,'" Epstein recalls, "primarily because clinicians, epidemiologists, and reporters perceived it through that filter, but secondarily because gay communities were obliged to make it their own."[32] Where medical solutions such as treatment or vaccination failed, strategies of prophylaxis addressed social behavior, sexual practices and dragged the issue of preventing AIDS, with all its contentious and uncannily intimate associations, into the wider public.[33]

While the relative success of declining infection rates at the end of the 1980s was commonly attributed to social change and political campaigns, the West remained blind to the emerging international scope of the pandemic. Cindy Patton has drawn attention to the globalization of AIDS not as an equal distribution of a single epidemic around the world, but as a system of classification in which AIDS reflected global structures of inequality. AIDS in Africa was perceived as a fundamentally different

---

[30] Steven Epstein, *Impure Science: AIDS, Activism, and the Politics of Knowledge* (Berkeley: University of California Press, 1996), 50, 186.

[31] David France, *How to Survive a Plague: The Story of How Activists and Scientists Tamed AIDS* (London: Pan Macmillan, 2016), 414.

[32] Epstein, *Impure Science*, 55.

[33] See, e.g., the following studies for narratives of how activist strategies were transformed into policy and public health strategies: Jennifer Brier, *Infectious Ideas: U.S. Political Responses to the AIDS Crisis* (Chapel Hill: University of North Carolina Press, 2009); Virginia Berridge, *AIDS in the UK: The Making of a Policy, 1981–1994* (Oxford: Oxford University Press, 1996); Peter Aggleton et al., eds., *AIDS: Safety, Sexuality and Risk* (London: Taylor & Francis, 1995); Paul Sendziuk, *Learning to Trust: Australian Responses to AIDS* (Sydney: University of New South Wales Press, 2003).

disease from the original American AIDS.[34] Shrouded by ecological controversy and abstracted images of the "African tragedy," as described by the *New York Times* in 1990, we have forgotten to engage with the "social concerns at the core of the AIDS epidemic" in South Africa, writes Didier Fassin.[35] Cultural anesthesia, he argues with reference to Allen Feldman and Theodor Adorno, is our capacity to render the Other's pain inadmissible, and simply forget about the catastrophe happening elsewhere.

The West's perception of AIDS as a remote crisis, embedded in the naturalized order of postcolonial global health and carried by what Paul Farmer described as "geographies of blame," was cemented when HAART became obtainable in 1995.[36] The availability of this treatment prolonged the lives of millions of infected patients and offered hope and optimism. What had been a disastrous epidemic, a return to the ages of catastrophic infectious diseases with the capacity to eradicate multitudes of people, became a chronic condition.[37] Already by the early 1990s infection rates could be controlled through practices of prevention, outbreaks could be regulated and prolonged through pharmaceutical intervention, while the phantasm of a general pandemic sweeping through society in the manner of plague and smallpox disappeared. The medical breakthrough of HAART enabled individuals, societies and nations that could afford to acquire and distribute treatment, to find themselves at the end of the twentieth century on a pathway of normalization.[38] With a steep decline in cases classified as AIDS from 1996 onward, the syndrome became practically unseen in the hospitals of North America and Europe.

---

[34] Cindy Patton, *Globalizing AIDS* (Minneapolis: University of Minnesota Press, 2002); Cristiana Bastos, *Global Responses to AIDS: Science in Emergency* (Bloomington: Indiana University Press, 1999).

[35] Didier Fassin, *When Bodies Remember: Experiences and Politics of AIDS in South Africa* (Berkeley: University of California Press, 2007), 273; Erik Eckholm, "AIDS in Africa: A Killer Rages On," *New York Times*, September 16, 1990.

[36] Paul Farmer, *AIDS and Accusation: Haiti and the Geography of Blame* (Berkeley: University of California Press, 2006); Paul Farmer et al., eds., *Reimagining Global Health* (Berkeley: University of California Press, 2013); Johanna T. Crane, *Scrambling for Africa: AIDS, Expertise, and the Rise of American Global Health Science* (Ithaca, NY: Cornell University Press, 2013).

[37] Compare the contributions to both collections, as the second presents critical commentary on the historical narrative presented in the first. Elizabeth Fee and Daniel M. Fox, eds., *AIDS: The Burdens of History* (Berkeley: University of California Press, 1988); Elizabeth Fee and Daniel M. Fox, eds., *AIDS: The Making of a Chronic Disease* (Berkeley: University of California Press, 1992).

[38] Rolf Rosenbrock et al., "The Normalization of AIDS in Western European Countries," *Social Science and Medicine* 50, no. 11 (June 2000), 1607–29.

Forgetting is another way of unseeing. In 2011, Christopher Castiglia and Christopher Reed published a provocative historical study, which described how our memory of AIDS is built on an unseen archive of the epidemic. *If Memory Serves* reflects on how we remember the past of AIDS and challenges a collective amnesia about its gay history. "Official memories," they write, "in the form of films, education, museum exhibitions, holidays, news reporting, and political speeches – constitute a potent form of forgetting even as they purport to traffic in memory."[39] The book's description of AIDS history exposes a strangely empty and largely sterile narrative in which "traumatic experience hovers, not forgotten but not remembered, on the edge of consciousness."[40] All too often, memory justifies the norms of our present, and aspects of AIDS – despite unswerving efforts to make what is invisible visible – remain unseen.

Part of a historian's craft is to define periods and moments of change and transformation. Even in the short history of AIDS, such points remain subject to exegesis and controversy. Did AIDS only fundamentally change when treatment reorganized the relationships between infected bodies, social politics and medical discourse?[41] Is a focus on this moment of pharmaceutical transformation to blame for the lasting invisibility of the epidemic within the unimagined communities, uncharted geographies and unseen networks of Sub-Saharan Africa?[42] Did a new time of AIDS only arrive, once discriminatory patent issues were in part resolved and generic medication became accessible?[43] Or should we follow a social history of activism in which the founding of ACT UP, the establishment of interdisciplinary international networks and the efforts of public health institutions are credited for containing the catastrophe?[44] Or do we attribute qualitative change to the artistic,

---

[39] Christopher Castiglia and Christopher Reed, *If Memory Serves: Gay Men, AIDS, and the Promise of the Queer Past* (Minneapolis: University of Minnesota Press, 2012), 2.

[40] Ibid., 11.

[41] Victoria Harden has recently published a historical account of AIDS from the perspective of the US NIH, which maintains the picture of the medical profession's pivotal agency in changing the face of AIDS: Victoria A. Harden, *AIDS at 30: A History* (Washington, DC: Potomac Books, 2012). For a critical account of how HIV treatment reconfigured the epidemic, see: Marsha Rosengarten, *HIV Interventions: Biomedicine and the Traffic between Information and Flesh* (Seattle: University of Washington Press, 2009).

[42] Robert Thornton, *Unimagined Community: Sex, Networks, and AIDS in Uganda and South Africa* (Berkeley: University of California Press, 2008); Epstein, *The Invisible Cure*; Mandisa Mbali, *South African AIDS Activism and Global Health Politics* (Basingstoke, UK: Palgrave Macmillan, 2013).

[43] Jeremy A. Greene, *Generic: The Unbranding of Modern Medicine*, 12.

[44] Theodore M. Brown, Marcos Cueto, and Elizabeth Fee, "The World Health Organization and the Transition from 'International' to 'Global' Public Health," *American Journal of Public Health* 96, no. 1 (2006), 62–72; Brandt, "How AIDS Invented Global Health."

cultural and theoretical interventions that changed perceptions, our mode of reflection and our thinking about the epidemic all along?[45]

The now-normalized idea that our epoch has somehow resolved the crisis of AIDS seems in need of a convincing narrative in which the notion of an *old* AIDS is successfully separated from the time of a *new* AIDS. The bygone time of AIDS is commonly characterized by a dramatic appearance of a mysterious and unusual immunodeficiency entangled with lifestyle and identity, a threat to social and cultural order, a traumatic loss of life and a tragic narrative of neglect, stigmatization and medical as well as political failure. *New* AIDS is described with sobered perception of the disease, or rather chronic condition, which is infectious – to some more than others – but can be pharmaceutically controlled. Given the financial and social resources, including a shared liberal notion of sexual networks and practices, the epidemic has simply ceased to be an epidemic. It is predominantly referred to through its causal agent: HIV. The combined acronyms of HIV/AIDS are widely used in medical circles and social sciences but what comes after the slash seems to be merely a reminder of a past that had once been the possible future of an infection.

While it is tempting to attribute such change in characterization to a single event in the history of scientific progress, to a decisive organization or network in the history of social transformation or to shifting cultural hegemonies, this book suggests a different way. With each edition of an AIDS atlas published from 1986 until 2008, AIDS was effectively separated into a time *before*, and a time *of*, the atlas. Each atlas attempted to clear up previous confusion, ambiguous definitions and open questions that had persisted up until *this* atlas was written. Revised from issue to issue, from one series to another, the announcement of a new AIDS presented through a distilled visualization of what mattered at the time was divorced from the growing archive of unseen versions of an old AIDS of the past. Rather than identifying a decisive moment in which AIDS substantially changed, I see the atlas as an ongoing commitment to medical progression. In other words, the atlas provides us with an archive that constitutes a cascade of norms between 1986 and 2008, a record of the persistence of medical authority during confusion. In consecutive collisions between historical traditions of medical seeing and the visualized politics of AIDS appear fragments of a history of the normalization of AIDS.

---

[45] Douglas Crimp and Adam Rolston, *AIDS Demo Graphics* (Seattle, WA: Bay Press, 1990); Gregg Bordowitz, *Imagevirus: General Idea* (London: Afterall Books, 2010); Currie, Trejo, and Goldin, *Gran Fury: Read My Lips*.

The AIDS Atlas

On first flush, scanning from one atlas edition to another, a story of AIDS's increasing complexity appears. The volumes tell a story of tireless research, expanding knowledge about manifestations on patients and insights into the virus' pathways and intricate mechanics. Closer observation refines this impression: Photographs dominate the earliest editions, seemingly the most trustworthy media in the first decade of AIDS, as they were essential touchstones with clinical signs on bodies in the initial confusion. Through each edition, hundreds of clinical photographs document the wide range of opportunistic infections that were thought to be related and therefore were classified within the rubric of AIDS, and that were strongly associated with the demographic groups in which the syndrome was appearing. Maps, the spatial diagrams of the epidemic, are sparsely scattered in the first editions, but would become the "face" of AIDS as the pandemic globalized in the 1990s. Maps promised to visualize the bigger picture. But they also risked turning a blind eye to the catastrophe of individuals who were amalgamated into datapoints. Models of HIV did appear in the first edition, and remained present in all subsequent editions, but it took until 1995 for the virus to take center stage. At this point, the atlas presents HIV as the agreed-upon, all-encompassing icon of the epidemic's original cause and its critical point of intervention. The viral model worked as synecdoche for a scientific- and evidence-based perception of the syndrome beyond its social, cultural and physiological appearance.

The atlas does not present an emphatic turning point or fissure when a previously unseen syndrome suddenly appeared in photographs of infected bodies. There is not a decisive point when pictures of individuals were replaced with cartographic representation of the AIDS space, or finally subsumed by the icon of HIV. Rather, it is through the editors' arrangement and ordering of the atlases' pictures in subtle configurations of references, shifting infrastructures of presentation and transforming visual economies that a collection of pictures becomes a visualization of AIDS. The historian and anthropologist of photography, Elisabeth Edwards, argued that "the material forms in which photographs are arranged . . . is integral to their phenomenological engagement, structuring visual knowledge."[46] In the atlas, editors positioned photographs in

---

[46] Elizabeth Edwards, *Raw Histories: Photographs, Anthropology and Museums* (London: Bloomsbury Academic, 2001), 16.

relation to maps and to virus models, added captions and sorted the images below headings and into groups to create a complex visualization of AIDS.

By convention, the genre of the medical atlas tends to be restricted to a medical specialty such as dermatology or oncology, complete representations of human anatomy or dedicated to single organs such as the brain. As they group diseases into classes, atlases are rarely dedicated to a single disease or syndrome.[47] The production of a new atlas for a new disease, maybe even a new genre of diseases, toward the close of the twentieth century, is a surprising, perhaps outmoded move. It not only emphasized the atlas as a dire call for medical authority to consolidate professional perspectives and practices regarding AIDS, it also established a specific structure of thinking through the syndrome. The atlas emphasized AIDS as a vulnerability to a long list of discrete disease entities that could be seen wreaking havoc over the patient body, and it encouraged the visualization of a syndrome that implicated different medical specialties. The atlas characterized AIDS as a rubric of other diseases.

When Rosenberg developed his well-known proposition that epidemics have a dramaturgic structure, he stressed the affinity of AIDS with older diseases. "AIDS has shown itself both a very traditional and a very modern sort of epidemic," he wrote, "evoking novel patterns of response and at the same time eliciting – and thus reminding us of – some very old ones."[48] It seems at times as if the ancient format and long-established authority of an atlas was sought in the second half of the 1980s to articulate an adequate response to the raging epidemic of signification, to control the epistemic anomaly and to establish a new infrastructure of knowledge.

Ludwik Fleck reminds us that the atlas – like the textbook – was once considered to be at the top of a hierarchy of written genres committed to knowledge production.[49] An atlas, Fleck argued, seeks to define the disciplines, negotiates understandings of facts and forms a collective thought-style as a consensual way of seeing.[50] The atlas' historical relationship

---

[47] The rare exception to this history is provided by two atlases on syphilis, both dedicated to the task of separating signs of syphilis from other dermatological diseases. Franz Mracek, *Atlas der Syphilis und der venerischen Krankheiten mit einem Grundriss der Pathologie und Therapie derselben*, Lehmann's Medicin. Handatlanten (München: J. F. Lehmann, 1898); Leo v. Zumbusch, *Atlas der Syphilis* (Leipzig: F. C. W. Vogel, 1922); Erich Langer, *Atlas der Syphilis* (Berlin: Berliner Medizinische Verlagsanstalt, 1949).

[48] Rosenberg, "What Is an Epidemic?," 3.

[49] Ludwik Fleck, *Genesis and Development of a Scientific Fact* (Chicago: University of Chicago Press, 1981), 161.

[50] Ilana Löwy, "Ways of Seeing: Ludwig Fleck and Polish Debates on the Perception of Reality," *Studies in History and Philosophy of Science* 39 (2008), 375–83.

to the foundations of objectivity and empirical sciences has been convincingly argued by Lorraine Daston and Peter Galison.[51] Atlases are "dictionaries of the sciences of the eye," they write, as each atlas collects, assembles and illustrates the state of current knowledge of its subject (as defined by its title). An atlas essentially teaches its readers how to see objectively.[52] Atlases of biology, astronomy, geology and anatomy offer objective cartographies of a field of knowledge, replicating those thoughts, hypotheses and facts that have become resistant to controversy within the field. In this way, atlases guarantee consistency and unity, while their authors tend not to be aspiring to produce divisive texts.

As an epistemological heavyweight, an atlas presents itself as a curated collection of valued and validated knowledge. It jealously guards its own immunity from the to-and-fro of discussion, critique and uncertainty. The ideal atlas teaches its student to recognize, and it taxes the eyes of the experienced expert. Yet, as Daston and Galison point out, the capacity of an atlas of gross anatomy to epitomize modern objectivity through the collective endeavor of anchoring visual information to unambiguous definitions and semantics did not always translate well into the realm of the pathological atlas. Atlases of disease were instead committed to present endless variety of pathological phenomena against the background of an established genre of visual anatomy, the reference norm.[53] Paradox and challenge were inevitable when the fastest-changing field of medicine was cataloged in a genre that heralds from a stable pillar of medical education.[54] But the representation of pathology in the AIDS atlas evidently needed to claim a different position of authority to that in the atlases of anatomy and natural science.

In the early nineteenth century, the appeal of a pathological atlas was not that it provided an account of archetypal disease species, ordered in abstracted tableaus of classes and systems in the tradition of German

---

[51] Lorraine Daston and Peter Galison, "The Image of Objectivity," *Representations*, no. 40 (1992), 81–128; Lorraine Daston and Peter Galison, *Objectivity* (Cambridge, MA: Zone Books, 2007).

[52] Daston and Galison, *Objectivity*, 22.

[53] Michael J. Ackermann, Judith Folkenberg, and Benjamin Rifkin, *Human Anatomy: Depicting the Body from the Renaissance to Today* (London: Thames & Hudson, 2006). Foucault, *The Birth of the Clinic*, 119.

[54] Carin Berkowitz, "The Illustrious Anatomist: Authorship, Patronage, and Illustrative Style in Anatomy Folios, 1700–1840," *Bulletin of the History of Medicine* 89, no. 2 (2015), 171–208, doi:10.1353/bhm.2015.0028; Eva Åhrén, "Figuring Things Out," *Nuncius* 32, no. 1 (January 1, 2017), 166–211, doi:10.1163/18253911-03201007.

Naturphilosophie. Influenced by the publications of the French pathologist Jean Cruveilhier, new empirical endeavors of the 1800s refused to follow aesthetic conventions of anatomical atlases, whose goal had been to capture the idealized human form in all its intricacy.[55] "It is no accident," Daston and Galison argue, "that pathological atlases were among the first to use characteristic images, for neither the *Typus* of the 'pure phenomenon' nor the *Ideal*, with its venerable associations with health and normality, could properly encompass the diseased organ."[56] Characteristic images of a disease do not aim for exactitude or completeness. Instead they capture an organ in its typical habitus with unusual lesions, manifestations of stigmata that bear some features of a typical appearance of a disease. This visualization is not the same as claiming a stable and ever-identical appearance but remains committed to a representation of a changing and shifting subject, or as Foucault described, disease appears in an "aleatory series."[57]

The first AIDS atlas was published in 1986, when the epidemic was five years old. Charles Farthing, leading the editorial team, was at that time a research registrar at St. Stephen's Hospital (today's Westminster Hospital) in London and an eminent doctor in the United Kingdom's early AIDS years. Farthing would go on to enjoy international recognition as a consultant for various international organizations working on AIDS policy. His co-editors were the dermatological consultant Richard Staughton and the clinical photographer Simon Brown. The same triumvirate of editors published the second edition of the atlas in 1988, entitled *The Colour Atlas of AIDS and HIV Disease.* Both editions were brought to press with the London-based publishing house Wolfe Medical Publications, which was known for its extensive repertoire of medical textbooks and clinical monographs.[58]

[55] Jean Cruveilhier, *Anatomie pathologique du corps humain ou descriptions avec figures lithographieés et coloriées des diverses altérations morbides* (Paris: Baillière, 1829); Lukas Engelmann, "Eine analytische Bildpraxis. Die pathologisch-anatomischen Zeichnungen Jean Cruveilhiers in ihrem Verhältnis zu klinischen Beobachtungen," *Berichte zur Wissenschaftsgeschichte* 35 (2012), 7–24; P. P. De Saint-Maur, "The Birth of the Clinicopathological Method in France: The Rise of Morbid Anatomy in France during the First Half of the Nineteenth Century," *Virchows Archiv* 460, no. 1 (2012), 109–17, doi:10.1007/s00428-011-1162-2.
[56] Daston and Galison, *Objectivity*, 82 (emphasis in original).
[57] Foucault has described the order of diseases in nineteenth century as an aleatory series, in which variations of a single disease became part of indefinite chain of references, whose studying trained the physician's eyes. Foucault, *The Birth of the Clinic*, 119.
[58] Charles F. Farthing et al., eds., *A Colour Atlas of AIDS (Acquired Immunodeficiency Syndrome)* (London: Wolfe Medical Publications, 1986); Charles F. Farthing, ed., *A Color Atlas of AIDS* (Chicago: Year Book Medical Publishers, 1988).

The second series of atlases was published in the United States at Saunders in Philadelphia. The chief editor of 1989's *Color Atlas of AIDS* was the renowned dermatologist and established expert on KS, Alvin E. Friedman-Kien. This was the doctor confident enough to see patients with the disease, introduced previously. He had been involved in AIDS research since its very first days in New York City. His perspective on the characteristics of AIDS and especially on the appearances of KS as part of AIDS was put down into atlas form. The purpose of his atlas was "[d]rawing the distinction between a benign condition and a dermatologic presenting sign of AIDS,"[59] and to this end he presented more than 200 photographs, predominantly detailing KS, the 1980s index disease of AIDS. The second edition in the same atlas series arrived seven years later in collaboration with Clay J. Cockerell, another dermatologist. In this updated work, Farthing, the first atlas editor, was put in charge of a new chapter on the "History of AIDS."[60]

A third series appeared in the United States, this time with Springer and initially under the editorship of Donna Mildvan, who would go on to lead three subsequent editions. Mildvan was also a clinician, but a specialist of infectious diseases. She had worked in AIDS research since the start of the epidemic. The first edition in her series appeared in 1995 as a volume of the *Atlas for Infectious Diseases* under the title *AIDS*. A second edition was published in 1997, co-edited by Gerald L. Mandell, after which the series became a stand-alone atlas in 2001, published by the same editors, as *Atlas of AIDS*. It was finally renamed and updated again in 2008 as the *International Atlas of AIDS*, edited solely by Mildvan and the last atlas on AIDS to date.[61]

Despite the authorship of the atlas, they were not niche texts for an interested few. Several of the atlases were translated into German, Spanish, Portuguese and Japanese.[62] Most of the editions received positive and enthusiastic reviews.[63] There were several specialized atlases that

---

[59] Alvin E. Friedman-Kien, ed., *Color Atlas of AIDS* (Philadelphia: Saunders, 1989), xv.

[60] Alvin E. Friedman-Kien and Clay J. Cockerell, eds., *Color Atlas of AIDS* (Philadelphia: W. B. Saunders, 1996), 1 ff.

[61] Donna Mildvan, ed., *AIDS*. Vol. 1. Atlas of Infectious Diseases (Philadelphia: Current Medicine, 1995); Donna Mildvan, *AIDS*, 2nd ed. Vol. 1. Atlas of Infectious Diseases (Philadelphia: Current Medicine, 1996); Gerald L. Mandell and Donna Mildvan, eds., *Atlas of AIDS*, 3rd ed. (Philadelphia: Springer, 2001); Donna Mildvan, ed., *International Atlas of AIDS*, 4th ed. (Philadelphia: Springer, 2008).

[62] Farthing's first atlas was translated to German and Japanese: Charles F. Farthing, ed., *AIDS: Erworbenes Immundefekt-Syndrom. Ein Farbatlas* (Stuttgart: Schwer, 1986); Charles F. Farthing, 広瀬俊一, and 松本孝夫, カラーアトラスAIDS (Tokyo: Igaku Shoin, 1987).

[63] Jeffrey S. Dover, "Review: Color Atlas of AIDS," *Archives of Dermatology* 125, no. 6 (1989), 857–8; John L. Ziegler, "Review: Color Atlas of AIDS and HIV Disease,"

focused on particular clusters of manifestations or affected organs, such as the ocular or oral manifestations of AIDS, each of which addressed a tightly circumscribed professional audience.[64] Also, a very different (but essential) companion was the extensive *London International Atlas of AIDS*, published by Blackwell and edited by three eminent geographers, Matthew Smallman-Raynor, Andrew Cliff and Peter Haggett from Cambridge, United Kingdom.[65] Equipped with a perspective and expertise distinct from the clinical and microbiologically motivated definitions of AIDS seen in other atlases, the geographic atlas did share similar aims: to arrive at an exhaustive picture of AIDS as a presence in time and space, but also to establish a coherent geographic critique of AIDS.

All clinical editors of the AIDS atlas had worked on the epidemic from its earliest days. Farthing studied dermatology at St. Stephens's hospital when he saw a pattern emerging among his patients who had rare skin conditions.[66] He joined the dermatological clinic in 1984, praised for having treated AIDS patients with respect rather than as pariahs. His inclusive practice contributed significantly to bringing AIDS out of "the shadows," as one who had encountered his ambition recalled in a recent obituary.[67] Patients, as well as their relatives, expressed their enduring gratitude for Farthing's courageous insistence on humane treatment of those cases dismissed by many as an uncontainable threat. Farthing, a gay doctor, dedicated his life to researching AIDS and HIV, and he influenced the slowly evolving British AIDS policy under Thatcher's conservative government in the 1980s. He worked on medical trials testing the feasibility of drugs such as AZT[68] at the end of the decade, before he moved to the United States to join the AIDS Healthcare

---

JAMA: The Journal of the American Medical Association 261, no. 24 (1989), 3621–2; Anita Grassi, "Review: A Color Atlas of AIDS," *Archives of Dermatology* 124, no. 1 (1988), 145; Ronald J. Marsh, "Review: A Colour Atlas of AIDS and HIV Disease," *British Journal of Ophthalmology* 74, no. 1 (1990), 64; "Review: Color Atlas of AIDS," *The Ulster Medical Journal* 58, no. 1 (1989), 118; Thomas Monson, "Review: International Atlas of AIDS," *JAMA: The Journal of the American Medical Association* 300, no. 5 (2008), 585–6.

[64] A nonexhaustive list of AIDS atlases with a narrower focus: Daniele Dionisio, ed., *Textbook-Atlas of Intestinal Infections in AIDS* (Milano: Springer, 2003); M. A. Ansary, ed., *A Colour Atlas of AIDS in the Tropics* (London: Wolfe, 1989); Abe M. Macher, ed., *AIDS: An Atlas of Cases for Diagnosis* (Baltimore: Williams & Wilkins, 1988); Sol Silverman, *Color Atlas of Oral Manifestations of AIDS* (Toronto and Philadelphia: Mosby, 1989); Elio Guido Rondanelli, ed., *Atlante Di Clinica e Laboratorio, AIDS, Clinical and Laboratory Atlas* (Pavia, Italy: Edizioni Medico-Scientifiche, 1989).

[65] Matthew Smallman-Raynor, Andrew Cliff, and Peter Haggett, eds., *London International Atlas of AIDS* (Oxford and Cambridge: Blackwell Publishers, 1992).

[66] Berridge, *AIDS in the UK*, 26, 75.

[67] Brian Gazzard, "Charles Farthing Obituary," *The Guardian*, May 11, 2014.

[68] For the history of early drugs like Azidothymidine (AZT), also known as Zidovudine see: Steven Epstein, "Activism, Drug Regulation, and the Politics of Therapeutic Evaluation

Foundation in 1991. Remarkably, he volunteered in controversial vaccine trials as a subject, and injected himself with a weakened strain of the
virus. His atlas emerged out of his early commitment to teach doctors
how to see and how to recognize AIDS and how to adapt their daily
routines to treat patients with AIDS. Most importantly, the atlas was
driven by Farthing's commitment to his patients, to those who presented
at the time of its publication when AIDS still had an almost 100 percent
mortality rate.

Friedman-Kien was already an established dermatologist and virolo-
gist at New York University's Medical Center when he encountered the
first unusual cases of KS in young gay men. He called the CDC and
published his findings of KS in 26 gay men in New York City, which was
eventually picked up by the *New York Times* running it under the
alarming, and by now infamous, headline: "Rare Cancer Seen in 41
Homosexuals."[69] Friedman-Kien developed a deep interest in the sexual
history of these unusual patients, admitting that this was an angle
"nobody ever taught me in medical school."[70] He resisted institutional
restrictions when hospitals tried to avoid being identified with the epidemic, he advocated against stigmatization and became a renowned
specialist in the epidemic's early years.

"Dermatologists' patients don't usually die," Friedman-Kien told *New
York Magazine* in 1987, "and with AIDS you see a young person destroyed. It's devastating."[71] His career acquired an even deeper profund-
ity in the company of this disease, and his research often returned to the
puzzling patterns of KS development in AIDS patients. He knew of other
KS appearances amongst the immunosuppressed (such as patients who
underwent organ transplants), he had seen cases in elderly patients
usually of Eastern European descent and he knew of cases in Africa.
But the specific appearance of KS in the presence of AIDS, affecting a
new geography and demographic, opened a research arena in which he
worked tirelessly.[72] Friedman-Kien's atlases bore dedications on their
title pages to his patients, reflecting perhaps how his systematic approach

in the AIDS Era: A Case Study of DdC and the 'Surrogate Markers' Debate," *Social
Studies of Science* 27, no. 5 (1997), 691–726.
[69] Alvin E. Friedman-Kien, "Disseminated Kaposi's Sarcoma Syndrome in Young
Homosexual Men," *Journal of the American Academy of Dermatology* 5, no. 4 (1981),
468–71; Lawrence K. Altman, "Rare Cancer Seen in 41 Homosexuals," *New York
Times*, July 3, 1981.
[70] Bayer and Oppenheimer, *AIDS Doctors*, 53.
[71] Janice Hopkins Tanne, "Fighting AIDS: On the Front Lines against the Plague," *New
York Magazine*, no. 12, February (1987), 16.
[72] Bayer and Oppenheimer, *AIDS Doctors*, 15 f.

to the task of clinical classification was complicated and challenged by queer encounters with sexual identities and practices.

Friedman-Kien's colleague and collaborator in New York was the infectious disease expert Donna Mildvan, responsible for the most recent atlas series. A crucial and striking case from her career that she often recalled was of a 33-year-old German who came under her care in 1980. This homosexual man had lived for three years in Haiti where he worked as a chef, arriving in New York after he was struck by unstoppable bloody diarrhea and subsequent emaciation. The usual antibiotic treatments against intestinal microbes and amoebic parasites were no help, and the patient's health deteriorated. When he started to lose his vision, Mildvan and her colleagues spent hours in the hospital's library searching for obscure diseases that might be responsible. Nothing suggested itself, and no treatments proved effective. Further virological analysis threw up cytomegalovirus (CMV) and herpes simplex as possibilities, but both viruses were unlikely to have produced the intense gastrointestinal symptoms this patient was experiencing. The German patient died just two months later, neurologically deteriorated and blind. Mildvan recalls how he "stopped talking to us, he curled up in a ball, staring blindly into the distance. He was incontinent. And he died."[73] The following year, Mildvan watched the declines of similar cases, and grew suspicious that she was witnessing the natural history of a new disease. She published an important paper on these initial encounters in 1982[74] and took part in the organization of early double-blinded trials on AZT efficacy. Here began a remarkable research career in HIV and AIDS.

Throughout the late 1970s, Mildvan had been studying sexually transmitted diseases with Dan William, a gay clinical colleague, and together they identified enteric diseases caused by pathogens that enter the body orally and travel through the gastrointestinal system.[75] In the late 1970s, particularly in 1978 and 1979, Mildvan had seen several patients in a cohort of sexually active gay men who presented with unexplainable lymphadenopathy, or unusually swollen glands. In hindsight, these were perhaps some of the earliest AIDS cases to be identified. Mildvan would

[73] Tanne, "Fighting AIDS: On the Front Lines against the Plague," 19.
[74] Donna Mildvan et al., "Opportunistic Infections and Immune Deficiency in Homosexual Men," *Annals of Internal Medicine* 96, no. 6 (1982), 700–4.
[75] Richard A. McKay, "Before HIV: Venereal Disease among Homosexually Active Men in England and North America," in *The Routledge History of Disease*, ed. Mark Jackson (Abingdon, UK: Routledge Handbooks Online, 2016), doi:10.4324/9781315543420. ch24.

come to remember these nascent years of the ensuing epidemic as "medieval,"[76] characterized as they were by a return to a forgotten time of infectious epidemics, a threat that modern industrial societies in the second half of the twentieth century seemed to have overcome.

For many, but not all the emerging specialist AIDS doctors, encounters with their patients opened a new era in pathology and care. Homosexual lifestyles, drugs, poverty and racial variation required doctors to foster liberal worldviews and to overcome institutional boundaries, or what Bayer and Oppenheimer have called "middle-class blinders."[77] The unofficial qualifying expertise for the AIDS atlas editorship, unlike atlases from other medical specialties, only partially derived from outstanding medical qualifications, prestigious careers and tireless commitment to research. Perhaps more crucially, these were doctors who were moved to become editors of an atlas dedicated to their patients, clinical practice and teaching thousands of other medical students and physicians to provide better care. Their personal encounters in the clinic – what they saw, as well as what their training had taught them to see down a microscope or on a graph – qualified them, through the interplay of words and images, to define what AIDS might be and how it should be seen. The atlas' authority did not always mirror the authority of the fast pace of scientific knowledge regarding the inner-mechanics of the syndrome, but was fundamentally grounded in medical practice, clinical diagnostics and the messy, frustrating and at times devastating encounter with the epidemic on the ground.

Medicine's Visual Histories

Medicine's long-standing visual traditions are powerful instruments to approach, integrate and stabilize new, unusual and unrecognized phenomena. Nineteenth-century genealogies of medical photography, geographical mapping and microbe visualization still inform contemporary approaches to tackling medical unknowns and have had tremendous influence in making sense of the crisis of AIDS. In other words, it appears that in times of epidemiological crisis, medicine's visual practices hold an archive of opportunity, open to appropriation and application against novel and uncertain entities. Visualizations in the AIDS atlas had to liaise between *synchronous* ways of seeing AIDS throughout society with the *diachronous* traditions of making disease visible in medicine.

[76] Bayer and Oppenheimer, *AIDS Doctors*, 63.   [77] Ibid., 53.

Today, photographs of patients with KS taken in the mid-1980s leave a strange impression. An audience in 2018 finds itself confronted with a picture of a person with AIDS, yet the photograph's purpose was likely to have been to capture the essence of some element of the syndrome. One can almost sense the now-historical urgency of its maker who circulated the image to better inform doctors. Such a photograph enfolds many layers of history: The photograph's subject has most probably succumbed to the severe infections and died. The panic and unfamiliarity attached to the sight of KS has long been absent from our public spaces in the West, and the mysterious significance of this cancer's appearance as a pathological sign has been resolved. KS has disappeared from our picture of the epidemic. The KS patient in the photograph has become a historical ruin of what it once signified, and the emotions it was once capable of provoking.

Derrida's reflections on a series of photographs of ruined Greek architecture in Athens are a surprisingly fitting counterpoint to capture the strange experience of seeing a now-defunct clinical photograph that has moved from the domain of AIDS medicine into the realm of AIDS history:

An original affect, an affect without pathos, surrounds the aura of these photographs: the sense of obsolescence [l'affect de la disaffection], precisely, the affect of the one affected by this disuse or obsolescence of technical objects, defunct signs of culture.[78]

We find not only ruins, as Derrida found in Bonhomme's photographs of classic Athens, but these medical photographs materialize the resistance of AIDS history to a flattening process that wishes to leave us with a series of lessons, reports and resolutions that can be assimilated and then forgotten. A KS photograph sustains melancholia for the traumatic epidemic, as well as maintains a surplus or rather a *punctum*, as Roland Barthes called it.[79] Not only the patient who has long passed away, but more so the impression of a useless medical visualization haunts the photograph.

The practice and study of visual history has evolved over the past 25 years from the so-called visual turn in the humanities and social sciences. This turn has been concerned with W. J. T. Mitchell's

---

[78] Jacques Derrida, *Athens, Still Remains: The Photographs of Jean-François Bonhomme*, (New York: Fordham University Press, 2010), 41.
[79] Roland Barthes, *Camera Lucida: Reflections on Photography* (New York: Farrar, Straus and Giroux, 1981).

provocative question: "What do pictures want?"[80] Mitchell argued emphatically for critical reflection on the relationship between the visual and the textual realms. He insisted on the productive contributions of pictures in science and argued for a science of images and pictures to be developed.[81] Visual history has left the niches of art history and cultural studies to carve deep impressions on traditional methods of historical scholarship.[82] The shape of the historical archive has been changed, integrating questions of affect and aesthetics, while elevating photographs, diagrams and "thinking-through-images" beyond the authority of written texts. A solid scholarship in the histories of medicine and science has emerged that internalizes Nicholas Mirzoeff's claim that when looking at a history of visual culture, one must concede that "visualizing had its most dramatic effects in medicine."[83]

Such new perspectives, to which this book is indebted for much of its methodological approach, emphasize the constructive and formative position of visual sources in the production of scientific and medical knowledge.[84] Today, pictures are rarely belittled as mere representations of historical events, protagonists or objects. Photographs, now the most prominent sources in medicine's visual history, have certainly ceased to be seen as mere windows onto a forgotten past. The majority of techniques in visual history stem, as Ludmilla Jordanova has repeatedly shown, from art history.[85] The art of description sets the foundation for systematic encounter with visual sources, and has recently received new

---

[80] W. J. T. Mitchell, "Showing Seeing: A Critique of Visual Culture," *Journal of Visual Culture* 1 (2002), 165–81.

[81] W. J. T. Mitchell, "Image Science," in *Science Images and Popular Images of the Sciences*, ed. Bernd Hueppauf and Peter Weingart (New York: Routledge, 2008), 55–68; Peter Galison, "Images Scatter into Data: Data Gather into Images," in *Iconoclash: Beyond the Image Wars in Science, Religion and Art*, ed. Bruno Latour and P. Weibel (Karlsruhe, Germany: Center for Arts and Media, 2002), 300–23.

[82] See, e.g., the following titles: Daniela Bleichmar, *Visible Empire: Botanical Expeditions and Visual Culture in the Hispanic Enlightenment* (Chicago and London: University of Chicago Press, 2012); Ludmilla Jordanova, *The Look of the Past: Visual and Material Evidence in Historical Practice* (Cambridge: Cambridge University Press, 2012); Jeanne Haffner, *The View from Above: The Science of Social Space* (Cambridge, MA: MIT Press, 2013). For an introduction into the mostly German debates on "image science" see: Gerhard Paul, ed., *Visual History. Ein Studienbuch* (Göttingen: Vandenhoeck & Ruprecht, 2006).

[83] Nicholas Mirzoeff, *An Introduction to Visual Culture* (Hove, UK: Psychology Press, 1999), 6.

[84] Lisa Cartwright, *Screening the Body: Tracing Medicine's Visual Culture* (Minneapolis: University of Minnesota Press, 1995); Jennifer Tucker, *Nature Exposed: Photography as Eyewitness in Victorian Science* (Baltimore: Johns Hopkins University Press, 2005); Hüppauf and Weingart, *Science Images and Popular Images of Sciences*; David Harley Serlin, ed., *Imagining Illness: Public Health and Visual Culture* (Minneapolis: University of Minnesota Press, 2010).

[85] Jordanova, *The Look of the Past*, 16.

historical interest.[86] Yet already in the late 1990s, the question was raised how to distinguish between pictures viewed as art, and pictures seen as medical objects, or objects of knowledge.[87] A dividing line to guarantee transhistorical indices of visual art versus visual science was widely rejected and ridiculed. Rather, the evidentiary character of any picture – its accepted capacity to represent not just itself but an external object of knowledge – is endowed by the specific historical and geographical context in which pictures are produced, circulated and perceived.[88] And perhaps nothing emphasizes the instrumental function of pictures for showing something besides themselves so forcefully as placing them in an atlas.

The editors' endeavors to arrive at consensual and uncontested visual representations of AIDS were embedded within a wider vibrant visual popular culture, in which AIDS was subject to extensive artistic, often agitprop, interventions, film treatments and journalistic visualizations.[89] Deciding how AIDS would be seen was a struggle in which medical and artistic, journalistic and activist visions collided, but also often collapsed. Forms of public, artistic and journalistic interpretation of the visual culture of AIDS find their way into the atlas, disrupting and subverting the editors' intention to achieve a normative and sanitized visual representation, purified from cultural and ideological contaminants, fit to show nothing but AIDS's very own nature. Instead, what the atlas editors delivered is a negotiation of medicine's visual tradition with the politicized visual culture of AIDS.

Campbell speaks of a visual economy of AIDS, a system of changing visual references to the epidemic.[90] This "economy" structured the field of the epidemic's public perception, and aesthetic conventions impacted how AIDS appeared and disappeared, and how visual politics brought previously unseen identities, geographies and disease agents into our

---

[86] Sharon Marcus, Heather Love, and Stephen Best, "Building a Better Description," *Representations* 135, no. 1 (2016), 1–21, doi:10.1525/rep.2016.135.1.1; Lorraine Daston, "Cloud Physiognomy," *Representations* 135, no. 1 (2016), 45–71, doi:10.1525/rep.2016.135.1.45.

[87] Caroline A. Jones and Peter Galison, "Introduction," in *Picturing Science, Producing Art*, ed. Caroline A. Jones and Peter Galison (London: Psychology Press, 1998), 12.

[88] Barbara Orland, "Repräsentation von Leben. Visualisierung, Embryonenmanagement und Qualitätskontrolle im reproduktionsmedizinischen Labor," in *The Picture's Image: Wissenschaftliche Visualisierung als Komposit.*, ed. Inge Hinterwaldner and Markus Buschhaus (München: Wilhelm Fink Verlag, 2006), 222–42.

[89] Crimp and Rolston, *AIDS Demo Graphics*; Currie et al., *Gran Fury: Read My Lips*; Bordowitz, *Imagevirus: General Idea*; Beate Schappach, *AIDS in Literatur, Theater und Film. Zur kulturellen Dramaturgie eines Störfalls* (Zürich: Chronos, 2012); Junge, *Art about AIDS*.

[90] Campbell, *The Visual Economy of HIV/AIDS*.

field of vision. Sander Gilman has provided early interpretations of the public visual representation of AIDS, asking how it impacted circulating attitudes and images about the disease.[91] Following Gilman's work, a small visual medical history of AIDS emerged in the last 10 years. Claudia Stein and Roger Cooter brought attention to the visual history of AIDS posters as a key transformation of public health propaganda, in which "visuality itself [came] into intellectual focus."[92] Posters drew the public gaze to the global archive, in which these visual artifacts were placed, used and archived. Critically revisiting Gilman's early thoughts on AIDS posters, Cooter and Stein remind us forcefully that one key capacity of the visual is to transgress lines of medical expertise, foregrounding journalistic or artistic purposes instead.[93]

Departing from posters as public health instruments, the history of visualizing AIDS cannot be told without acknowledging the work of the most influential artistic collectives for US AIDS activism. General Idea and Gran Fury left a profound mark on the history of both urban cultures and "guerrilla marketing." Arresting visual statements have encouraged and attracted analysis of the aesthetics of AIDS outside of medical institutions. A visual history of AIDS would also be unthinkable without the impact of film and video practices, transformative interventions that not only brought forth narratives of those living with AIDS, but were also essential nodes for community building, mediating mourning and presenting an archive of "animation" of those lost in the trenches.[94] Many such expressions were driven by a desire to craft a visual language, where words had proved blunt tools. There was a desire to engage with the experience and subject of AIDS, by escaping the monopoly of the

---

[91] Sander L. Gilman, "AIDS and Syphilis: The Iconography of Disease," in *AIDS, Cultural Analysis, Cultural Activism,* ed. Douglas Crimp (Cambridge, MA: MIT Press, 1988), 87–107; Sander L. Gilman, "The Beautiful Body and AIDS: The Image of the Body at Risk at the Close of the Twentieth Century," in *Picturing Health and Illness: Images of Identity and Difference* (Baltimore: Johns Hopkins University Press, 1995), 115–83.

[92] Roger Cooter and Claudia Stein, "Coming into Focus: Posters, Power, and Visual Culture in the History of Medicine," *Medizinhistorisches Journal* 42, no. 2 (2007), 182.

[93] Claudia Stein and Roger Cooter, "Visual Objects and Universal Meanings: AIDS Posters and the Politics of Globalisation and History," *Medical History* 55 (2011), 85–108.

[94] M. Crewe and P. Brouard, "Film as an Educational Medium – A Review of Four HIV/ AIDS Films: Continuing Education," *AIDS Bulletin* 3, no. 3 (1994), 12–13; Jim Hubbard, "Fever in the Archive," *GLQ: A Journal of Lesbian and Gay Studies* 7, no. 1 (2001), 183–92; Jim Hubbard, *United in Anger: A History of ACT UP,* Documentary (2012); Schappach, *AIDS in Literatur, Theater und Film*; Chris Tedjasukmana, *Mechanische Verlebendigung. Ästhetische Erfahrung im Kino* (Paderborn: Wilhelm Fink Verlag, 2014).

medical gaze that had structured so many problematic aspects of how AIDS was perceived.[95]

But again, what is a representation of AIDS that is not medical? How, and to what end, can we ever define ways of seeing that free the subject of AIDS from the clinic? Does not every act of making AIDS visible contribute to the distinction of the disease, the epidemic or the microbe from what is normal and healthy? In the atlas, this distinction between the normal and the pathological enables professionals to understand and differentiate diseases, communicate between medical practitioners and represent medical authority. The apprehension of disease, one could argue, is an essential translation of the appearance and occurrence of strange, unusual and painful experiences into tables, charts and index cases. To shift what has presented itself to the doctors' eyes into words, which can be shared and scrutinized, translates the visible into discourse. To arrive at meaningful perceptions that leave behind general apprehension of the dire reality of illness, to form classes and species of disease, is the medical art of visualization. A doctor's flair for diagnosis means possession of a "speaking eye," Foucault writes, an eye that translates its sights into knowledge, that sees and speaks a diagrammatic of pathological signs.[96]

Structure

Each of the three chapters in this book situates a visual genre in its particular relevance to AIDS. It places photography, mapping and modeling of HIV in their own time of AIDS history and interrogates how each mode of seeing enabled the atlas to distill a medical vision of AIDS, and how it mitigates the notion of AIDS as an epistemological crisis. Each chapter can be read on its own and provides a coherent essay on AIDS photography, AIDS mapping and HIV modeling to those interested in the particulars of a visual configuration of AIDS/HIV. But the history of the epidemic's normalization emerges only in the unruly and inconsistent relationships drawn between these visualizations' appearance and successive fading.

---

[95] Robert Atkins, "Difficult Subject: Photographing AIDS," *Village Voice*, June 28, 1988; Jan Zita Grover, "OI: Opportunistic Identification, Open Identification in PWA Portraiture," in *Over Exposed: Essays on Contemporary Photography*, ed. Carol Squiers (New York: New Press, 1999), 105–22; Engelmann, "Photographing AIDS."

[96] Foucault, *The Birth of the Clinic*, 149; Volker Hess, *Von der semiotischen zur diagnostischen Medizin. Die Entstehung der klinischen Methode zwischen 1750 und 1850* (Husum, Germany: Matthiesen, 1993), 103.

The first chapter is dedicated to photography and follows the perspectives of clinicians regarding embodied experiences. It engages the controversies around the politics of representing the person with AIDS. Clinical photography guided the medical eye through an assortment of unusual diseases, framing them as opportunistic infections and symptoms of a new, poorly grasped underlying syndrome. These photographs bore witness to the fact that something terrifying but nevertheless biomedical was happening. Photography connected the suffering bodies through a shared identity, or as the earliest CDC report – the epidemic's birth certificate – put it, these individuals shared "some kind of homosexual lifestyle or disease."[97] Tapping into a rich archive of medical photographic practices developed since the nineteenth century, the tradition of clinical photography was reinvented to frame AIDS as a diagnostic category that relied on clustered visualizations of discrete disease entities (such as KS and Pneumocystis pneumonia [PCP]) in combination with a social and sexual identity. Today, these photographs are an archive of a chapter of AIDS history, which facilitates a reconstruction of how the rules of seeing AIDS were once set up around the "mysterious male homosexual text" to empower a clinical discourse about AIDS.[98]

The chapter rests on eminent scholarship on the medical histories of photography that reaches from photographic representations of medical practice to portraiture of disease in the nineteenth and twentieth centuries to the conceptualization of the "camera medica."[99] Jennifer Tucker

---

[97] Center for Disease Control, "Pneumocystis Pneumonia – Los Angeles," *Morbidity and Mortality Weekly Report* 30 (June 5, 1981), 250–2.

[98] Treichler, "AIDS, Homophobia, and Biomedical Discourse," 42.

[99] A nonexhaustive list of significant works on the history of medical photography influential to the perspective in this book includes: K. Aterman and J. A. Grimaud, "The Brothers Lumière: Pioneers in Medical Photography," *The American Journal of Dermatopathology* 5, no. 5 (October 1983), 479–81; Joel-Peter Witkin and Stanley Burns, eds., *Masterpieces of Medical Photography: Selection from the Burns Archive* (Pasadena, CA: Twelvetrees Press, 1987); Daniel M. Fox and Christopher Lawrence, *Photographing Medicine: Images and Power in Britain and America since 1840* (New York: Greenwood Press, 1988); Bettyann Kevles, *Naked to the Bone: Medical Imaging in the Twentieth Century* (Reading, MA: Addison-Wesley, 1998); Mike Barfoot and A. D. Morrison-Low, "W. C. M'Intosh and A. J. Macfarlan: Early Clinical Photography in Scotland," *History of Photography* 23, no. 3 (September 1, 1999), 199–210, doi:10.1080/0308 7298.1999.10443322; Erin O'Connor, "Camera Medica," *History of Photography* 23, no. 3 (September 1, 1999), 232–44, doi:10.1080/03087298.1999.10443326; Marta Braun and Elizabeth Whitcombe, "The Photography of Pathological Locomotion," *History of Photography* 23 (1999), 218–23; Didi-Huberman, *Invention of Hysteria*; John Harley Warner, *Dissection: Photographs of a Rite of Passage in American Medicine, 1880–1930* (New York: Blast Books, 2009); Kirsten Ostherr, *Medical Visions: Producing the Patient through Film, Television and Imaging Technologies* (Oxford: Oxford University Press, 2013); Jose Van Dijck, *The Transparent Body: A Cultural Analysis of Medical Imaging* (Seattle: University of Washington Press, 2015); Beatriz Pichel, "From Facial

interrogated the conditions under which the authority of photographic evidence was established to structure representations of nature in the nineteenth century.[100] Daston and Galison have paved the way for an understanding of photography as a technique of mechanical objectivity, controlled and substantiated through a once-common concern about the researcher's subjectivity.[101] The history of medical photography has left the confines of Western institutions and has been explored through medical and anthropological inquiries, expeditions and imperial and colonial encounters.[102] Collections and archives of photographs have been scrutinized in their materiality and shown to impact on how medical photographs align and resist the archival grain.[103]

By the end of the 1980s, AIDS decentered the bodies of Americans, and with them the American body politic, to expose its African origins and forge new trajectories in global health.[104] AIDS became the subject of new maps. The second chapter traces this new global vision of the epidemic and reconstructs the rationale of epidemiologists, public health advocates and geographers in the production of a new spatial order of AIDS. An original purpose of AIDS maps was to disrupt simplified patterns and models of the disease's early years, diversify the epidemic's picture and structure a new pandemic global order. A threat to social structures, national borders and illusions of global equality in healthcare

Expressions to Bodily Gestures: Passions, Photography and Movement in French 19th-Century Sciences," *History of the Human Sciences* 29, no. 1 (February 1, 2016), 27–48, doi:10.1177/0952695115618592; Christos Lynteris and Ruth J. Prince, "Anthropology and Medical Photography: Ethnographic, Critical and Comparative Perspectives," *Visual Anthropology* 29, no. 2 (March 14, 2016), 101–17, doi:10.1080/08949468.2016.1131104; Katherine Rawling, "'She Sits All Day in the Attitude Depicted in the Photo': Photography and the Psychiatric Patient in the Late Nineteenth Century," *Medical Humanities* 43, no. 2 (June 1, 2017), 99–100, doi:10.1136/medhum-2016-011092.

100 Tucker, *Nature Exposed*.   101 Daston and Galison, "The Image of Objectivity."

102 Ari Larissa Heinrich, *The Afterlife of Images: Translating the Pathological Body between China and the West* (Durham, NC: Duke University Press, 2008); Lynteris and Prince, "Anthropology and Medical Photography"; Ruth J. Prince, "The Diseased Body and the Global Subject: The Circulation and Consumption of an Iconic AIDS Photograph in East Africa," *Visual Anthropology* 29, no. 2 (2016), 159–86, doi:10.1080/08949468. 2016.1131517.

103 Edwards, *Raw Histories*; Elizabeth Edwards, "Photographic Uncertainties: Between Evidence and Reassurance," *History and Anthropology* 25, no. 2 (March 15, 2014), 171–88, doi:10.1080/02757206.2014.882834; Branwyn Poleykett, Niccolas H. A. Evans, and Lukas Engelmann, "Fragments of Plague," *Limn*, March 4, 2016, limn.it/fragments-of-plague/; Lukas Engelmann, "What Are Medical Photographs of Plague?," *REMEDIA*, January 31, 2017, https://remedianetwork.net/2017/01/31/what-are-medical-photographs-of-plague/.

104 Thomas Yingling, *AIDS and the National Body* (Durham, NC: Duke University Press, 1997); Patton, *Globalizing AIDS*; Bastos, *Global Responses to AIDS*.

access, maps of AIDS vectors cast the world into a geography of crisis. Maps provided transformative snapshots of counted and estimated cases, which showed where politics, medicine and science had failed to intervene, treat and cure. Today, many maps and their patterns of AIDS, like photographs, have become part of the historical archives. To our eyes they reveal the astonishingly ephemeral nature of the epidemic's transgressions. But they also visualize theories that guided geographers' and epidemiologists' attempts to make sense of the spaces taken over by AIDS, before the epidemic found its current stronghold in Sub-Saharan Africa.

The longer history of disease mapping has been carved out most notably by Tom Koch, and his two extensive monographs provide a rich resource for the chapter. From as early as the seventeenth century, Koch describes how maps were analytical instruments, experimental systems and ways of thinking – rather than merely representing diseases on the ground.[105] Other important contributions to the history of medical geography – to name just a few – have touched on the legacy of cholera in London and its resolution, touched on the geographical imaginary in Chinese history of bubonic plague, and extended the cartographic perspective onto viral cartographies.[106]

However, in the mid-1990s, the shape of AIDS shifted once again. Having zoomed out from the individual body of the patient to the diagram of the epidemic's global ecology, the field of vision homed onto the virus that had created many visual traces of its presence. My third chapter engages the "unseen enemy," its invisible presence in the period of clinical latency, the condition that is not yet AIDS, in models and symbols of the virus. These pictures of HIV would eventually undermine all other visualizations to become iconic of a past, present and future of

---

[105] Tom Koch, *Cartographies of Disease: Maps, Mapping, and Medicine* (Redlands, CA: ESRI Press, 2005); Tom Koch, *Disease Maps: Epidemics on the Ground* (Chicago: University of Chicago Press, 2011); on the history of medical geography, see also: Nicolaas A. Rupke, ed., *Medical Geography in Historical Perspective* (London: Wellcome Trust Centre for the History of Medicine at UCL, 2000); Frank A. Barrett, *Disease and Geography: The History of an Idea*. Vol. 23 (York: York University Press, 2000); A. D. Cliff and P. Haggett, *The Geography of Disease Distribution*, ed. R. J. Johnston and Michael Williams (Oxford: Oxford University Press, 2003); Melinda S. Meade, *Medical Geography* (New York: Guilford Press, 2010).

[106] See, e.g., Kari S. McLeod, "Our Sense of Snow: The Myth of John Snow in Medical Geography," *Social Science and Medicine* 50, no. 7 (2000), 923–35; Marta Hanson, *Speaking of Epidemics in Chinese Medicine: Disease and the Geographic Imagination in Late Imperial China* (New York: Routledge, 2012); Johanna T. Crane, "Viral Cartographies: Mapping the Molecular Politics of Global HIV," *BioSocieties* 6, no. 2 (2011), 142–66.

the epidemic. Electron micrographs and computerized models convince us today that in these portraits of HIV we glimpse the essence of AIDS. This disease agent seems to make visible an unseen nature. As schematized graphics of HIV circulated through the media, public health campaigns, illustrating scientific papers as well as books on gender, race and stigma in AIDS, these icons of the virus leave a strange representation of the epidemic: A picture displaced from affected bodies, immune to social unrest and eerily distilled from the worldly appearances of AIDS as a crisis. Most crucially, it provided a vision that never had a temporal dimension and that never became an archive. Pictures from 1983 seem to be as accurate a visualization of AIDS today as they were back at the point of their earliest production.

Many have worked on the history of technological visualization of invisible worlds inhabited by unseen microbes.[107] An extensive German scholarship examined the significance of mechanical visualization of early bacteriology, in which Robert Koch famously deemed photographs sometimes more important than the suspect specimen.[108] The visualization of viruses, as Brigitte Weingart has shown,[109] attracted wide fascination, drawing artists' critical interrogations to the lifeless, artificial and techno-scientific representations of these objects of microbiological research.[110] Hans-Joerg Rheinberger's work on microbes is of great significance as he describes their visualization to be an integral element of the experimental systems in which new entities such as viruses emerge. He argues that visualizations are traces of the research process, and the

[107] Tucker, *Nature Exposed.*

[108] Thomas Schlich, "'Wichtiger als der Gegenstand selbst' – Die Bedeutung des fotografischen Bildes in der Begründung der bakteriologischen Krankheitsauffassung durch Robert Koch," in *Neue Wege in der Seuchengeschichte*, ed. Martin Dinges and Thomas Schlich, Medizin, Gesellschaft und Geschichte (Stuttgart: Franz Steiner Verlag, 1995), 143–52.

[109] Brigitte Weingart, "Viren visualisieren: Bildgebung und Popularisierung," in *Virus! Mutationen einer Metapher*, ed. Ruth Mayer and Brigitte Weingart. Vol. 5, Cultural Studies (Bielefeld, Germany: transcript Verlag, 2004), 97–130.

[110] Ibid.; Andrea Sick, "Viren 'bilden.' Visualisierungen des Tabakmosaikvirus (TMV) und anderer infektiöser Agenten," in *Sichtbarkeit und Medium. Austausch, Verknüpfung und Differenz naturwissenschaftlicher und ästhetischer Bildstrategien*, ed. Anja Zimmermann (Hamburg: Hamburg University Press, 2005), 257–87; Thomas Baechi, "Visualisierung von Viren? 'Seeing Is Believing,'" in *VirusExpress. Rendez-Vous im Überall*, ed. Matthias Michel and Isabelle Köpfli (Zürich: Edition Museum für Gestaltung, 1997), 30–1; Angela N. H. Creager, *The Life of a Virus: Tobacco Mosaic Virus as an Experimental Model, 1930–1965* (Chicago: University of Chicago Press, 2002); Nicolas Rasmussen, *Picture Control: The Electron Microscope and the Transformation of Biology in America, 1940–1960* (Stanford, CA: Stanford University Press, 1999).

resulting icon thus processes a historiality that contributes in turn to their status as epistemic things.[111]

As far as visualizations of AIDS have been essential to the articulation of a medical, social and cultural apprehension of the epidemic, sufficient attention has not been paid to the role of fading images, the unremembered but not quite forgotten bodies and spaces, through which the disease was once experienced, understood and seen. What is left behind in the archive of the atlas is a series of visual ruins, pictures that were once used to make sense of AIDS's appearance, maps that have been drawn to emphasize a threat or an overlooked trajectory, and electron micrographs that caught undifferentiated particles, which only later were recognized as the viral agent of the disease. In these ruins of AIDS's visual history an archive of the unseen is buried. By unearthing these sights, we reclaim a history of how the emergence of an epidemic crisis was resolved through methods that were first and foremost visual.

---

[111] Rheinberger, "Experimental Systems."

1   Seeing Bodies with AIDS

The literary theorist Thomas Yingling asked a haunting question after experiencing the first decade of AIDS: What might it mean "to be a person with AIDS?" What did it mean, Yingling wrote, to secure a subjectivity for the person with AIDS that was not simply an erasure of his or her previous subjectivity, that "simply did not read the illness as the end of meaning"?[1] Losing a body, losing an identity, losing collective and spatial grounds for an open sexual, political and cultural subjectivity characterized the experiences of many living with AIDS in early years, and beyond.

Grasping, defining and seeing the "person with AIDS" was the single most important way to perceive the epidemic in its first decade. It matters, of course, that this was not a random kind of person, but from a particular population. From the first official acknowledgment of the syndrome in 1981, AIDS was a disease of gay men. And, male homosexuality became the frame through which AIDS was seen as a disease.[2] In the following years, this much-discussed conflation of sexual identity with AIDS was rejected, criticized, reworked, redefined, destabilized and normalized. Even though male homosexuality is not the dominant picture of AIDS anymore, this socio-medical conflation has a fixed position in the historical narrative of AIDS. Its history is enshrined in a wide range of questions pertaining to politics of identity in the photographic archive of the epidemic.

Photography was deeply enmeshed into the complex politics of representation of the person with AIDS. The person with AIDS was perceived by the public and doctors alike as a risk to a general, heterosexual, public health.[3] A melancholy associated itself to losing the lightheartedness of a

---

[1] Thomas Yingling, *AIDS and the National Body* (Durham, NC: Duke University Press, 1997), 22.

[2] Centers for Disease Control, "Pneumocystis Pneumonia – Los Angeles," *Morbidity and Mortality Weekly Report* 30 (June 5, 1981), 250–2.

[3] Catherine Waldby, *AIDS and the Body Politic: Biomedicine and Sexual Difference* (London: Routledge, 1996), 77 f.

lifestyle that had – once again – been overtaken by medical categories, to the extent that, as Leo Bersani commented, the foundations of sexual identity and masculinity were in peril.[4] Prompted by this abundant visual politics, Douglas Crimp characterized the struggle of identity in times of AIDS to be torn between forces of mourning and calls to militancy; a struggle driven by repeated questioning as to whether the body of a person with AIDS can be imagined – and visualized – as "still sexual?"[5]

Such questions were not a guiding concern for the atlas editors who selected and laid-out photographs in the first AIDS atlas from 1986 (Fig. 1.1).[6] This page shows sections of a male body covered in pigmented patches. The photograph's restricted views do not confide information about the identity or biography of the patient. The body's presentation in fragments – a flexed arm, the side of a face – leaves the reader in no doubt that the pictures were not intended to deliver a portrait of a person, but rather to visualize what was happening on its surface. The position of the arm and the way it has been cropped in the second picture directs attention to the discolored patches and thus to the significant phenomenon around which the design and argument of the photographs center. The caption to both photographs calls these "typical lesions of Kaposi's sarcoma in patients with AIDS."[7] While the reader might have assumed they were seeing signs of a disease on different body parts of one patient, the caption's use of the plural form asks us to believe that these pictures are from two different people with AIDS who both show typical lesions of its characteristic skin cancer. The patterned distribution of the lesions, their linearity, is described as a "common appearance," suggesting the experience of the reading doctor's eye.[8]

Both photographs are presented as classical examples of clinical photography. The editors included them to visualize exemplary signs of a condition, to allow for better recognition and understanding of the disease in the medical community by learning from such ideal cases.

[4] Ann Cvetkovich, "Legacies of Trauma, Legacies of Activism," in *Loss: The Politics of Mourning*, ed. David L. Eng, David Kazanjian, and Judith Butler (Berkeley: University of California Press, 2003), 427–57; Deborah B. Gould, *Moving Politics: Emotion and ACT UP's Fight against AIDS* (Chicago: University of Chicago Press, 2009); Leo Bersani, "Is the Rectum a Grave?," in *AIDS, Cultural Analysis, Cultural Activism*, ed. Douglas Crimp (Cambridge, MA: MIT Press, 1988), 197–222.

[5] Douglas Crimp, "Portraits of People with AIDS," in *Melancholia and Moralism: Essays on AIDS and Queer Politics*, ed. Douglas Crimp (Cambridge, MA: MIT Press, 2002), 91.

[6] As with most photographs in this and the following editions, the origin of photographs is not explicitly given, but the co-editor and clinical photographer Simon Brown has probable taken some of the pictures. Charles F. Farthing et al., eds., *A Colour Atlas of AIDS (Acquired Immunodeficiency Syndrome)* (London: Wolfe Medical Publications, 1986), 24.

[7] Ibid.   [8] Ibid.

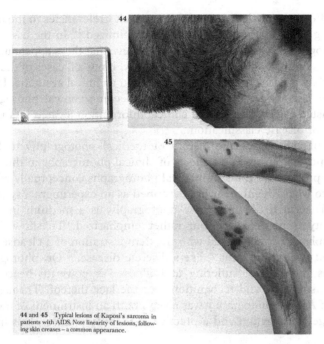

44 and 45 Typical lesions of Kaposi's sarcoma in patients with AIDS. Note linearity of lesions, following skin creases – a common appearance.

Fig. 1.1 A page from Farthing's 1986 atlas with two photographs showing "typical lesions of KS." The photographs were used to draw attention to the morphology of clinical signs while the editors cropped out details that would allow the recognition of personal identities. *Source:* Charles F. Farthing, Simon E. Brown, Richard C. D. Staughton, Jeffrey J. Cream, and Mark Mühlemann, eds., *A Colour Atlas of AIDS: Acquired Immunodeficiency Syndrome* (London: Wolfe Medical Publications, 1986), p. 24. Permission granted by Elsevier.

According to recent guidelines, a clinical photograph, a specific genre within the broader category of medical photography, should have two key features.[9] First, the sign of disease must be presented to enhance its recognizability in a day-to-day clinical setting. Second, the photograph

[9] While medical photography could be understood as a genre in which photographs are concerned with the wide range of medical phenomena, ranging from medical practice, to epidemiological mappings, anthropological inquiries and to portraits of institutions and hospitals, the clinical photograph was and is focused on the portrayal of symptoms comparable to the clinician's gaze at the bedside. To some extent clinical photography is solely concerned with the depiction and definition of diseases. See Engelmann, *Picturing the Unusual, Medical Photography as Experimental System*, forthcoming in 2019; Engelmann, *A Source of Sickness, Mapping Plague in 1900 Honolulu*, forthcoming in 2019; Christos Lynteris, *Ethnographic Plague: Configuring Disease on the Chinese-Russian Frontier* (London: Palgrave Macmillan, 2016).

should offer an analytical perspective in which irrelevancies to the task of visualizing and isolating the disease are minimized.[10] In the case of the two photographs here, we are invited to believe that these appearances of KS lesions on the two bodies resemble many, if not all, cases of the same class. This is what could tentatively be called a clinical aesthetic. Photographs of persons suffering from illness become clinical photographs when trusted as visualizations of clinical information located in an atlas, textbook or disease classification.

This chapter revisits the history of medical photography to better understand the purpose and effects of clinical photographs in the AIDS atlas.[11] I propose we think of medical photographs conceptually with an analogy to what Rheinberger has described as an experimental system.[12] I use this term to describe how photography is a medium in which uncertainty is not resolved but rather emphasized. To show AIDS, photographs are either tasked with the demonstration of a cleansed and abstracted "epistemic thing," like a discrete disease.[13] Or, photographs persist as portraits of suffering and illness, as powerful beacons of empathy, solidarity and recognition – or the lack thereof. Through the history of AIDS, photography was always both an instrument of medical knowledge visualization and a practice of identity politics. This history

[10] J. R. Nayler, "Clinical Photography: A Guide for the Clinician," *Journal of Postgraduate Medicine* 49, no. 3 (September 2003), 256–62.

[11] The literature on the history of photography is extensive. For the argument developed here, I have focused on scholarship that has deliberated the ways in which photographs acquire meaning through their contexts and material configurations in archives, albums, publications and atlases. Of particular interest has been Elizabeth Edward's work on uncertainty in photographic archives. Ryo Morimoto has recently described photographs as messages without a coda, as a by nature antisemiotic medium, which requires cultural domestication to make sense. I prefer a more pragmatic approach to photography, in which a certain indeterminacy never disappears but a pictures' relationship to the history it bears witness of remains in the center of its cultural, social and political perception. Closer to the problems and intricacies of medical photography discussed in this chapter is perhaps Barthes's view on photography and its perpetual that-has-been effect. Here, each photograph has created a vision of the past, in which the *studium* yields to a readability of a past event captured in the picture, while the *punctum* embodies a rather haunting nature of an indeterminable past. Elizabeth Edwards, "Photographic Uncertainties: Between Evidence and Reassurance," *History and Anthropology* 25, no. 2 (March 15, 2014), 171–88, doi:10.1080/02757206.2014.882834; Ryo Morimoto, "Message without a Coda: On the Rhetoric of Photographic Records," *Signs and Society* 2, no. 2 (September 1, 2014), 284–313, doi:10.1086/677923; Roland Barthes, *Camera Lucida: Reflections on Photography* (New York: Farrar, Straus and Giroux, 1981).

[12] Hans-Jörg Rheinberger, "Experimental Systems: Historiality, Narration, and Deconstruction," in *The Science Studies Reader*, ed. Mario Biagioli (New York: Routledge, 1999), 417–29.

[13] Hans-Jörg Rheinberger, *Toward a History of Epistemic Things: Synthesizing Proteins in the Test Tube* (Stanford, CA: Stanford University Press, 1997); Rheinberger, "Experimental Systems."

questions what counts as medical photography as much as it asks how to imagine a person with AIDS.

The "camera medica," as Erin O'Connor has written, is a medium of naming and identifying, of repeatedly raising the question: "What is it?"[14] Conversely, most photographs of AIDS have provoked the question "who is it?" or indeed, "who is at stake?" Clinical photography integrated the perception of homosexual men into clinical ways of seeing AIDS, using "who" as a frame to visualize the "what." But artistic and journalistic photographs were also accused of falling prey to this clinical gaze by superimposing the portraits of homosexual men ("who") with indices of disease and despair ("what").[15] I argue that photography continuously failed to provide satisfying answers to either of these questions. Rather, photography's key outstanding significance is to be found in its capacity to sustain the relationship of "who" and "what" in enduring uncertainty.

The chapter begins with an outline of photographic practices in the early years of AIDS. It continues with the question of how photography contributed so-called characteristic pictures of diseases to the AIDS atlas. Through the history of medical photography, the chapter's central concern is to address how photographs acquired authority where language and extant medical categories failed to provide clarity and certainty. With rigorous interrogation of the relationship between disease morphology and patient identity, I ask how photography catalyzed to their entangled appearances. How, if at all, did the placement, arrangement and captioning of photographs in the atlas succeed in separating signs of diseases from persons and cases?

Medical photography owes its visual faculties – its authority in making diseases visible – to two different historical genealogies. On the one hand, after photography was invented in the mid-nineteenth century, when this new visual technology entered the clinic, it adapted and integrated

---

[14] Erin O'Connor, "Camera Medica," *History of Photography* 23, no. 3 (September 1, 1999), 235, doi:10.1080/03087298.1999.10443326.

[15] This is a point raised by almost every scholar who had worked on photographs of people with AIDS, as particular explicit examples see: Simon Watney, "Photography and AIDS," in *The Critical Image: Essays on Contemporary Photography*, ed. Carol Squiers (Seattle, WA: Bay Press, 1990), 173–92; Jan Zita Grover, "Visible Lesions: Images of PWA in America," in *Fluid Exchanges: Artists and Critics in the AIDS Crisis*, ed. James L. Miller (Toronto: University of Toronto Press, 1992), 23–52; Jan Zita Grover, "OI: Opportunistic Identification, Open Identification in PWA Portraiture," in *Over Exposed: Essays on Contemporary Photography*, ed. Carol Squiers (New York: New Press, 1999), 105–22.

elements of the centuries-old tradition of medical illustration.[16] Visualizing knowledge rather than mirroring observed occurrence, illustrations had provided visual abstractions, diagrams of symptoms and drawings of signs, reimagined through the eyes of the experienced physician. Illustrations and medical drawings provided exemplary visualizations in which observations from a series of cases were drawn together into a characteristic single visual reference.[17] Photography, by comparison, was perceived by physicians as a medium of mechanical objectivity and was almost exclusively attached to the single case. On the other hand, and unlike illustration, doctors used photography in the decades after its invention to document unique, spectacular and often-monstrous cases. The extant archives show how extreme appearances and bodily deformities spiked the curiosity of doctors, collectors and a fascinated public.[18] For representations to be useful to clinicians, photography had to combine an illustrative function with an expression of spectacular appearance. In photography, the visualization of pathological commonplaces was combined with the visual documentation of those appearances that seemed to have left the realms of well-known pathology.[19] Medical photographers had to prove they could make knowledge about diseases visible, while also making documentations of what was previously unseen and remained unknown and unusual.

Both genealogies of visualizing disease positioned medical photography to be a fitting medium for documenting AIDS in the mid-1980s. Photographs could usefully visualize the incidence of already-known diseases such as KS and herpes simplex, as well as commonplace signs such as lymphadenopathy. Photography married this familiarity with the notion of a radically new syndrome appearing in a highly unusual

---

[16] Carin Berkowitz, "Introduction: Beyond Illustrations," *Bulletin of the History of Medicine* 89, no. 2 (2015), 165–70, doi:10.1353/bhm.2015.0057; Domenico Bertoloni Meli, "The Rise of Pathological Illustrations: Baillie, Bleuland, and Their Collections," *Bulletin of the History of Medicine*, 89, no. 2 (2015), 209–42, doi:10.1353/bhm.2015.0034.

[17] Elke Schulze, "Zeichnung und Fotografie – Statusfragen. Universitäres Zeichnen und Naturwissenschaftliche Bildfindung," *Berichte zur Wissenschaftsgeschichte* 28 (2005), 151–9.

[18] Gunnar Schmidt, *Anamorphotische Körper. Medizinische Bilder vom Menschen im 19. Jahrhundert* (Köln: Böhlau, 2001).

[19] Canguilhem described the notion of monstrous representations in the nineteenth century as a fascination for those obscure and extreme natural phenomena that did not fit into the defined ranges of normal appearances as a challenge to systems of normativity in biology and physiology. Photographs of monstrous appearances similarly engaged with something that had left the realm of normality, while its real existence also contributed to an extension of what was previously considered as normal. Georges Canguilhem, "Monstrosity and the Monstrous," trans. Therese Jaeger, *Diogenes* 10, no. 40 (December 1962), 27–42, doi:10.1177/039219216201004002.

demographic and social circumstance. The two photographs introduced in the preceding text, and thousands like them, performed two simultaneous tasks in 1986: They showed a skin cancer, training the eye of the doctor or the medical student to recognize the shape of the lesion, its discoloration and specifically its diagnostic qualities. And, they presented an unusual appearance of the cancer on a previously healthy young man. Only by bringing the new and unusual habitat of the skin cancer to light, the photographs showed AIDS.

Still Sexual

In every AIDS atlas published between 1986 and 2008, photographic representations remained loyal to similar clinical aesthetics. Images appeared in series, often spread across two pages, tied together by a caption or title, to name the disease in question. Beginning with the first atlas from 1986, 137 clinical photographs filled 70 pages to catalog rare occurrences, such as a rash resulting from co-trimoxazole treatment in patients with late-stage PCP, to unusual gastrointestinal complications and oral cavity disease, while the main body of photographs was dedicated to skin diseases that seem to have appeared in patients with AIDS. Dermatitis, xeroderma, extensive folliculitis and shingles, among others, were captured in three to four pictures each, attached to a brief but far from exhaustive description of the frequency of the disease's occurrence, with added notes about treatment experiences.[20] Among these skin diseases, the most prominent condition with its own dedicated section is KS. After the first page of this section, discussed previously, the atlas featured a further 50 photographs of this rare skin cancer. Pictures detailed lesions' appearance on the patient's face, in the mouth, on the tip of the nose as well as on the penis. Some photographs also show relative success and failure of treatments.[21] The atlas's second edition in 1988 gives a similar impression, using many of the same photographs. Categories such as pediatric cases were adjusted and photographs were added where none had been available in 1986, such as in the case of bilateral parotid swelling in two little girls with HIV.[22]

---

[20] For example, on the appearance of Herpes Zoster the editors argue: "Shingles is very common, occurring in some 25% of patients with AIDS and ARC. Clinically its course does not appear to be more severe and dissemination is rare. High dose oral acyclovir is helpful if given early." Farthing et al., *A Colour Atlas of AIDS* (1986), 63.

[21] Ibid., 24–43.

[22] Charles F. Farthing, ed., *A Color Atlas of AIDS* (Chicago: Year Book Medical Publishers, 1988), 89 f.

In the manner of a catalog of opportunistic infections, the atlas provided a long series of possible clinical appearances of patients with AIDS. To this end the body of photographed patients were never shown in their entirety. Visual references to the same signs were repeated on different, fragmented bodies, as the atlas editors seem to stress that their subject was disease and infection, not the patient. But the series of photographs hardly qualifies as a "cleansed" picture of a disease, which would be ideally presented at a remove from ambiguities, uncertainties and unsolved problems. Fragmented and scattered, distorted and anonymized, the identity of the photographed persons haunts this presentation of the range of diseases characteristic for AIDS. But was a cleansed picture of AIDS ever the aim of Farthing and his colleagues?

In the history of science and medicine objects of knowledge are often discussed as appearing through a process of cleansing. The cohesiveness of any object of inquiry in the sciences is not a given, Bruno Latour has argued, but instead emerges through practices of dividing and of organizing appearances into well-defined objects. "Sorting out the kernel of science from the chaff of ideology" was necessary to differentiate objects of nature from perspectives of culture.[23] New objects, such as a new disease or syndrome did accordingly never appear in a sudden emanation from the past. But the separation of phenomena that were considered relevant to a scientific investigation from elements which shrouded and clouded its appearance was a necessary step to arrive at a solid body of knowledge about an emerging epidemic.[24] But instead of seeking a cleansed, separated entity, it is useful here to consider the work of Karin Knorr-Cetina. Her anthropology of scientific labor unmasked rather a rationale for "making things work," a rationale that governs the laboratory as much as the atlas production as a social space.[25]

As a historian too, it is impossible to define transhistorical and globally pervasive patterns in which science or medicine make things work, intellectual and material dimensions are clearly distinguished and the

---

[23] Bruno Latour, *We Have Never Been Modern* (Cambridge, MA: Harvard University Press, 2012), 35.

[24] See, e.g., the structure and development of cluster studies in early AIDS epidemiology conducted in San Francisco to identify "patient 0," critically discussed by Richard McKay, or see Oppenheimer's reflections on the sorting of social practices in AIDS epidemiology. Gerald M. Oppenheimer, "In the Eye of the Storm: The Epidemiological Construction of AIDS," in *AIDS: The Burdens of History*, ed. Elizabeth Fee and Daniel M. Fox (Berkeley: University of California Press, 1988), 267–300; Richard A. McKay, *Patient Zero and the Making of the AIDS Epidemic* (Chicago: University of Chicago Press, 2017).

[25] Karin Knorr-Cetina, *Epistemic Cultures: How the Sciences Make Knowledge* (Cambridge, MA: Harvard University Press, 1999).

physical world is separated from the world of ideas. What once counted
as intellectual dispute may have become the inventory of contemporary
research routines: As Donna Haraway has shown so well, the metaphors
of the past are routinely transformed into the hardware of the present.[26]
So too did doctors, editors and research scientists perhaps share the
objective to make AIDS appear as an epistemic thing, a cleansed object
observable to the sciences, redeemed of its ideological ballast, surrounding stereotypes and complicated relationship to social and sexual identities. But in the 1986 atlas, driven by clinical rather than scientific
concerns, AIDS did not seem cleansed and sorted out but was still
embroiled in a subject governed by metaphors, stereotypes and many
unknowns. The epidemic was witnessed *in actu*, a yet-developing disaster
far from resolution. Nonetheless, this impure and ambiguous mode of
representation still seemed to make things work. Just as the Hippocratic
recognition of *krisis* was supposed to enable a prediction of a disease's
inevitable course, the atlas allowed its readership a first sighting of the
scope of what was still a rapidly developing AIDS crisis.[27]

In the 1980s, the atlas was by far not the only place in which the
medical visualization of persons with AIDS took place. For a time, there
was no social or cultural space in which such pictures did not risk
becoming medicalized. In his detailed analysis of photojournalistic coverage of the epidemic between 1981 and 2007 David Campbell mapped a
shifting visual economy of AIDS. Journalistic framings in the first half of
the epidemic were most concerned with capturing the disease in pictures
of patients, focusing on symptoms of diseases, such as KS, and medical
signs, such as emaciation. But even when a close-up zoomed onto the
face of a person with AIDS, refraining to reveal immediate signs of
disease and illness, the larger framing as an AIDS photograph tended,
as Bethany Ogdon has argued, to "facify" the disease rather than show
anything about the individual, such as his or her immediate social context
or biographical experiences.[28] According to Campbell, this trail of visual

---

[26] Haraway has coined this phrase in her reading of Harry Harlow's monkey studies:
Donna Haraway, *Primate Visions: Gender, Race and Nature in the World of Modern
Science* (New York: Routledge, 1989).

[27] Michel Foucault, *Psychiatric Power: Lectures at the Collège de France, 1973–1974* (New
York: St. Martin's Press, 2008), 243.

[28] Ogdon cites Deleuze to engage with the close-up as a cinematic practice in which the
individual is removed from its context, in which individualization resembles also a
process of decontextualization that inevitably yields to depolitization and a lesser
perception of the photographed individual as political subject but overarching as a
victim of a terrible disease. Bethany Ogdon, "Through the Image: Nicholas Nixon's
'People with AIDS,'" *Discourse* 23, no. 3 (2001), 75–105; Gilles Deleuze, *Cinema 1: The
Movement-Image* (London and New York: Bloomsbury Publishing, 2005).

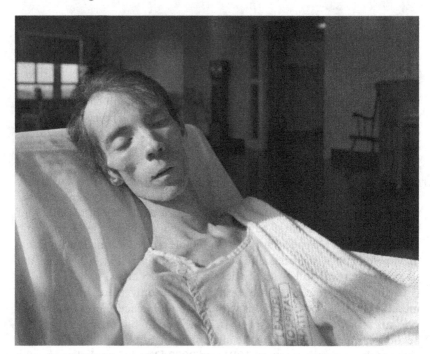

Fig. 1.2 Photograph of Tom Moran, a person with AIDS in "Pictures of People" by Nicholas Nixon from 1987. Although produced with the liberal motive of "giving AIDS a face," the exhibition and portraits like this came under scrutiny by ACT UP and others, as they were accused of presenting the person with AIDS as isolated, desexualized and ravaged by disease.
Source: Courtesy of the artist, Nicholas Nixon.

representations presented the issue of AIDS to the public as a medicalized one, regardless of the publication in which they appeared, from newspapers, journals, galleries to medical publications.[29]

On September 15, 1988, the photographer Nicholas Nixon opened an exhibition at the New York Museum of Modern Art (MoMA), called "Pictures of People."[30] The celebrated curation of portraits (Fig. 1.2) gave an insight into America's private life, bringing hidden worlds and marginalized experiences to center stage. Among the portraits was a series of pictures of people dying from AIDS: Intent on bringing

[29] David Campbell, *The Visual Economy of HIV/AIDS*, 2008, www.visual-hivaids.org.
[30] Nicholas Nixon et al., *Nicholas Nixon: Pictures of People* (New York: Museum of Modern Art, 1988).

individual suffering into the frame, Nixon's black-and-white aesthetic leaves a moving impression of the hopelessness AIDS inflicted on individuals like Tom Moran, which had remained largely unseen by the American public. Nixon's motivations were liberal and humanitarian, but his exhibition and the controversy that ensued showed the complexities of any naïve endeavor to "give AIDS a face." The political representation of those affected by a deadly epidemic was at stake in this photography. In AIDS's first decade, photographs of persons with AIDS became a subject in which the morally and politically astute way of seeing the person with AIDS was deliberated, exhibited, analyzed and, by some, fiercely rejected.[31]

While Nixon's photographs were praised by the media, art critics and politicians, AIDS activists staged a protest at the exhibition's opening. Douglas Crimp lists the criticisms raised by the activists in his analysis, when he argues that the photographs decontextualized the persons suffering from AIDS, isolated them and thus catalyzed fear of AIDS and those who carried the virus, instead of diminishing the fear. To Crimp, the exploitation of isolated and individualized personal experiences of AIDS for public spectacle was bound to the extermination of a public, social, cultural and political responsibility for the epidemic crisis. "[T]he privacy of the people portrayed is both brutally invaded and brutally maintained."[32] In Crimp's view, these photographs should be understood as "phobic images, images of the terror at imagining the person with AIDS as still sexual."[33] By representing the person with AIDS as marked by traces of emaciation and cancer, their personality, history, social existence and, in particular, desires were rendered unseen. In Nixon's photographs, Crimp argued, the person with AIDS became not only the face of the disease but also a powerless patient and a sign of the disease.[34]

Sander Gilman has described the photography of patients with visible stigmata of disease as a public practice of demarcation in which the difference between health and disease is played out as a social, cultural

---

[31] Grover, "Visible Lesions: Images of PWA in America"; Grover, "OI: Opportunistic Identification, Open Identification in PWA Portraiture"; Ogdon, "Through the Image: Nicholas Nixon's 'People with AIDS'"; Crimp, "Portraits of People with AIDS"; Sophie Junge, *Art about AIDS, Nan Goldin's Exhibition Witnesses: Against Our Vanishing* (Berlin: De Gruyter, 2016), doi:10.1515/9783110453072.

[32] Crimp, "Portraits of People with AIDS," 90.   [33] Ibid., 106.

[34] Similar criticism on the exhibition has been raised by other authors on artistic and journalistic photography of people with AIDS, see: Robert Atkins, "Difficult Subject: Photographing AIDS," *Village Voice*, June 28, 1988; Grover, "Visible Lesions: Images of PWA in America"; Grover, "OI: Opportunistic Identification, Open Identification in PWA Portraiture."

and moral distinction. "The construction of the image of the patient," he wrote in 1988 reflecting on AIDS photographs, "is thus always a playing out of this desire for a demarcation between ourselves and the chaos represented in culture by disease."[35] In the mid-1980s, photographs of people with AIDS were foundational to ongoing debates about how the epidemic was to be perceived, how the problematic history of the medical politics of lifestyle were to be reconciled and how a person with AIDS was imagined and seen. In the case of Nixon's portraits, they seem to have failed to reveal a political person as they were broadly conceived to exhibit a clinical gaze. Broadly defined as the visualization of disease rather than individual illness experience, this gaze was blamed for structuring the predominant visual regime of AIDS photography at that time. The professional practice of medical photography in turn was thought to be the origin of a way of seeing disease in which personal crisis, the social struggle and the political movements remained unseen.[36]

Photography was used by doctors and by artists in and out of the clinic to craft a representation of AIDS as an embodied condition, which begs the question what it is that sets apart a photograph of a person with AIDS in an artist's exhibition from a medical perspective applied in an AIDS atlas? To reiterate a prominent question that has been raised before, how do we decide which photograph counts as artistic representation or as an object for scientific and biomedical analysis?[37] What exactly qualifies a photograph to be bound to the ideas, practices and institutions of the clinic? If the dense entanglement of disease morphology and patient identity is to be seen as an overarching feature of all photographic representations of people with AIDS, how is a singular photograph categorized as an artistic, a journalistic or a medical picture?

The MoMA's press statement praised Nixon's photographs for their humanizing capacities. While his photographs sought to bring the audience closer to human suffering, "[T]hey also draw us to the person as an individual, not as an anonymous victim."[38] Artistic as well as journalistic portraits were supposed to individualize and hint at the subject's fate and

---

[35] Sander L. Gilman, *Disease and Representation: Images of Illness from Madness to AIDS* (Ithaca, NY: Cornell University Press, 1988), 4.

[36] Watney, "Photography and AIDS," 181.

[37] Caroline A. Jones and Peter Galison, "Introduction," in *Picturing Science, Producing Art*, ed. Caroline A. Jones and Peter Galison (London: Psychology Press, 1998), 16.

[38] MoMa Press Release, August 1988, www.moma.org/momaorg/shared/pdfs/docs/press_archives/6579/releases/MOMA_1988_0082_83.pdf?2010.

draw an audience to the patient behind the visible stigmata of disease.[39] In contrast, the task of an AIDS atlas seems to be to bring the disease to the foreground, to isolate its repeating patterns by hiding the patient's individuality and rendering the patient's body an anonymous canvas for the spectacle of recurring symptoms. A first conclusion would be: While the personal and individual proved problematic for visualizing the disease, the abstract notion of pathology posed an obstacle for successful emphatic portraiture. Yet this simplified dichotomy of pictures of disease versus affected persons does not apply to the way medical photography appeared in the first decade of AIDS; to what end was this genre used in the atlas to demonstrate the characteristics of AIDS? Furthermore, one could ask, how far does such a distinction between photography of AIDS in art, journalism and medicine make sense at all, as the shared endeavor was to capture characteristic pictures of a disease in and through portraits of people with AIDS.[40]

A Characteristic Picture of AIDS

Characteristic medical photographs taken to visualize common, typical and obvious signs of disease, but not the patient, comprised Farthing's *Colour Atlas of AIDS* in 1986. The atlas was published as a culmination of the clinical experience of Farthing and his colleagues at Westminster Hospital in London as the epidemic was officially five years old. The number of infections had been constantly rising in the United States and the majority of Europe, while preliminary counts suggested an onset of the epidemic in the southern half of Africa.[41] The only available and partially effective treatment was AZT, approved and introduced a year later, while social profiling of risk groups was still focused on the four Hs: homosexual men, heroin users, Haitians and hemophiliacs. Disputes about the nature of the virus suspected to be the etiological agent were unresolved amongst several research teams, which argued for their chosen pathogenic candidate. Against this backdrop, the atlas editors attempted to produce the first total vision of the epidemic to date, made

[39] Rosalind Solomon, *Portraits in the Time of AIDS*, ed. Grey Art Gallery & Study Center (New York: Grey Art Gallery & Study Center, New York University, 1988); Junge, *Art about AIDS*.

[40] Lukas Engelmann, "Photographing AIDS: Capturing AIDS in Pictures of People with AIDS," *Bulletin of the History of Medicine* 90, no. 2 (2016), 250–78.

[41] Jonathan M. Mann et al., "Surveillance for AIDS in a Central African City: Kinshasa, Zaire," *JAMA* 255, no. 23 (1986), 3255–9, doi:10.1001/jama.1986.03370230061031; Centers for Disease Control, "HIV Surveillance – United States, 1981–2008," *Morbidity and Mortality Weekly Report* 60, no. 21 (2011), 689–93.

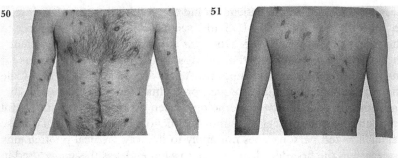

50 to **53** Widespread Kaposi's sarcoma in different
patients with AIDS.

Fig. 1.3 A page from the section on KS in Farthing's 1986 atlas
of AIDS. The design of the page emphasizes again the focus on a
characteristic appearance of widespread KS lesions on two different
bodies, each positioned in an anatomical position to maximize the
visible surface.
Source: Charles F. Farthing, Simon E. Brown, Richard C. D. Staughton,
Jeffrey J. Cream, and Mark Mühlemann, eds., *A Colour Atlas of AIDS: Acquired
Immunodeficiency Syndrome* (London: Wolfe Medical Publications, 1986), p. 26.
Permission granted by Elsevier.

vivid as a characteristic rather than a definitive picture to its medical
audience predominantly through photography.

In the mid-1980s, the state of knowledge about the epidemiology,
immunology and virology of AIDS was sparse. Information given
throughout the atlas remained vague, speculation is scattered throughout
the chapters and many questions they posed remained unanswered. In
this state of uncertainty, the resulting atlas appears more like bricolage
than a systematized topology. But this seems to have been sufficient to
fulfill the atlas's aim to be a functional diagnostic instrument.

The photographs in the 1986 atlas were not included to strengthen a
public empathy with persons who had developed AIDS, nor was their
purpose to raise public awareness of the disastrous effects of the disease.
As this example (Fig. 1.3) shows, bodies of different patients were
depicted as an exchangeable canvas for similar lesions of the sarcoma.
To guarantee anonymity, faces were cropped, patients were asked to
assume an "anatomical position," maximizing exposure of the body's
surface to the camera.[42] Clearly, the photographs do not follow aesthetic
conventions of portrait photography: The face is absent unless it is

[42] Farthing et al., *A Colour Atlas of AIDS* (1986), 26.

directly affected. Where photographs showed lesions on the facial area, thick black lines were used to provide and secure anonymity for the patients. The background of almost every picture is white, the lighting even and bright and all are, as the title of the atlas promises, in color. Few of the photographs are anchored with a caption, and even if some specific background on what is seen in the photographs is given, no information is offered about the patients, their biography, their location or even their – at this stage improbable – chance for survival. Speculations about homosexual practices and lifestyles were not absent from the atlas but remained disconnected to individual photographs and could be found, for example, in the section on epidemiology.[43]

At the time of Farthing's atlas production, the available method of analyzing blood samples (enzyme-linked immunosorbent assay [ELISA]) was complicated, expensive and sometimes unreliable.[44] Diagnosing the immunodeficiency was often done by bedside clinical methods, and the occurrence of opportunistic infections were caught by the knowing eyes of doctors. Replicating the doctor's trained gaze, the atlas's photographs show the reader common diseases including KS, herpes, lymphoma and PCP. All these established diseases, however, now appeared in an unusual social group of bodies, unusual circumstances and, crucially, an unusual frequency and geographical density. These diseases were tied to a milieu in which most of them had never been seen before. The atlas's first aim was to present a series of cases in which these known diseases had appeared out of their usual place.

This presentation of AIDS was almost exclusively dermatological. It builds on a long legacy of adequate representation of discrete patterns and unique shapes of symptoms on the exterior of the skin.[45] The gaze rested, to use a Foucauldian phrase, largely on the surface of the body.[46]

---

[43] Ibid., 13.

[44] Bill D. Roberts, "HIV Antibody Testing Methods: 1985–1988," *Journal of Insurance Medicine* 26 (1994), 13–14.

[45] It is noteworthy, that much of the late nineteenth century of dermatology and in particular dermatological illustration was dedicated to the separation of the field of common skin diseases from those that became increasingly known as venereal diseases. See: Franz Ehring, *Hautkrankheiten. 5 Jahrhunderte wissenschaftlicher Illustration – Skin Diseases* (Stuttgart: Fischer, 1989); W. H. Neuse et al., "The History of Photography in Dermatology: Milestones from the Roots to the 20th Century," *Archives of Dermatology* 132, no. 12 (December 1996), 1492–8; Richard Barnett, *The Sick Rose, Or, Disease and the Art of Medical Illustration* (D.A.P./Distributed Art Publishers, 2014); Anne R. Hanley, *Medicine, Knowledge and Venereal Diseases in England, 1886–1916* (New York: Springer, 2016).

[46] Michel Foucault, *The Birth of the Clinic: An Archaeology of Medical Perception* (New York: Pantheon Books, 1973), 139 ff.

It replicates those occurrences that catch the eye immediately and it catalogs the signs that everyone can see. The characteristic picture is construed through series of photographs, presentations of cases to the eyes of interested clinicians and students. The picture series mirrors the structure of the early World Health Organization (WHO) classification of AIDS, published in 1985.[47] It provided a catalog of opportunistic infections and diseases, clustered into important, frequent and other signs of the immunodeficiency. Each sign was given a number, pneumopathy scored 2 while chronic or relapsing herpes were considered a 4. With several infections present reaching or exceeding a score of 12, the diagnosis of AIDS was established. According to the 1985 classification, generalized KS was counted on its own as 12. In the following years, the classification scheme was widely criticized for its shortcomings and vagueness and was replaced in 1994 with an updated international standard for the diagnosis of AIDS, now heavily reliant on serostatus.[48]

But photographs did more than just replicating the contested classifications of the time. Photography promised the benefit of an impartial perspective, a sober observation of clinical signs and the maintenance of an apparent indifference to the contested terrains of theory about causes, underlying ecologies and epidemiological profiles – the at-the-time-widely-popular investigation into the idea of patient zero, for example, is absent from the atlas.[49] Contrary to Nixon's photographs in the MoMA exhibition, the atlas's series of clinical photographs were designed to visualize only specific aspects and effects of the syndrome. The underlying condition causing the symptoms to appear in the first place was implied as a diagnostic category; it remained a rubric that at this stage could only appear through long series of scattered signs. The clinical photographs did technically not show AIDS, but just isolated aspect of the syndromes disastrous effects.

Susan Sontag has called this absence of a unique signifier of AIDS an "inference." Diseases like cancer and syphilis served as metaphorical reservoirs to help describe and interpret the new syndrome, indeed

[47] World Health Organization, "Workshop on AIDS in Central Africa" (Bangui, Central African Republic: World Health Organization, October 22, 1985), 15, www.who.int/hiv/strategic/en/bangui1985report.pdf?ua=1.

[48] Alison D. Grant and Kevin M. De Cock, "HIV Infection and AIDS in the Developing World," *British Medical Journal* 322, no. 7300 (June 16, 2001), 1475–8, doi:10.1136/bmj.322.7300.1475.

[49] Richard A. McKay, "'Patient Zero': The Absence of a Patient's View of the Early North American AIDS Epidemic," *Bulletin of the History of Medicine* 88, no. 1 (2014), 161–94, doi:10.1353/bhm.2014.0005.

"the very definition of AIDS requires the presence of other diseases."[50] Instead of appearing as a radically new disease, yielding to unknown and unprecedented symptoms, AIDS instead acquired its unique quality by being a disposition of deficiency that lays the body vulnerable to a series of infections and diseases, and therefore is only accessible as an object of knowledge through the application of a new order of these known diseases and their appearances. The AIDS atlas's editors used photography to act out this "inference" of AIDS, turning the unseen condition into something visible through a catalog of photographs of manifestations of discrete diseases that can then be seen as references to AIDS.

Another conclusion as to what photography had to offer medical knowledge production in the epidemic's first decade offers itself here: Through photographs, Farthing's atlas did not only express the unique shape of AIDS, but his commitment to clinical observation also reinstated medical authority where certainty and expertise were scarce. While the atlas's first section is about the epidemiology of AIDS, which covered virology, immunology and practical details on accessible test kits, the body of the publication was concerned with a doctor's bedside encounter with the patient. Rather than detailed descriptions about the agent's biomedical structure, and in the absence of sufficient epidemiological data or distribution models, photographs seemed to allow a step back from the clamor and to ask its spectator to see rather than to speculate. Photography served as a first layer of careful abstraction, in which the repeated observation of cases was captured and recorded in an emphatically neutral or, rather, clinical way.

The Clinical Close-Up

A year after Farthing's atlas was published, Paula Treichler delivered her famous essay on the "epidemic of signification." Confronted with an unending stream of interpretations, beliefs and accusations against the populations at risk, she used this phrase to describe the vast distribution of suggested meanings for AIDS. These conjectures circled around the figure of the hypersexual homosexual male and inscribed those affected by implicating their lifestyle in theories of causation and guilt. By focusing on the continuum between biomedical practices and popular discourses, Treichler cites numerous theories that had at one time been shored up by biomedical knowledge. From the destructive power of sperm, or female immunity against infection, to lethal bacterial cocktails, acquired through many sexual encounters, debate about the true nature

---

[50] Susan Sontag, *AIDS and Its Metaphors* (New York: Farrar, Straus and Giroux, 1989), 16.

of AIDS was heated, despite broad agreement on a viral cause as of 1983. "We cannot therefore look 'through' language," Treichler concludes, "to determine what AIDS 'really' is."[51]

Yingling, by comparison, claimed that the epidemic threatened the fabric of knowledge reaching far beyond the immune systems of risk groups.

The material effects of AIDS deplete so many of our cultural assumptions about identity, justice, desire, and knowledge that it seems at times able to threaten the entire system of Western thought – that which maintains the health and immunity of our epistemology.[52]

Steven Epstein subsumed his analysis of these first years of the epidemic under the header "politics of lifestyle," as the vast majority of medical knowledge on AIDS was acquired through epidemiological analysis of those affected, while biomedical interrogation lacked convincing explanations for the full range of appearances and occurrences associated with AIDS. Epidemiologists working on AIDS in the 1980s, as Oppenheimer argues, tended to conceptualize the syndrome as complex social phenomenon, inextricably linked to vague social behavior such as "promiscuity," relations, networks and perceptions of communities.[53] Lifestyle, sexual identity and communities became embroiled into equally vague definitions of the syndrome, exposing a toxic environment for stigmatization, exclusion and ignorant bigotry toward those considered at risk and perceived as a risk.[54]

In the eyes of many critics, language had provided inadequate to grapple with the emergence of AIDS; words seemed to fall short in the face of such an extent of individual, bodily loss enfolded within a social disaster, political crisis and with little progress in medical understanding. Or as Crimp summarized the crisis in 1987: "AIDS intersects with and requires a critical rethinking of all of culture: of language and representation, of science and medicine, of health and illness, of sex and death, of the public and private realms."[55] The perpetual crisis of AIDS led to a

---

[51] Paula A. Treichler, "AIDS, Homophobia, and Biomedical Discourse: An Epidemic of Signification," in *AIDS, Cultural Analysis, Cultural Activism*, ed. Douglas Crimp (Cambridge, MA: MIT-Press, 1988), 31.

[52] Thomas Yingling, "AIDS in America: Postmodern Governance, Identity and Experience," in *Inside/Out: Lesbian Theories, Gay Theories*, ed. Diana Fuss (New York: Routledge, 1991), 292.

[53] Oppenheimer, "In the Eye of the Storm: The Epidemiological Construction of AIDS," 269.

[54] Brigitte Weingart, *Ansteckende Wörter, Repräsentationen von AIDS* (Frankfurt am Main: Suhrkamp, 2002), 41.

[55] Douglas Crimp, "AIDS: Cultural Analysis/ Cultural Activism," in *AIDS: Cultural Analysis, Cultural Activism*, ed. Douglas Crimp (Cambridge, MA: MIT Press, 1987), 15.

stream of metaphors of AIDS, which foregrounded racist stereotypes, conspiracy theories and religious angles alongside competing medical theories that rejected a viral cause.[56] Looking back, Treichler would call her own collection of AIDS essays, published in 1999, "How to Have Theory in an Epidemic?" to emphasize the complicated ethical challenges of theorizing a disease of such devastating and deadly proportion. By even daring to speak of theory, cultural constructions or explanatory frameworks in the face of those dealing with the epidemic's overwhelming demands, the immediacy of empirical approaches was appealing in and outside medicine.[57]

Social theory, cultural studies and literature were not the only places in which language seemed to fail grasping the epidemic. Farthing's atlas is filled with indications and gestures of uncertainty. His captions reflect discussions about the commonality of certain symptoms and the frequency of their appearance. The reason for increased immunoglobulin production, for example, is described as "uncertain,"[58] "progressive weight loss may be extremely marked in some patients,"[59] "the reason for the seborrheic dermatitis is as yet unclear"[60] and the reason for the significant prevalence of KS in homosexual men with AIDS is "unknown."[61]

Alex Preda has described the ubiquitous practice of calling the appearance of KS and PCP "unusual" and "uncommon" in the early medical publications on AIDS. But for Preda the notion of unusualness and uncommon appearance is not an indication of the authors' perplexity. Rather he suggests these notions of doubt served as instruments to enable new explanatory models, "signaling novelty and unusualness, redirecting the production of medical knowledge."[62] And KS was presented in almost every early report and publication as the disease, whose unusual appearance and uncommon occurrence provided the framework to assume an underlying immunosuppression as its cause. In other words, Preda makes us aware that seeing KS and PCP in these new unusual appearances was the condition under which AIDS could be seen as an "unusual usual" syndrome.[63] Photographs, which do not

[56] Seth C. Kalichman, *Denying AIDS: Conspiracy Theories, Pseudoscience, and Human Tragedy* (New York: Springer Science, 2009).

[57] Paula A. Treichler, *How to Have Theory in an Epidemic: Cultural Chronicles of AIDS* (Durham, NC: Duke University Press, 1999).

[58] Farthing et al., *A Colour Atlas of AIDS* (1986), 8.   [59] Ibid., 50.   [60] Ibid., 57.

[61] Ibid., 24.

[62] Alex Preda, *AIDS, Rhetoric, and Medical Knowledge* (Cambridge: Cambridge University Press, 2005), 61.

[63] Ibid., 58.

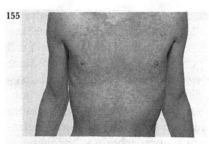

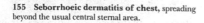

155 **Seborrhoeic dermatitis of chest,** spreading beyond the usual central sternal area.

156 Close-up of patient in **155**, showing follicular accentuation.

Fig. 1.4 Two photographs of seborrhoeic dermatitis of chest from Farthing 1986. The close-up amplifies the gesture of abstraction with which clinical photography aims to arrive at characteristic representations of the unusual extent of the clinical sign of this skin disease that has been seen in patients with AIDS.
Source: Charles F. Farthing, Simon E. Brown, Richard C. D. Staughton, Jeffrey J. Cream, and Mark Mühlemann, eds., *A Colour Atlas of AIDS: Acquired Immunodeficiency Syndrome* (London: Wolfe Medical Publications, 1986), p. 58. Permission granted by Elsevier.

feature in Preda's study of medical rhetoric, resembled this classification practice and presented the unusual appearances as a sign of AIDS.

A useful example of how photographs addressed uncertainty and unusualness is one of the many clinical close-ups from Farthing's atlas (Fig. 1.4).[64] Displayed in a diptych conformation a first photograph demonstrated the unusual extent of seborrhoeic dermatitis, spread across the patient's chest, who is similar to the preceding picture (Fig. 1.3) positioned in an anatomical posture, while the second picture zoomed in to detail the follicular accentuation. The closer the lens got to the patient's body, the less the patient appears a person and becomes instead a canvas. With higher magnification the appearance of follicles seemed removed from the individual body, from a person's experience of illness and the dramatic development of the epidemic. Where the first picture tells of a posture of a person, at least partially naked and vulnerable to a frightening disease, the second picture has erased these affective residues of the portrait. Furthermore, the spread of skin disease is captioned as unusual, having moved beyond the commonly affected areas. In the process of cropping, arrangement and caption, these two photographs seem to move successfully from the unusual and confusing appearance of

[64] Farthing et al., *A Colour Atlas of AIDS* (1986), 58.

this skin disease to the representation of a disease, which has been marked as indicative of AIDS through its unusual patterns. The depiction "facifies" the symptom in the way that Ogdon describes the close-up as an isolation of the enhanced detail from social, historical and cultural circumstance.[65] The closer the lens gets, the less contextualized appears the object in front of the camera.

For O'Connor, clinical photography's concern with superficial occurrences of pathology extends to a visualization practice as an "Art of Truth," which alludes to the impression the photographs present "things as they are." But this is less a description of the camera's accuracy than a representation of the camera's capacity to conflate surface and substance, to present visual clarity as the key to the deep truth of disease.[66] For cases deemed exemplary of the ongoing epidemic, photographs gave a way of seeing AIDS that made the abundance of its metaphoric meanings and the uncertainty and resistance of AIDS as an object of medical knowledge for a while unseen. In this particular sense, clinical photography offered a way of seeing AIDS that moved beyond the epidemic of signification and provided an order in which uncertainty and unusualness were sustained rather than resolved.

With this use of photography, the AIDS atlas was built on an old fantasy of medicine, which put faith in an account of pathological phenomena free from speculation, assumption and theory. These photographs appeared to be the products of pure observation as well as accurate case description. Photography as "eyewitness" had been long trusted to translate observation into publication.[67] In this way, the atlas photographs showed the clinician's eye applied to AIDS and lent that same way of seeing to the reader. Committed to physical morphology and willfully impervious to the raging "epidemic of signification," the atlas revealed AIDS as a series of discrete entities of medical knowledge appearing in a new order. To encounter the new epidemic through seeing familiar signs and diseases allowed for the rapid assertion of medical authority.[68]

But how exactly did clinical photography acquire this capacity to assert such authority in the absence of refined categories of AIDS epidemiology or any fundamental understandings of HIV and its microbiological mechanics? The longer history of visualizing disease in illustrations and

---

[65] Ogdon, "Through the Image: Nicholas Nixon's 'People with AIDS,'" 85.

[66] O'Connor, "Camera Medica," 235.

[67] Jennifer Tucker, *Nature Exposed: Photography as Eyewitness in Victorian Science* (Baltimore: Johns Hopkins University Press, 2005).

[68] Preda, *AIDS, Rhetoric, and Medical Knowledge*, 54.

photographs offers some indication as to how photography emerged as a unique professional medical practice. While it is tempting to see photography as part of the history of the empirical gaze applied to medical phenomena, such an approach forecloses other influences on the photographic picture of disease. Particular modes of analytical and diagnostic seeing were adapted by photography from the older genre of medical illustration, and what could tentatively be called a tradition of diagrammatic reasoning in medicine.

Analytical Visualization in the History of Medicine

The rejection and condemnation of theory was a recurring topic in medical thinking throughout the long nineteenth century. Already the pathologist and atlas-producer Jean Cruveilhier was concerned about systems, concepts and theories in the minds of the physicians around him in the 1820s as he favored an empirical account of disease entities, based on observation and illustration of clinical appearances. In this spirit, Cruveilhier declared the illustrations in his epic atlas to be timeless imprints of nature, resistant to the "back and forth of systems of thinking."[69] Instead of reading pedantic descriptions of skin rashes, he believed that seeing illustrations provided immediate and lasting impressions of the diseases in their actual state.[70]

Daston and Galison discuss concern about authorial subjectivity, part of which rested in the limited capacities of language to capture the spectacle of diseases in dense descriptions. To trust descriptions as accurate translations of appearances seen on a patient's body became contested throughout the nineteenth century. Language was seen as untrustworthy, as it was perceived of leaning toward preconceived images and theoretical abstractions such as the archetype in German *Naturphilosophie*.[71] Not paying due diligence to techniques of observation and shrouding the doctor's judgment, written words were conceived

---

[69] Cruveilhier wrote in his introduction: "[U]n dessin fidèle est éternel comme la nature, et à l'abri des vacillations des systèmes: il reproduit incessamment la même image, rappelle à l'un ce qu'il a déjà vu, apprend à l'autre ce qu'il ne connait pas, dispense de fastidieuses lectures, et laisse dans l'esprit des impressions aussi profondes que durables." Jean Cruveilhier, *Anatomie pathologique du corps humain ou descriptions avec figures lithographiées et coloriées des diverses altérations morbides* (Paris: Baillière, 1829), IX.

[70] Lukas Engelmann, "Eine analytische Bildpraxis. Die pathologisch-anatomischen Zeichnungen Jean Cruveilhiers in ihrem Verhältnis zu klinischen Beobachtungen," *Berichte zur Wissenschaftsgeschichte* 35 (2012), 7–24.

[71] Lorraine Daston and Peter Galison, *Objectivity* (Cambridge, MA: Zone Books, 2007); Volker Hess and J. Andrew Mendelsohn, "Case and Series: Medical Knowledge and Paper Technology, 1600–1900," *History of Science* 48, no. 161 (2010), 287–314.

as obstacles to the clinicians' ability to see and recognize the disease before their eyes.

Cruveilhier's introduction to his atlas in 1824 provides an interesting starting point for situating illustration in the field of pathological anatomy. His rejection of language and appreciation of illustration as inerrable representation paved the way for the epistemic obstacles photography had to address half a century later. His atlas, the by-then largest collection of illustrations of pathological anatomy was published in 40 consignments between 1829 and 1842 in a design largely influenced by the Paris School of Medicine. Its wide distribution around Europe left a profound imprint on medical visualizations. The order of diseases did not follow abstract tables and classifications but was crafted around the anatomical location of pathological specimen within the human body. The atlas thus further established a way of thinking about disease based not on clusters of disparate signs across the body, but rather on the place of each appearance within or on the body's surface.[72]

Cruveilhier's stunning illustrations enhance their depth of meaning through weighted lines, careful coloring and exquisite detailing. Different types of melanoma, which comprised a large portion of the diseases included in the atlas, seem to almost pop out from the page, acquiring vividness and therefore achieving a lifelike truthfulness even to later audiences at the end of the twentieth century.[73] Letters and numbers were integrated into the fine lines of the drawings and provided anchor points for references in accompanying texts, which delivered detailed description of the particular case history and the diagnosis, such as the names of patients and the circumstances of their arrival at the Hôpital Hôtel-Dieu. Cruveilhier's drawings focused on the pathological forms and appearances, in the foreground of the pictures, while the surrounding normal anatomy occasionally appeared as a faded background. The malignant tumor depicted in "Maladies des Nerfs Ganglionnaires" (Fig. 1.5) draws particular attention to the color of the tissue, the morphology of the unusual growth and the position within the anatomy of the neck. The healthy anatomy appeared generic and exchangeable, through

---

[72] Moncef Berhouma, Julie Dubourg, and Mahmoud Messerer, "Cruveilhier's Legacy to Skull Base Surgery: Premise of an Evidence-Based Neuropathology in the 19th Century," *Clinical Neurology and Neurosurgery* 115, no. 6 (June 2013), 702–7, doi:10. 1016/j.clineuro.2012.08.005; P. P. De Saint-Maur, "The Birth of the Clinicopathological Method in France: The Rise of Morbid Anatomy in France during the First Half of the Nineteenth Century," *Virchows Archiv* 460, no. 1 (2012), 109–17, doi:10.1007/ s00428-011-1162-2.

[73] K. Denkler and J. Johnson, "A Lost Piece of Melanoma History," *Plastic and Reconstructive Surgery* 104, no. 7 (December 1999), 2149–53.

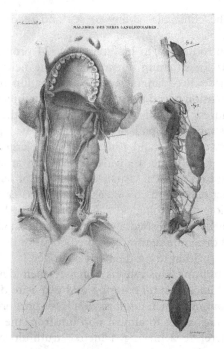

Fig. 1.5 Plate from the section "Maladies des Nerfs Ganglionnaires" in Cruveilhier's atlas of pathological anatomy from 1824. The characteristic style of Cruveilhier pulls attention to the pathological specimen by drawing it in its place within a generic human anatomy.
Source: Jean Cruveilhier *Anatomie pathologique du corps humain, ou descriptions, avec figures lithographieés et coloriées, des diverses altérations morbides* (Paris: Baillière, 1829–42), Liv. 1, Plate III. Courtesy of the Staatsbibliothek zu Berlin.

the absence of color, faded edges and the almost unnatural viewpoint. While the disease is displayed in its figural individuality, the physiological space is brought in as a repeatable background, like a generic stage set.

Cruveilhier's illustrations were rooted in the tradition of case description as well as the long history of visual anatomy.[74] The ways in which cases have been described in medicine has been subject to much research in recent years, exposing a deep level of formalization in the translation of observation into text and illustration. Prudent observation enabled exhaustive description, which then meant the clinician could turn to systems and classes to compare practice with theory and forge new

[74] Michael J. Ackermann, Judith Folkenberg, and Benjamin Rifkin, *Human Anatomy: Depicting the Body from the Renaissance to Today* (London: Thames & Hudson, 2006).

nosologies throughout the eighteenth and nineteenth century.[75] But these new empirically based techniques of observation constantly confronted the problem of distinguishing between significant and random signs. When should an observed detail be considered as pertinent to the disease described? How might this decision be made and by whom, as depictions could not always rely on classes and theories of knowledge that preexisted the observation of appearances on a particular body?[76] Cruveilhier's visual contribution was precisely tuned to this problem. He wanted his illustrations to be concerned with capturing a characteristic impression of the disease, independent of the back and forth of the "Systèmes."[77]

The first step in Cruveilhier's analytical drawing method derived from Philipp Pinel's commitment to disease observation.[78] Pinel translated visible signs into exact written replica. The resulting text should be closely tied to what is seen, as if the disease could reveal itself, speaking its own, "native" language through the conduit of the describing clinical observer.[79] Pinel's method relied on an exchangeable relation between descriptive language and visual perception of symptoms. This suggested an economy of medical language that could include everything of relevance without losing significant details in its account of the visible stigmata of a disease. This ideal appealed to a stable and exact relation between what is seen and what is said, as Foucault described it for the early-nineteenth-century medicine. Knowing and seeing had become one in this endeavor and doctors imagined themselves to be naturally equipped with a "speaking eye."[80] Volker Hess wrote about this as the formation of a grammar of the language of diseases, in which the disease acquired a medical meaning only in the way in which it was enabled to

---

[75] Lauren Kassell, "Casebooks in Early Modern England: Medicine, Astrology, and Written Records," *Bulletin of the History of Medicine* 88, no. 4 (2014), 595–625, doi:10.1353/bhm.2014.0066; Hess and Mendelsohn, "Case and Series: Medical Knowledge and Paper Technology, 1600–1900"; Volker Hess and Andrew Mendelsohn, "'Sauvages' Paperwork: How Disease Classification Arose from Scholarly Note-Taking," *Early Science and Medicine* 19, no. 5 (2014), 471–503.

[76] Christiane Frey, "Am Beispiel der Fallgeschichte. Zu Pinels 'Traité médico-philosophique sur l'aliénation,'" in *Das Beispiel: Epistemologie des Exemplarischen*, ed. Jens Ruchatz, Stefan Willer, and Nicolas Pethes (Berlin: Kulturverlag Kadmos, 2007), 263–78.

[77] Cruveilhier, *Anatomie pathologique du corps humain*, v.

[78] Philippe Pinel, *Nosographie philosophique; ou La méthode de l'analyse appliquée a la médecine* (Paris: J. A. Brosson, 1818).

[79] Foucault, *The Birth of the Clinic*, 78.   [80] Ibid., 149.

reveal itself.[81] Reflecting on Pinel's shortcoming, Cruveilhier criticized this analytical method as a theoretical deformation of the disease. He intervened by providing visualizations of pathological anatomy, which sought to capture nature as it really was.

Through his drawings he could address a most pressing problem of his time. Toby Gelfand described it in the following words: "Formal accounts did not (and could not if they wished to be of finite length and comprehensible) attempt a total picture of disease, replete with the multiple variations which occurred."[82] The pathological could not be displayed by using the normative visual practice applied in anatomy atlases: The individuality of cases and appearances and their instances could not be so readily flattened into something so recognizable as a perfected "normal." Cruveilhier used illustrations to establish the idea of a characteristic picture, a drawing that relies on a single case while it argues that this particular case should be seen as an exemplary case. Where anatomical atlases enjoyed an easy relationship to the individual bodies that might have served as models or templates to arrive at an average, the atlas of pathological anatomy needed to appreciate and integrate the notion of the single case. In its commitment to an empirical account of diseases, Cruveilhier's drawings bore traces of mistrust to both the formal accounts of nosological tables and archetypical visual traditions of anatomy. The drawings established a way of visualizing pathology that lay somewhere in between, and Daston and Galison refer to Cruveilhier's drawings as a unique way of arguing visually about diseases in which his approach resembled "a hybrid of the idealizing and the naturalizing modes."[83] The pathological object was kept as an individual object but related to a class of things placed in an atlas. This reinvented depicting of pathology at Cruveilhier's time was needed, as neither the visual tradition of anatomy with its idealistic visualizations, nor the representation of an archetype, or pure phenomena were considered appropriate modes of seeing when it came to diseases.[84] Intended to heavily supplement or even replace a language-based system, which had failed as a *Grammatik* of the disease, illustrations established a diagrammatical way of seeing and understanding pathological appearances.

---

[81] Volker Hess, *Von der semiotischen zur diagnostischen Medizin. Die Entstehung der klinischen Methode zwischen 1750 und 1850* (Husum, Germany: Matthiesen, 1993), 103.

[82] Toby Gelfand, "A Clinical Ideal: Paris 1789," *Bulletin of the History of Medicine* 51 (Fall 1977), 397–411.

[83] Lorraine Daston and Peter Galison, "The Image of Objectivity," *Representations* no. 40 (1992), 94.

[84] Ibid.

After photography's inception, illustration did by no means become an outdated technique of clinical visualization. It was and remained an artful diagrammatic of the pathological that embraced empirical yet structured accounts of the observed phenomenon. Similarly to how observations and descriptions were considered first orders of abstraction instead of preconditions for classification, did the art of illustration serve as a translation between the visible lesions and their systematic understanding as signs of disease.[85]

Illustration foreclosed the chance of seeing the unseen in visual representations. The pictures did not include the excess, the information discarded by the clinician's eye. The unintended, accidental and overseen elements and aspects that might perhaps relate to the disease were routinely excluded from their visualization. Consequently, the reader of these drawn images could not expect to make additional discoveries and could not use the image to interrogate the visualized disease in its multifaceted shape. The viewer had to accept the illustration as the visual representation of an analytical gaze; someone had already decided what was significant for seeing a particular disease.

The AIDS atlas, published 150 years later, was also structured by an analytical perspective comparable to Cruveilhier's publication. Editorial decisions had been made to include prominent opportunistic infections like KS, PCP, herpes, psoriasis, but not all. Photographs were taken of patients, whose cases had been decided to be characteristic appearances; these photographs were then cropped and captioned to make only those elements visible that were necessary to see the current picture of AIDS. Finally, the comparatively brief paragraphs of text throughout the atlas gave further guidelines for readers to learn how to see and recognize the syndrome in a certain way, but refrained from engagement with larger, contested matters in any systematic way.

However, unlike the illustration, a photograph cannot be so tightly controlled. The use of photography left room for other pictures to emerge. Most importantly, it allowed inclusion of uncertainty, of the unusualness of the appearance of infections in these particular bodies, and freed up an integration of the many unseen assumptions, theories and speculations about the young epidemic, although the overall impression was apparently somber and clinically neutral. Clinical photography was well-suited to present AIDS precisely for its faculty of offering a disease both as a standardized object of knowledge and as an excess of

[85] Hess and Mendelsohn, "Sauvages' Paperwork."

norms, classes and theories. This visual technology emphasized AIDS as crisis of medical knowledge while indicating the stability of medical authority.

Photography and Illustration

The history of clinical photography is still widely unwritten. Studies have analyzed representations produced by the medical use of photography as examples in larger arguments about the visual history of medicine, but no scholar has engaged systematically with this genre at large. Clinical photography's history remains overshadowed by scholarship on the representation of medicine in society, on specific photographic practices in psychiatry in the case of Charcot and on the history of photography of physiological movement.[86] Clinical photography has often been loosely included in the wider corpus of scientific photography, as researched by Tucker and others.[87] But these perspectives tend to overlook a crucial point about clinical photography: As a visualization technique it is intimately attached to the portraiture of the pathological and thus deeply bound to the history of the clinician's gaze. This gaze is not identical with the perspective of a biologist or a chemist and must be treated within deliberation of the normal and the pathological instead of wrestling objects of nature from systems of culture.[88] Clinical photography was neither fully committed to eye-witnessing natural phenomena, nor did it work as a pure visualization of nosological knowledge, tables and categories or diseases.

---

[86] Gilman, *Disease and Representation: Images of Illness from Madness to AIDS*; Georges Didi-Huberman, *Invention of Hysteria: Charcot and the Photographic Iconography of the Salpetriere* (Cambridge, MA: MIT Press, 2003); Tanya Sheehan, *Doctored: The Medicine of Photography in Nineteenth-Century America* (University Park: Pennsylvania State University Press, 2011); Sander L. Gilman, *Illness and Image: Case Studies in the Medical Humanities* (Piscataway, NJ: Transaction Publishers, 2014); Beatriz Pichel, "From Facial Expressions to Bodily Gestures: Passions, Photography and Movement in French 19th-Century Sciences," *History of the Human Sciences* 29, no. 1 (February 1, 2016), 27–48, doi:10.1177/0952695115618592; Katherine Rawling, "'She Sits All Day in the Attitude Depicted in the Photo': Photography and the Psychiatric Patient in the Late Nineteenth Century," *Medical Humanities* 43, no. 2 (June 1, 2017), 99–100, doi:10.1136/medhum-2016-011092.

[87] Tucker, *Nature Exposed*; Kelley E. Wilder, *Photography and Science*, Exposures (London: Reaktion, 2009); Ann Thomas and Marta Braun, eds., *Beauty of Another Order: Photography in Science* (New Haven, CT: Yale University Press, 1997); Daston and Galison, *Objectivity*.

[88] Foucault asked for all historical inquiry into the practices of the life sciences to consider two parallel dichotomies: one of the formation of biological concepts of things and facts and the other grounded in the bipolarity of health and disease, normalcy and pathology. Foucault, *The Birth of the Clinic*, 42.

Just months after the invention of the daguerreotype, the earliest form of photography in 1835, the first medical images were taken. In 1852 Berend published photographs that focused on orthopedic diseases, Squire colored photographs in 1864 to show dermatological textures and in 1893 the first comprehensive handbook for medical photography, *La photographie medicale* was published in France. That year the first issue of the new journal *Internationale Medizinisch-Photographische Monatsschrift* was published, which taught doctors and photographers alike how to take medical photographs. Photography had become a successor to earlier "visual concepts of pathology" and provided a radical new "medium of seeing" disease.[89] By the middle of the twentieth century, photography had become the most important medium for the increasingly visual basis of medical diagnostics.

However, this was not a smooth progression to prominence unhindered by resistance, critique and protest. The physician William Keiller expostulated his concern about the craze for medical photography in the 1894 issue of the *New York Medical Journal* that the "excellence and cheapness of the recent methods of reproducing photographs by photoengravings has driven the majority of medical illustrators photo-mad." He continued, "How many text-books and articles are spoiled by beautiful photo-engravings which teach absolutely nothing, where simple diagrams would have been most instructive!"[90] Similar concerns were raised in the *British Medical Journal*, where authors complained about the overall lack of detail in photographic visualization.[91] These outspoken photography protests were not representative of the majority of the medical profession. But many doctors, editors and publishers remained skeptic about the instructive faculty of photography. What was it about a photograph that provoked these concerns, and what ways were found to overcome the epistemic obstacles that forged clinical photography into a genre that could – as in the case of AIDS – express both the stability of medical knowledge and the appearance of a new, poorly understood and mysterious disease?

Moritz Kaposi, who identified and subsequently named the skin cancer that would become an index marker for AIDS, refused to use the new medium. As one of the best-known dermatologists of his time, Kaposi represented the dermatology school of Vienna. Between

[89] Tucker, *Nature Exposed*, 239.
[90] William Keiller, "The Craze for Photography in Medical Illustration," *New York Medical Journal* 59 (1894), 788–9.
[91] Daniel M. Fox and Christopher Lawrence, *Photographing Medicine: Images and Power in Britain and America since 1840* (New York: Greenwood Press, 1988), 24.

1898 and 1900, Kaposi published the *Handatlas der Hautkrankheiten für Studierende und Ärzte*, which relied exclusively on watercolor illustrations, using wax moulages as templates.[92] In his preface, Kaposi claimed that the atlas not only collected all significant clinical pictures for dermatology, but visualized the different appearances of the most significant diseases, such as syphilis. He did not give explicit reason for ignoring the half-century history of medical photography, which had already been used in other dermatological atlases.[93] Instead, he expressed his admiration for the "superior art" of illustration. The atlas consists of hundreds of beautifully painted aquarelles, which depict the then-known dermatological diseases, affixed with short captions.[94] Beyond the brief preface, no textual commentary is found in the atlas. The authorial medical voice had disappeared from the text or rather taken up residence in the drawings that were fully trusted by Kaposi to transmit knowledge and his clinical perspective in the intended form.

Historically, photographs were mistrusted by physicians because they showed too much. It was not always easy to find particularly poignant cases, photograph them in the right way and crop the resulting picture in a manner that the disease can take center stage. While medical metaphors traveled to conventional portrait photography in the nineteenth century, to lend authority and professionalism to the urban studio photographer, the medical photographer was concerned that his practice would bear too much resemblance to classic portraiture.[95] The overarching presence of a person, rather than the symptom, was particularly difficult to contain when diseases appeared in the face.

When KS occurred in patients with AIDS, one of the unusual aspects was its manifestation throughout the patient's body. Classically, in the cancer's appearance before the time of AIDS, KS lesions were usually to be found along the lower limbs. But the AIDS related appearance of lesions in patient's faces provided new problems for the atlas editors and photographers. As could already be seen in the first example of this chapter (Fig. 1.1), photographing lesions on and close to the face challenged not only the anonymity that was guaranteed to the volunteering patients, but in regard to the visualization of a disease, it made it significantly more difficult to make the person behind the KS lesion unseen.

---

[92] Moritz Kaposi, *Handatlas der Hautkrankheiten für Studierende und Ärzte* (Wien: Braumüller, 1898).

[93] Ehring, *Hautkrankheiten.*

[94] On the history of watercolors in dermatology, see: Mechthild Fend, *Fleshing Out Surfaces: Skin in French Art and Medicine, 1650–1850* (Oxford: Oxford University Press, 2016).

[95] Sheehan, *Doctored: The Medicine of Photography in Nineteenth-Century America,* 3.

But KS in persons with AIDS often appeared in the face, and it was partly for that reason that it was the most visible and immediately recognizable sign of AIDS at the time. This prominence exceeded the doctor's vision, as the facial KS lesion became a spectacle, working as AIDS's index sign in popular culture, film and television.[96] But it was still important to draw attention to the unusual facial location, so doctors knew exactly where to look. Ethical considerations and the heated political conflicts around AIDS compelled the editors to maximize anonymity. Their answer in the 1986 atlas was to crop as much of the surrounding visage as possible, to reveal just enough to enable clinical recognition of the signs; to this end the editors were prepared to manipulate pictures extensively.

But securing a photograph's message to be concerned with disease and not a personal portrait was far more challenging, if the disease did not present through characteristic lesions. In the photograph discussed at the beginning of this chapter (Fig. 1.1), we not only see lesions of KS at the edge of the man's beard but also another striking feature: The facial hair around the chin has become gray.[97] Graying hair might have been indicative of another process, which was vague in its definition and even more problematic to visualize: the acceleration of appearing old. At the end of the atlas's section on clinical presentations, the editors drew reader's attention to AIDS-related signs of "rapid aging." Two photographs, taken on two separate occasions with an interval of two years, demonstrate the progress of "premature greying, frontal recession and thinning of hair, loss of facial fat with hollowing of contour."[98]

The photographs look like standard portrait photographs or passport pictures, but two black lines, forming a T-shape, were intended to ensure patient anonymity while enabling the usability of the photograph (Fig. 1.6). Many facets of these pictures are puzzling. The AIDS manifestation described here as "rapid aging" is difficult to define in detail. The overall impression of aging is hard to condense into a comprehensive list of indicators. Where does aging become medical? What excess of aging is too much, and how is this measured? This overall impression is captured in the familiar arrangement of a before-and-after depiction of

---

[96] Paul Sendziuk, "Philadelphia or Death," *GLQ* 16, no. 3 (2010), 444–9; Beate Schappach, "AIDS-Bilder – Zur Bedeutung des Kaposi Sarkoms im AIDS-Diskurs," in *Bild und Gestalt. Wie formen Medienpraktiken das Wissen in Medizin und Humanwissenschaft?*, ed. Frank Stahnisch and Heiko Bauer (Hamburg: Wilhelm Fink Verlag, 2007), 199–210.

[97] In the second edition of Farthing's atlas from 1988, the photograph is further cropped and the spot of gray beard remains unseen. Farthing, *A Color Atlas of AIDS* (1988), 65.

[98] Farthing et al., *A Colour Atlas of AIDS* (1986), 70.

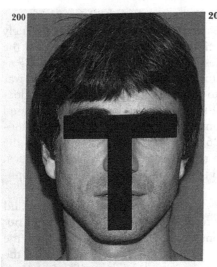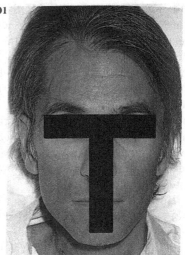

200 and **201** **Rapid ageing.** These photographs were taken with an interval of two years. Premature greying, frontal recession and thinning of hair, loss of facial fat with hollowing of contour contribute to this appearance.

Fig. 1.6 Two photographs selected to demonstrate the process of rapid aging as a symptom of AIDS in the 1986 atlas by Farthing. The black lines guarantee anonymity but also turn the portrait photographs into functional representations, supposed to reveal recognizable signs of aging without compromising the privacy of this person with AIDS. *Source:* Charles F. Farthing, Simon E. Brown, Richard C. D. Staughton, Jeffrey J. Cream, and Mark Mühlemann, eds., *A Colour Atlas of AIDS: Acquired Immunodeficiency Syndrome* (London: Wolfe Medical Publications, 1986), p. 58. Permission granted by Elsevier.

the person's face. The premature graying, also present in the KS photograph in the preceding text (Fig. 1.1), the thinning of hair and absence of facial hair is captured in the second shot, but so are other features. The unusual blue background on the left picture suggests it to be perhaps an older prepathological, personal photograph, while a changing haircut hints at the movement of fashion, styles and taste and a sense of the facial expression – in both pictures serious and performing an emphatic neutrality – makes these photographs, despite the editorial gesture of anonymity, particularly vulnerable to be seen as a portrait of a person.

Despite the black lines' questionable success in keeping the identity of the patient protected, they made these photographs a clinical picture.

Among the practices that photographers, editors and designers applied throughout the atlas, this might be one of the most intrusive and obstructive to the readers' gaze, hindering a recognition of the person and guiding to an analytical observation of the signs of aging listed in the caption. The black lines practice an abstraction through which the photographs were intended to become readable as a vessel of clinical information. Such practices of taming the photographs' content have a long tradition. Draping, covering and hiding unnecessary aspects to guide the reader's gaze to substantial features contributed to the very act of turning a photograph into a medical photograph, by establishing it as an analytical perspective.

Clinical photography adopted these practices from illustration. But it also owes much of its conventions to the wax moulage. In reverse, at the end of the nineteenth century the art of moulage became increasingly dependent on photography. The fragile wax models were photographed for distribution far beyond the hospitals that stored them for teaching purposes. The *Atlas der Hautkrankheiten. Mit Einschluß der wichtigsten venerischen Erkrankungen für praktische Ärzte und Studierende,* published in 1903 by Eduard Jacobi, used photography exclusively as reproduction of wax moulages, rather than as a technique to capture cases in vivo.[99] The editor of this dermatological atlas, reissued until the 1920s, gave some hints about why he chose photographed moulages. His reasons were partly based on technical problems. But he also emphasized the advantage of photographed moulages, as they maintained the idealized perspective of the doctors and artists, produced in such perfection, to exactly resemble the disease in the living patient.[100] Jacobi emphasized that he relied on photographs of moulages as representations of typical diseases, and he expressed no interest in the contemporary trend of bringing monstrous or "interesting" cases to the fore.[101] That his atlas

---

[99] Eduard Jacobi, *Atlas der Hautkrankheiten: Mit Einschluß der wichtigsten venerischen Erkrankungen für praktische Aerzte und Studierende* (Berlin and Wien: Urban & Schwarzenberg, 1903).

[100] Moulages were preferred by many dermatologists to illustrations, as they allowed textures to be copied, and could be used in teaching as robust demonstrations of the living body. Each moulage represents a characteristic sign of a disease, identified by an experienced and attentive physician, transferred into a three-dimensional wax model, which uses different colors to mimic the disease in its natural appearance. The art of creating the models, their conservation and the utility of collections in medical teaching were considered essential to teaching pathology throughout the nineteenth century. Schnalke argues that this technology reached its zenith between the 1880s and 1940s before being replaced by color photography. Thomas Schnalke, "Moulagen und Photografie," *Photomed* 2 (1989), 21–4; Thomas Schnalke, *Diseases in Wax: The History of the Medical Moulage* (Chicago: Quintessence Publications, 1995).

[101] Jacobi, *Atlas der Hautkrankheiten*, 4.

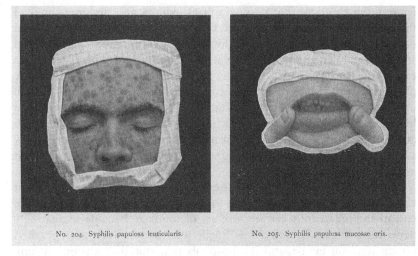

No. 204. Syphilis papulosa lenticularis.   No. 205. Syphilis papulosa mucosae oris.

Fig. 1.7 Two photographed moulages in a chapter on Syphilis in Jacobi's dermatological atlas from 1903. While the moulages were too fragile to be widely circulated, photographic reproduction made these three-dimensional and lifelike illustrations of diseases widely accessible.

Source: Eduard Jacobi, *Atlas der Hautkrankheiten. Mit Einschluß der wichtigsten venerischen Erkrankungen für praktische Aerzte und Studierende* (Berlin and Wien: Urban & Schwarzenberg, 1903), plate 112. Courtesy of the Wellcome Collection.

illustrated typical clinical pictures, he saw the utmost value in guided visual representations so that the practicing physician or the student of dermatology would profit most from reading the atlas.[102]

Syphilis was at that time the central topic of dermatology and venereology. Many publications used visual sources to establish a canon of referential images, and Jacobi dedicated a long chapter of his atlas to the pressing problem of a widely distributed syphilis epidemic. He recalled the history of isolating the syphilis infectious agent, the *spirochaeta pallida*, and listed the visible and invisible clinical signs of its presence in a patient's body. Detailed and vivid descriptions of lesions, their characteristic appearance and their usual places on a body were briefly referenced by Jacobi in the text but were also visualized through illustrations of so-called Schleimhautpappeln (papulosa).

Two photographic reproductions of moulages (Fig. 1.7) showed the face, or rather a portion of the face. The moulage had been modeled in

[102] Ibid.

detail to create a lifelike appearance, emphasized by details like the fingers that pull down the lip to make the lesions visible. As with photography, lifelike impression was the key element that led many doctors to trust the moulage as a teaching instrument. As the moulages' immobility and fragility were impractical for dissemination and expensive to reproduce and to store, their circulation through photography was of immense value. The act of cropping and draping stands in for the clinician's analytical perspective, guiding the gaze to the significant details. Cropped into diagnostic certainty, the moulage offered standardized clinical pictures, ready to be widely distributed through photography.

Returning to the AIDS atlas, a resemblance between the aesthetic of Jacobi's photographed wax moulages and the persons with AIDS in, for example, the pictures of aging (Fig. 1.4) is uncanny. In both cases, we see lifelike representations of the symptoms on patient's bodies, body parts moved to reveal the symptom in its entirety and a series of pictures of bodies juxtaposed to render the individuality of patients, the arbitrary appearance of symptoms in single cases unseen. Cropping and captioning the photograph was a practice modeled on the historical example of illustration and moulage to process diagnostic certainty, so that photographed patient bodies in the AIDS atlas would seem no more than wax models. The point of focus was artfully crafted through a doctor's speaking eyes, the established medical authority that in turn allowed the pictures to be trusted as instruments of comparison and teaching to recognize actual cases. Drawing on the diagrammatic faculty of the illustration, photographs needed to be tamed, pictures needed to be turned into structured representations of lesions to show a disease.

It is a commonplace that a photographs' content becomes visible through their material arrangements. "[H]ow they are printed and viewed, as albums, lantern slides, or mounted prints, is integral to their phenomenological engagement, structuring visual knowledge."[103] But as Edwards has argued further, while arrangement makes the photograph a readable entity and structures our reading of its content, the photograph's picture can never fully be disclosed, its meaning is never quite secure and its vision never firmly anchored: The "photograph awakens a desire to know that which it cannot show."[104] Showing a lesion, to visualize a rash as it manifests on a person's body, might be achieved through the material arrangement and manipulation of a photograph in

---

[103] Elizabeth Edwards, *Raw Histories: Photographs, Anthropology and Museums* (London: Bloomsbury Academic, 2001), 16.
[104] Ibid., 62.

an atlas. But for the photograph to work as a visualization of AIDS, it must do more. It is here where the unseen surplus of the photograph becomes important, where precisely that which illustration cannot show acquires importance and where the relationship of signs of a disease and the person depicted moves to the center.

Here, a second historical genealogy of clinical photography is apparent. Distinct from the diagrammatic capacities of illustrations and wax moulages, photography could bring something new to disease visualization: It showed disease in the contingent individual and singular shape that resisted formal account and abstraction. Skeptical to the idea of solid disease entities, classes and tableaus, the photograph contributed in the late nineteenth century to a new appreciation of disease as an excessive state of life. Precisely because photography was able to integrate the individual picture of disease into the crafting of formalized accounts, it enfolded attraction as a visual representation of pathology as both an abstract entity and a lived reality.

Morphology and Identity

Farthing's atlas had worked through the process of what Preda had called "making up the rules of seeing."[105] Making photographs to show AIDS required extensive framing and manipulation; photographs needed to adapt qualities usually associated with its predecessor genres, illustration and wax moulages. But using photographs could also emphasize the uncertainty and the unusualness of the appearance of diseases in the new habitat of mostly young homosexual men. According to Preda, this notion of unusualness served generally as a condition to see AIDS. And as much as photography could exert a medical authority, where language couldn't, its key contribution was not to remove but to visualize uncertainty and unusualness as a medical characteristic of the epidemic.

Clinical photographs, I argue here, should be seen as a contribution to persistent ambiguity between the population in which the diseases appeared and the new immunodeficiency syndrome. In other words, seeing AIDS through clinical photographs had the advantage to show the vaguely disclosed, never quite visible, never fully hidden social identity of those, who were part of the demographic, perceived to be hosting AIDS at that time. Rather than aiming for a clear distinction between a

---

[105] Preda, *AIDS, Rhetoric, and Medical Knowledge*, 48.

disease morphology and a patient's identity, clinical photography could present the underlying syndrome through a series of pictures of discrete diseases, bound together through the social group in which they appeared.

The conflation of gay male identity and KS became more than an underlying subtle theme in Friedman-Kien's atlas. First published in 1989, this second series operated differently from its predecessor volume by Farthing and colleagues, who contributed a chapter on the history of AIDS to the new atlas. This updated and newly conceptualized book was preoccupied almost exclusively with KS, or rather with the representation of an "AIDS-related epidemic KS" as a specific disease entity. The majority of photographs in this volume either visualize the characteristic skin cancer or show "clinical simulators." In more than 200 photographs, this AIDS atlas began with a detour, which introduced classic and African cases of KS. The first 40 photographs visualize a wide variety of cases of KS in elderly men in the United States and extreme cases of KS in Africa. These photographs presented a picture of the rare skin cancer as it might have been perceived before the emergence of AIDS. The rest of the atlas was then dedicated to visualizing the variety of KS appearances in people with AIDS, separating different stages – plaque, ocular and nodular – each with about five photographs. Of particular interest is the section on clinical "simulators," other skin cancers and harmless rashes that share a course of appearances similar to KS but in fact might not share any relation to AIDS. The remaining portion of the atlas is concerned with microscopic and ultrastructural presentations of KS, before a final section with another 50 photographs lists other cutaneous signs of people with AIDS or AIDS-related complex (ARC). Among these conditions are those previously visualized in Farthing's atlas with prominent presentations of shingles and candidiasis. Only the very last chapter of the 1989 atlas discusses cutaneous appearances of HIV infections, presenting three photographs among microscopic visualizations of the quite unusual and rare appearances in the syndrome's clinical latency. Throughout the atlas, each photograph is given a short description, classification and diagnostic judgment from the editors, which points in terms of definition and depth of description well beyond Farthing's work. These texts are significant because they effectively turn each photograph into a singular representation of a case that has been chosen as exemplary.

According to the atlas's rationale the social identity of the patient achieved yet further significance. Photographs of classical KS, according to how the sarcoma was considered and classified before AIDS emerged, tend to be captioned by identity placeholders such as "elderly Ashkenazi

Jewish male" or "75 year old Italian male."[106] The second category of "African Endemic KS" was shown on what the editor understood to be African bodies: These are bodies of different ages, sexualities and gender and with different disease histories as far as can be gleaned, but similar only in regard to their common African heritage. The third and largest category included photographs that look similar to those used by Farthing (Fig. 1.8), which here demonstrated the epidemic AIDS-related KS in bodies of "a 44 year old otherwise healthy, homosexual male ..., A 23 year old homosexual male. ... A 39 year old homosexual male."[107] What was an implicit, almost silent connection made in Farthing's atlas two years earlier became an explicit observation deemed crucial for differentiating and classifying the AIDS-related variant of KS. In a summary of the first decade of AIDS, Friedman-Kien reflected, that: "One of the most intriguing epidemiologic observations is that 95 percent of all cases of AIDS-associated Kaposi's sarcoma in the United States have been diagnosed among homosexual and bisexual men."[108]

The introduction of the atlas claimed that KS is "truly one of mother nature's puzzle games." AIDS was no longer understood as a primarily homosexual disease, and by 1989, as the editor notes, its prevalence among gay communities was indeed declining, the atlas aimed to teach a valuable lesson:

AIDS is not yet a common disease, and many physicians have a limited personal experience with it. The rapidly increasing incidence and spread to the heterosexual population will soon present the general physician with many diagnostic problems. This text will provide a valuable visual course on the cutaneous manifestations of AIDS.[109]

The atlas was founded upon the task of visualizing this transition and expected distribution of the epidemic beyond its already familiar occurrence in homosexual men. In a way, Friedman-Kien aimed to correct the silent – and all too often quite tangible – assumption that AIDS only appeared within the confines of a particular sexual identity. As the introduction to this atlas demonstrates, the notion of unusualness, typical for AIDS's early years, had taken on a tone of warning. Although the appearance of epidemic AIDS-related KS is shown predominantly on the bodies of homosexual males, Friedman-Kien sought to demonstrate how

---

[106] Alvin E. Friedman-Kien, ed., *Color Atlas of AIDS* (Philadelphia: Saunders, 1989), 15, 18.
[107] Ibid., 25.   [108] Ibid., 31.   [109] Ibid., xvi.

Clinical Manifestations of Kaposi's Sarcoma

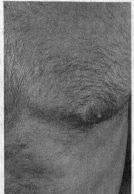

Figure 2–39. Epidemic Kaposi's sarcoma. Patch stage.
This totally asymptomatic faint pink macular lesion of Kaposi's sarcoma spontaneously appeared on the side of this patient's chin. Similar patch-stage lesions developed at distant sites on the patient's body at about the same time.

Figure 2–40. Epidemic Kaposi's sarcoma. Patch stage.
A 44 year old otherwise healthy, homosexual male with a single flat red macule of Kaposi's sarcoma on his lower chest.

Figure 2–41. Epidemic Kaposi's sarcoma. Patch stage.
An elongated flat lesion on the trunk, which varied in color from pink to red, was initially ignored because the patient thought that this "spot" represented a minor bruise. As this skin lesion became darker in color, other macules developed at distant sites. The patient sought medical attention at that time.

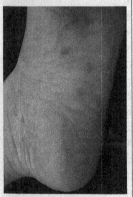

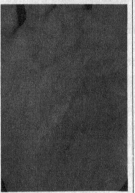

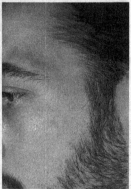

Figure 2–42. Epidemic Kaposi's sarcoma. Patch stage.
A 23 year old homosexual male with multiple flat, tawny pink lesions on the sole and ankle of the foot. Initially, the lesions were thought to represent secondary syphilis. There were several other cutaneous lesions of a similar nature widely disseminated over the rest of his body.

Figure 2–43. Epidemic Kaposi's sarcoma. Patch stage.
A single light brown flat macular lesion on the palm of the hand. The biopsy confirmed the diagnosis of Kaposi's sarcoma.

Figure 2–44. Epidemic Kaposi's sarcoma. Patch stage.
Multiple patch-stage lesions on the temple and bearded areas of the face. The lesions were slightly irregular in shape and widely dispersed over the rest of the body.

Fig. 1.8 Page with photographs of people with AIDS-related epidemic KS in Friedman-Kien's atlas from 1989. The editor disclosed the age and sexual identity of the depicted cases to point to the persistent prevalence of KS among homosexual men with AIDS. But rather than crudely conflating AIDS and sexual identity, this arrangement suggests an analytical separation.

Source: Alvin E. Friedman-Kien, ed., *Color Atlas of AIDS* (Philadelphia: Saunders, 1989), p. 25. Permission granted by Elsevier.

AIDS had become a familiar sight for some while it was still uncommon to the wider population, where it was assumed to eventually arrive. As a result, many more doctors needed to become fluent with what AIDS might look like. The threat of an impending pandemic seemed to have structured the urgency behind this edition of an AIDS atlas.

By 1989, when Friedman-Kien turned his extensive research on KS into an atlas, the epidemic had become the primary reason for death in the US population between the ages of 25 and 44. The challenge was to overcome a previously established way of seeing, which had proven catastrophic to those who were stigmatized as being the cause for the epidemic. But even according to the US Surgeon General, such outdated perception of a homosexual disease became a public health risk, as it transpired a false sense of security to the rest of the population.[110] What becomes visible, therefore, in Friedman-Kien's atlas is an attempt to separate an abstract notion of AIDS and how it worked from the concrete appearance of KS in homosexual men. Clinical photography still contributed to the parallel presence of disease morphology and patient identity but was used in this atlas as a visualization method that aimed for distinction and comparison rather than conflation.

When Friedman-Kien presented sexual identities in the captions of cases in the atlas, he turned an implicit practice of AIDS's first decade into an explicit exercise. The "rules of seeing" were already established and provided a frame through which the observation and perception of AIDS arrived at new classifications and structures. Friedman-Kien laid out an archive of the epidemic's appearances and the prevalence of KS in homosexual men. Although this suggests a mere confirmation of the early years in which the entanglement of sexual identity and disease were guiding principle, the arrangement of pictures in the 1989 atlas points to a different mode of perception. Where each photograph tends to entangle morphology of disease and the unseen identity of the depicted patient, Friedman-Kien provided a detailed definition of their relationship, rather than leaving that relationship ambiguous and open to misinterpretation. Each photograph becomes a representation of a particular case, the individual history of which is added through the caption, but in doing so the visualization lost some of its capacity to demonstrate uncertainty and the unusualness described previously regarding the case of Farthing's work.

---

[110] Koop C. Everett, *Surgeon General's Report on Acquired Immune Deficiency Syndrome* (Washington, DC: US Public Health Service, 1986).

This practice is indebted to the editor's mission to arrive at a new disease entity, AIDS-related epidemic KS. Based on a revision of cases from the first decade and his presentation, KS left the territory of unusual and unexpected appearances. Against the background of the editor's explicit warning that a common pandemic might be imminent, his visual archive of KS in homosexual men was not intended to work as an indeterminable conflation of sexual identity and disease morphology. Instead he drew the reader's attention to the problematic implications of such an identification. In other words, adding information on homosexuality and age to the captions of pictures representing AIDS cases retrieved the sexual identity from the depth of etiological uncertainty.

Photographing AIDS as a Disease

Clinical photography transformed the perception of the epidemic through its first decade, but the genre struggled to arrive at abstract representations of the syndrome. Initially a medium prone to conflate identity and morphology to make AIDS visible, it only hesitantly became a technique tasked with separating the notion of the abstract entity of AIDS from the portraits of persons who contracted it. Increasingly, in the late 1980s, photography was supposed to make their entanglement unseen to perceive the one as a disease and the other as a generic, interchangeable body hosting a virus. But was it ever possible to capture the disease as an abstract entity on a photograph? Or is a photograph of a disease inescapably a medium of semantic transgression?

Sander Gilman considered the visualization of AIDS through photographs as a continuous encounter with uncertainty and an "indeterminable universe" of illness that required control, boundaries and the construction of a stable difference between health and disease.[111] The photograph of the patient created difference, as it served as a vehicle to achieve an initial understanding about the assumed social nature of the disease.[112] To many physicians in the early 1980s, homosexuality prompted suspicion and susceptibility for AIDS.[113] The notion of AIDS

[111] Gilman, *Disease and Representation: Images of Illness from Madness to AIDS*, 2.
[112] Sander L. Gilman, "AIDS and Syphilis: The Iconography of Disease," in *AIDS, Cultural Analysis, Cultural Activism*, ed. Douglas Crimp (Cambridge, MA: MIT Press, 1988), 89.
[113] Likewise, many physicians developed their approach to the epidemic as members of the gay community contributing substantially to the successful implementation of safer sex. See: David France, *How to Survive a Plague: The Story of How Activists and Scientists Tamed AIDS* (Stuttgart: Pan Macmillan, 2016); Ronald Bayer and Gerald M. Oppenheimer, *AIDS Doctors: Voices from the Epidemic* (Oxford: Oxford University Press, 2000); Gerald Oppenheimer and Ronald Bayer, "An Epidemic of Unknown

as a homosexual disease, or as a disease implicated in homosexual lifestyles, disallowed its characterization as a viral disease divorced from social prevalence, and foregrounded an image of transmission through sexual practices at the cost of seeing other routes of spread. Clinical photography, one could argue therefore, foregrounded the perception of AIDS as a disease of homosexual lifestyle and identity, simply because it failed to present AIDS as an abstract entity.

A visual precedent of this perception, Gilman argues, can be identified in the history of syphilis. Here, a sexually transmitted disease was bound to a long-standing history of visualizing sexual transgression. The appearance and spectacle of the disease was part of an iconography of punishment.[114] Seeing the photograph of the diseased body reassured the healthy viewer's impression that this illness was deserved and fit to unseen moral failures of the person. The carrier of the disease and the photograph represented the boundaries of the epidemic, isolating the threat to particular persons and identities, while bolstering the image of immunity and safety for everyone else.

On an aesthetic level, photography of people with AIDS – within and beyond the medical AIDS atlas – was, of course, occupied by traces of decay, symbolism of doom and icons of bodily crisis. The disintegration of the body, the destruction of political subjectivities and the annihilation of sexual identities structured the visual language of AIDS photography throughout the epidemic's first decade. Following Gilman's arguments, Watney directs attention to the fact that it was fairly surprising to use photography at all, given that AIDS was understood as a diagnostic category of several different and not always visible opportunistic infections. Choosing to frame the appearance of AIDS as a "discrete illness rather than a conceptual diagnostic category" attracted significant success to craft an image of the AIDS carrier as a person who is understood to be qualitatively different from the majority of the population.[115] The victim was perceived as threat to public health and safety and is ostracized through the frame of difference. Furthermore, as Grover notes, almost everyone pictured in circulating photographs of AIDS in the early 1980s was destined to die and had most probably died, leaving us with images of their "visible lesions."[116]

Proportions: The First Decade of HIV/AIDS," in *HIV/AIDS in the Post-HAART Era: Manifestations, Treatment, and Epidemiology*, ed. John C. Hall, Clay J. Cockerell, and Brian J. Hall (Sheldon, CT: PMPH-USA, 2011), 3–19.

[114] Gilman, "AIDS and Syphilis: The Iconography of Disease," 93.
[115] Watney, "Photography and AIDS," 178.
[116] Grover, "Visible Lesions: Images of PWA in America."

Call it stigmatization, isolation or the framing of difference, photographs of illness continued to distinguish the subject from what was assumed to be healthy, normal and morally correct. Sontag took up the perception of the Other's suffering to argue at length about the effects of identification with depicted pain that guarantees spectatorship immune from what they were witnessing.[117] Judith Butler has also worked extensively on the frames of war, in which an economy of grief is visually organized, demarcating deserving lives from those less deserving of our empathy.[118] Both arguments resonate with ACT UP's calls for action, the activist's struggle for visibility and particularly the "Ashes Actions," when activists and relatives of people who died of AIDS threw their ashes on the lawn of the White House, demanding their recognition with ultimate means.[119] Both Sontag and Butler point to the uncontrollable resonances of visual representations of a body in crisis, and that visualizations of suffering bodies do not necessarily encourage a humane response or provoke emphatic identification. If we consider these effects to inevitably accompany a photographic representation of AIDS, how could – if at all – photography be used to encourage a sober and abstract representation of AIDS that is safely removed from perception of lifestyle and sexual identity?

Monstrous Photography?

This characteristic quality of AIDS photography to carry vague signs of identity into representations of diseases attaches these images to another tradition of medical photography from the later nineteenth century. A close look onto this history illuminates the attraction medical photography had in the early years of AIDS but will also explain how the genre lost most of its appeal after the epidemic's first decade.

In the late nineteenth century, many medical photographs were collected in private or public collections, traveled with "freak shows" and presented as trophies of nature's experimentations to a morbidly fascinated public. These images earned a reputation for visualizing a quality in its awe-inspiring distance from health, normality and society. This visual regime of extreme pathological signs and exceptional anomalies must be regarded as a second quality of clinical photography, which bears no

---

[117] Susan Sontag, *Regarding the Pain of Others* (New York: Farrar, Straus and Giroux, 2003).
[118] Ibid.; Judith Butler, *Frames of War: When Is Life Grievable?* (London: Verso, 2009).
[119] Jim Hubbard, *United in Anger: A History of ACT UP*, Documentary, New York, 2012.

direct relation to the tradition of pathological illustration, but is deeply embedded in late-nineteenth-century fascination for the idea of the monster.

As already discussed, photography was swiftly praised for overcoming the weaknesses of illustration and for providing representations based on empirical observation. Medical photography was often contrasted with the subjective and imprecise genre of drawing as it moved away from *ideal* representations in favor of exemplary and characteristic cases. Grounded in the "real" by the end of the nineteenth century, medical photography sometimes left the realm of classifying diseases and became the focus of efforts to collect, expose and curate archives of biologically grotesque appearances, abnormal tumors and spectacular deformations. Long series of photographs showed disfigured fetuses, collections of inoperable tumors and unthinkable deformations. Public appreciation for the extreme forms and shapes made medical photography a recording practice for the unpresentable, never-before-seen and unthinkable aspects of human life and death.[120] While the taste for the grotesque and monstrous surely had a longer history than photography, medical photography took part in making the aesthetic of the ugly and abject widely available.[121]

Photographs of spectacular appearances reflect shifts in European medical thinking that rejected understanding diseases as species that were bound to their own ontologies. The most influential interventions came from Rudolf Virchow, a German proponent of cell theory and social medicine, who argued in 1847 that diseases could not be thought of as autonomous organisms or parasites that entered and attacked the human body. Rather, diseases were more akin to various forms of life. So rather than being different in kind, they could be understood as excessive forms of physiology. The French physician Claude Bernard, famous for his work on experimental medicine, also argued that "physiology and pathology are intermingled and are essentially one and the same thing."[122] Canguilhem followed Bernard's and Comte's reasoning about the identity of disease and human life, arguing for a late-nineteenth-century medicine, which considered diseases to be a mere quantitative excess of human life, rather than its opponents.

---

[120] Gunnar Schmidt, "Todeszeichen. Zu literarischen und medizinischen Bildern im 19. Jahrhundert," in *Bildkörper. Verwandlungen des Menschen zwischen Medium und Medizin*, ed. Marianne Schuller, Claudia Reiche, and Gunnar Schmidt (Hamburg: Lit Verlag, 1998), 64.

[121] Schmidt, *Anamorphotische Körper*, 78.

[122] C. Bernard, 1877, cited in Georges Canguilhem, *On the Normal and the Pathological* (Dordrecht, the Netherlands: Reidel, 1978), 67.

"The existence of monsters," Canguilhem wrote, "throws doubt on life's ability to teach us order."[123] The notion of the monstrous, which emerged in the late nineteenth century, was both intimately bound to the idea of organic organization as much as it posed a substantial challenge to understanding the norms that governed organic life forms. Proponents of this approach rejected ontologist theories that considered diseases as natural entities. Instead, the focus rested on lumps, tumors, swellings and spectacular disfigurements. A medical photography of the spectacular, monstrous and excessive physiological form presents an opportunity for Canguilhem's thoughts to be extended into visual history. Photography offered a visual instrument with which the pathological was interrogated as nature's experiments, a form in which the radical identity of disease and human life was constantly performed.[124]

To use photography as an instrument to frame life's excess contributed to its rejection by those physicians who disliked the idea of disease as a continuum of pathological and physiological states. Doctors and atlas editors who were more interested in visualizing characteristic and archetypical states of pathology, as in the cases of Jacobi and Kaposi, refused outright the usefulness of spectacular or interesting cases to be presented to the atlas's audience.[125] Photography of "monsters" stirred common understandings about health and disease and prompted questions about the validity of disease categories. The practice contributed to an ongoing and contingent documentation, an archive of the unclassifiable. The genre did not present clinical signs as a discrete aspect of a nosological entity, a class or abstract table of a disease, but visualized disease as an erratic and poorly differentiated situation along the spectrum of life. This mode of photographic visualization was more akin to the appearance of enormous tumors as excess to the body's own tissue than to the idea of an infection by a foreign microorganism. Due to this association with excess rather than difference, photography was distrusted as a productive instrument for stabilizing classes of disease but assumed prevalence as a portraiture of spectacular cases that pointed to the limits of classification and the borderlines of medical knowledge.

The KS photography in Friedman-Kien's atlas confronts us with a combination of representational modes of the person with AIDS and the diseases indicative of AIDS. Rows and rows of pictures neither fully

---

[123] Canguilhem, "Monstrosity and the Monstrous," 27.
[124] For Virchow, diseases were thought of as spectacles of a Darwinian nature, in which the infinite capacities of human physiology were demonstrated and tested. Rudolf Virchow, "Ueber die Standpunkte in der Wissenschaftlichen Medicin," *Archiv für Pathologische Anatomie und Physiologie* 1 (1847), 3–19.
[125] Jacobi, *Atlas der Hautkrankheiten*, iii.

engaged with the discrete entity of an opportunistic infection and its symptoms, nor did they commit clearly to the social profile of the infection or the epidemiology of the immunodeficiency syndrome. The atlas uses photography of single cases, grouped together to reveal different social settings of KS, to deliver an argument of how AIDS-related KS was separated from African KS and Classic KS. Photographs in this atlas worked as portraits of individual cases rather than indeterminate visualizations of a syndrome. They illustrated the appearance of a disease in a group defined through sexual practice. Both the patients as well as the disease appeared in Friedman-Kien's atlas as discrete entities, begging the question of how their relationship has defined the short history of AIDS. The photographs seem almost to "illustrate" the history of how AIDS came into view, rather than contributing to the task of solving problems and open questions.

Beyond its instructive and demonstrative faculty, clinical photography was always also bound to such an illustrative capacity, adding the unique value of individual cases to the definition of diseases. Where this capacity of photography made pictures of monstrous appearances and spectacular cases to desirable objects for collection and exhibition it also added a new level to what Fox and Lawrence describe as photography's "visual concepts of pathology."[126] Photography could contribute a visible representation of disease based on "people who suffered afflictions."[127] The ways in which these visualizations came to be convincing instruments in textbooks and atlases are complicated, as "photography did not replace drawing to depict morbid anatomy until new conventions were created to represent tissues and tissue change."[128] Partly based on the diagrammatic tradition of drawings and moulage, photography also introduced a radically new element to the textbook, atlases and instructive publications of medicine: The appearance of individual and exemplary patients was no longer dependent on narratives, case descriptions and personal remarks, but could be represented through photographic reproductions of the patient's bodily appearance.

An exemplary account of the gradual introduction of unmasked portrait photographs of cases is given by yet another dermatologist, a contemporary of Jacobi called Edmund Lesser.[129] He published his *Lehrbuch der Haut- und Geschlechtskrankheiten für Studierende und Ärzte* between 1886 and 1887 at F. C. W. Vogel in Leipzig; it was a well-known dermatologist's

---

[126] Fox and Lawrence, *Photographing Medicine*, 28.   [127] Ibid., 23.   [128] Ibid., 24.
[129] Günter Stüttgen, "Edmund Lesser and the International Congress on Dermatology," *International Journal on Dermatology* 27 (1988), 269–73; Joachim J. Herzberg, "Edmund Lesser und seine (vergessene) Schule," *Der Hautarzt* 39 (1988), 598–601.

handbook and was distributed widely with 14 new editions before 1927. It was used both as an atlas and as a textbook, in which diseases were described through detailed texts as well as visualized in photography.[130] The familiar tone of a textbook dominated Lesser's teaching instrument and photographs remained subsidiary; predominantly used to "illustrate" the detailed written accounts of diseases and dermatological abnormalities.

Take, for example, the chapter on Herpes tonsurans. Accompanying the dense descriptions are four pictures: a magnified picture of the fungus *Trichophyton tonsurans* at 300:1, a visualization of Herpes tonsurans in the skin, a visualization of a herpes infection on the side of a bearded face and a microscopically enhanced picture of a fungus infection within hair structures.[131] The text in Lesser's atlas stayed vague about the conditions of the pictures, and none is contextualized in detail but used as a secondary illustration, anchored in the text through markings and reference numbers but not integral to the image that the book conveyed. Photographs were added as complementary add-ons to emphasize details explained in the narrative of the written description. They stabilized and made evident what is known and described about herpes tonsurans through repetition in a subsidiary visual means. This demoted inclusion of photographs in the atlas represents a fundamentally different way of using visual media compared to the earlier atlas of Cruveilhier, or to the "silent" illustrations used by Kaposi.

This pattern was repeated in a remarkable photograph of a male patient that visualized a "papulo-ulceroeses Syphilid" (Fig. 1.9). The photograph appears near the end of Lesser's book in an addendum of photographic plates. The picture has been taken in accordance with aesthetic norms of portrait photography of the time, in its visual arrangement intent on guiding the viewer's gaze to the syphilitic symptoms on the forehead, biceps and forearm of the patient. In contrast to Cruveilhier's more abstract depiction of the patient's body, or to the draped sections of patients' bodies presented in moulages, this photograph gave a full upper-body view of the patient and his face. The posture, the facial expression and the disease-stricken body became part of the visualization of the clinical picture. The disease was not revealed through visual isolation of its signs or analytical close-ups; instead its signs were shown

---

[130] Ehring, *Hautkrankheiten*, 222.

[131] Edmund Lesser, *Lehrbuch der Haut- und Geschlechtskrankheiten für Studierende und Ärzte* (Leipzig: F. C. W. Vogel, 1888), 272–80. This typical assemblage of different types of visualization is found throughout most of the chapters of the book. The intricate effect of the combination of these different genres is the standard way used in the later AIDS atlases.

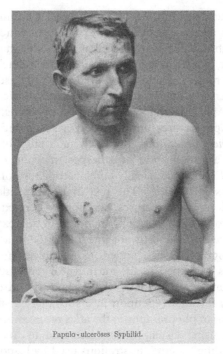

Papulo-ulceröses Syphilid.

Fig. 1.9 Portrait of a patient with syphilis in Lesser's dermatological handbook from 1890. Instead of guiding the readers gaze directly to clinical signs, this photograph emphasized the embodied nature of the disease, illustrating the abstract definition of the disease with a singular case.
Source: Edmund Lesser, *Lehrbuch der Haut- und Geschlechtskrankheiten für Studierende und Ärzte* (Leipzig: Vogel, 1886), Appendix, Plate III. Courtesy of the Wellcome Collection.

as part of a larger composition of the suffering patient. The medically significant part, the syphilitic rash on the arm and the face, was emphasized using captions and by anchoring the photograph to the chapter on syphilis.

Photographs such as this do not display a picture of disease in the way Kaposi's atlas or Jacobi's moulages did, nor do they seek to isolate a disease entity from the patient's body. A characteristic picture is not revealed – nor is it the photograph's purpose – but the picture illustrates agreed-upon knowledge with visual references to patients and their suffering. Photographs like this one ground the abstract disease category of syphilis in a particular case, which demonstrates to a medical audience the impact and crisis that comes with the development of the disease. The photographed disease is illustrated through the single case, neither bound to an analytical gaze (there is no draping, cropping or covering), but relies on an emphatic and affective impression of a person enduring the affliction. Such pictures visualize specific disease in its entanglement with the person affected, and they require a more complex and extensive anchoring in descriptive and analytical text, as their contribution lies in the translation of knowledge into visibility instead of vice versa.

This example suggests that photography cannot be understood as the simple successor to, or improved version of, medical illustration. Yet it would also be a mistake to understand the sidelining of visual practices in Lesser's atlas as a rehabilitation of written clinical pictures at the end of the nineteenth century. Photography presented a classic epistemological obstacle, as Bachelard put it, when set to the task of establishing a visual clinical picture.[132] Photography pointed to the limits of delivering characteristic pictures based on the single case, as well as to potential for delivering a new way of seeing the pathological. Photography's novelty allowed the pathological to be appreciated as a structured appearance that maintained an arbitrary, contingent and irreducibly undefined element.

Photographic Illustration of Cases

The work of Edinburgh-based clinician Byrom Bramwell and his *Atlas of Clinical Medicine*, published in three volumes between 1892 and 1896, is further illuminating to understand the clinical integration of exemplary photographic case portraits. Lacking both preface and introduction, the work shows unusual as well as typical cases in the voluminous atlas, which covered a broad range of medical specialties. It is remarkable that most of the pictures were visualized through both photography and watercolor illustrations side by side. Both strategies of visualization were further complemented by detailed descriptions and structured case histories. The clinical presentation of a case, along with two pictures, was described in the following way: "The case which is depicted in Plates XII and XIII presented all the symptoms characteristic of chronic progressive bulbar paralysis, in its advanced stage."[133] The patient, a 50-year-old

---

[132] Gaston Bachelard, *The Formation of the Scientific Mind* (Manchester, UK: Clinamen, 2002).
[133] Byrom Bramwell, *Atlas of Clinical Medicine, Volume I* (Edinburgh: Constable, 1892), 104.

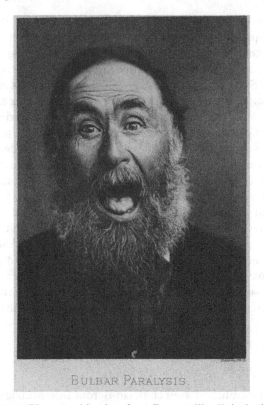

Fig. 1.10 Photographic plate from Bramwell's clinical atlas from 1892.
In combination with the watercolor detail of the tongue, this
photograph contributes to the appearance of an embodied and
personalized case; a characteristic example for a well-defined disease,
supported by the aesthetic appearance of a "carte visite."
Source: Byrom Bramwell, *Atlas of Clinical Medicine* (Edinburgh: Constable,
1892), vol. I, p. 118. Courtesy of the Wellcome Collection.

peasant, died by the time the atlas was published. The "characteristic"
photograph (Fig. 1.10) is an aesthetic portrait of an aged man sticking
out his tongue. The accompanying description emphasized the great pain
that sitting for this photograph would have caused the patient, as well as
noting how the disease developed rapidly and how many of the crucial
features of this clinical picture could not possibly be communicated
through a photograph.

On the next page, the photograph is contrasted with a colored illustration that magnified one part of the photograph, the tongue, to

reveal its "uneven, wrinkled, 'hob-nailed' condition."[134] The author explained that:

This Plate shows the exact appearance of the tongue in the case of chronic progressive bulbar paralysis described above. The furred, uneven (atrophic) and yet oedematous condition of the organ is admirably shown. The water-colour drawing, from which the plate is copied, was made on October eighteenth, 1891 – the same day that the patient presented himself at the author's clinique.[135]

The photograph served a different function to the illustration, as in the author's reflection it seemed to hide, rather than reveal the diseases key features. The photograph fits easily in the conventions of nonmedical portrait photography, deviating only in its facial expression. Bramwell perhaps attempted to show the disease in its larger environment to demonstrate its occurrence in ordinary people, whereas the illustration maintains its abstract and analytical function, especially in its coloring, which was supposedly drawn directly from the original case. At the end of the nineteenth century, a clinical atlas problematized the authenticity of photographs as media too close to aesthetic norms, while the illustration is included to deliver a characteristic and exemplary visualization of disease.

Lesser's choice to sideline photographs in his handbook, the absence of photography in Kaposi's atlas and the combination with illustrations in Bramwell's atlas all account for a belief that photography could not alone deliver what was required for atlases and handbooks. If used at all, photography's function was to individualize, portray or illustrate the otherwise abstract notion of diseases, given by text or illustrations. In other words, photography introduced a way of seeing disease as an ever-embodied form in which the endeavor of separating the experience of disease from abstract classes of thinking and knowing diseases was questioned. Photography thus adopted a position in medical knowledge production that had previously been inhabited by case histories.[136]

Photography has since its inception posed a challenge to the idea that there can be a clear line between health and pathology. These simplistic categories of normalcy and disease fade, and in their place the liminal, unsolved and *unusual* appears. A photograph can document what is not, or not yet, known, classified and ordered whether as a monstrous extreme or an arbitrary individual case. In photography a disease cannot appear as an isolated clinical sign but as a poorly differentiated situation

[134] Ibid., 118.   [135] Ibid., 119.
[136] Hess and Mendelsohn, "Sauvages' Paperwork"; Kassell, "Casebooks in Early Modern England."

of life. In Canguilhem's approach, photography could be seen as an instrument of observation and interrogation in which diseases are not isolated and defined in their own ontologies, but where disease is inescapably presented as an embodied entanglement with life. I propose to see the significance and the success of clinical photographs of AIDS therefore to be essential for setting up a kind of experimental system in which the process of separation, the strategies of isolation and the methods of visualization of a disease could be seen, rather than the disease.

It is crucial to understand that photographs always denied doctors the chance to exercise tight control over categories, classes and genres of diseases. This challenge to authority and definition suggests a rationale for photograph's marginalized position, occasional absence or their extensive visual anchoring through illustrations in medical publications in the late nineteenth century. None of the atlas editors from this bygone century relied on photographs to speak for themselves or teach an audience in the way illustrations and moulages had been entrusted. Photographs carried a certain mistrust because of their excess of signification and because the visibility of personal element made the pictures liable to distract the less experienced observer. But photography's contribution to medicine was also not exclusively bound to a visualization of unusual singularity.[137] As I have shown previously, photography was also used to reproduce characteristic visions by distributing mechanical reproductions of illustrations and moulages. As a medical tool, photography could both be useful in showing new and previously unseen singularities, and by distributing subjective accounts of characteristic images more widely than ever before. By the 1980s, it had become the perfect genre equipped

---

[137] In his recent dissertation Alexander Moffett points to another enterprise in which photography was used to create characteristic pictures of diseases by visualizing the average picture of diseases. Against the background of collective investigations by the British Medical Association in the 1880s, protagonists began to discuss possible ways in which photography could be used to combine many single cases into one picture. The investigations were based on examination cards used to assemble and sort thousands of opinions from clinicians throughout the country on pneumonia, TB, and other diseases, while photographs were taken in cooperation with Francis Galton and used in the same way that he used to deliver composite images of criminals. By superimposing hundreds of photographs of phthisis, a composite portrait of the disease's physiognomy was to be achieved. See: Francis Galton and F. A. Mahomed, "An Inquiry into the Physiognomy of Phthisis by the Method of 'Composite Portraiture,'" *Guy's Hospital Reports* 25 (1882), 475–93; Alun D. Hughes, "Commentary: 'On the Cards': Collective Investigation of Disease and Medical Life Histories in the Nineteenth Century," *International Journal of Epidemiology* 42, no. 3 (June 1, 2013), 683–8, doi:10.1093/ije/dyt062; Alexander Moffett, "Generic Images of Disease: The Uses of Collective Investigation, 1880–1900." Talk given at AAHM 2015, New Haven, CT, 2015.

to visualize an impending crisis, as well as renewing a traditional medical authority in absence of clarity and reliable medical understandings.

The epistemic tension of photography between the patient's illness and an abstract definition of disease that was set up in the late nineteenth century continued through the twentieth century. Peter Hansell, photographer at the Department for Medical Photography in London's Westminster Hospital argued just after World War II for a timely transformation of medical photography. He hoped it could become a method of knowledge dissemination rather than mere recording.[138] Despite an increase in professional education he demanded the installation of standardized archives and the inclusion of arrows, labels and scales within the pictures to regulate medical photography as a useful and exploratory tool of modern clinical practice.[139] Similar ideas have been articulated by Brian Stanford, who argued for clinical photographs to "provide an absolute image to the mind of a doctor who has never seen the patient before; they must even provide an absolute image to a doctor who has never seen a similar complaint before."[140] He demanded standardization and broad institutionalization of clinical photography to "evoke a real image"[141] of the disease, and not just mere partial glimpses of illness, pain and affliction.

Mifflin has recently pointed out that this entanglement between photographic records and spectacular diseases could again today be of use in medical teaching to demonstrate illnesses, symptoms and full-blown disease pictures in their original, untreated stages that have never been seen by most medical students or doctors.[142] The photographs of people with AIDS work similarly today compared to the 1980s, as pictures of full-blown AIDS that is rarely seen in contemporary clinics or even publications. The emerging epidemic was photographed in its early years, when its complicated, confusing and sensitive appearance was best captured by the historically developed practice of a clinical photography: It provided a way of seeing, that remained on the surface, both individually and regarding the epidemic's unresolved etiology. The spectacle of

---

[138] Peter Hansell and Robert G. W. Ollerenshaw, "Applied Photography: Relation of the Photographic Department to the Teaching Hospital," *The Lancet* 250, no. 6479 (November 1, 1947), 663–6, doi:10.1016/S0140-6736(47)90689-2. Originally published as volume 2.

[139] Peter Hansell, "Medical Photography: A Review," *The Lancet* 248, no. 6418 (August 31, 1946), 296–9, doi:10.1016/S0140-6736(46)90799-4.

[140] Brian Stanford, "The Hospital Photographic Department," *The Lancet* 248, no. 6418 (August 31, 1946), 299, doi:10.1016/S0140-6736(46)90800-8.

[141] Ibid., 300.

[142] Jeffrey Mifflin, "Visual Archives in Perspective: Enlarging on Historical Medical Photographs," *The American Archivist* 70, no. 1 (2007), 41.

newness, unusualness and rarity could be captured to illustrate what was known about the threatening epidemic, while teaching how it was to be seen so to reestablish medical authority in face of an epistemic crisis.

The End of AIDS Photography

In 1983, the author and enthusiastic bodybuilder Stephen Greco wrote a contribution to the gay magazine *The Advocate*.[143] Meditating on the rising number of gym memberships in New York's gay community since the epidemic begun, he wondered if a stronger body would bring protection. He shared with his readers a particularly insightful anecdote about a community AIDS briefing, set up to inform about the latest advances in understanding the new disease, which was probably held at the Gay Man's Health Center in New York. Casually, he described the despair, the shared experience of AIDS cases that almost everyone in his vicinity had seen and described the grim benefits resulting from the high prevalence of KS:

There have been so many recent cases of Kaposi's in New York that the doctors who throw these grim parties no longer need use as illustrations those outdated slides showing the so-called classic cases of the disease as manifested in older Jewish and Italian men. Now we have our own cases and what appear before us in darkened auditoriums 10 times life size are pictures of our own bodies. It makes you think.[144]

He goes on to recall the effect of a particular image, a photograph of a young man's chest, bearing lesions typical for KS, but unlike what one might expect from a clinical photograph, in this case the lesions had appeared on the "most carefully inflated pectorals imaginable."[145] The audience, Greco remembers, gasped, and he found himself contending with a sudden flash of sexual desire directed at the body, projected at the wall. But how to reflect on this attraction, Greco asks, when the body before you was projected to instill awareness through its visible signs of a deadly skin cancer to promote sexual modesty and restraint?[146]

The medical framing of this photograph from Greco's anecdote could not eradicate the patient's body as one which is still sexual. The presence of obvious clinical signs of KS, the setting of the briefing organized by doctors like Farthing or Friedman-Kien (with the latter even possibly

---

[143] I'm indebted to Richard McKay for pointing me in the direction of this very fitting source: Stephen Greco, "Strong Bodies Gay Ways," *The Advocate*, July 7, 1983, 20–3.
[144] Ibid.   [145] Ibid., 22.
[146] On the wider discussion of desire and pathological portraits in AIDS, see: Crimp, "Portraits of People with AIDS."

being the attending medic of the mentioned event), could not prevent the photograph from working as a call to desire, contradicting the original intent, that led to the production, circulation and projection of the photograph. Instead of a warning, instead of delivering a shocking pathological appearance, a monstrous disfiguration of a once-healthy body, the photograph appeared to allow identification with the person depicted as a desirable body. What became unseen in this particular configuration was the disease, not the patient.

Farthing's atlas contains many traces that threatened to operate in the same kind. Visualizing KS on the face of a patient (Fig. 1.1), tracing the spread of unusual skin diseases (Fig. 1.4) or attempting to formalize a visual representation of "rapid aging" (Fig. 1.6); the fate, the story and the personalities of these disease representations continue to haunt the atlas' mission. A gray spot of hair, a posture, a changing hairstyle and facial expressions humanized the catalog of opportunistic infections. But it would be a mistake to address these affective residues as a failure of the atlas in its attempt to discipline its photographs into medical representations. On the contrary, the photographs do their medical work through linking the appearance of diseases on real cases, as these individuals lent their authenticity to the intended impression of urgency and inescapable sense of unusualness; something drawn illustrations and photographs of wax moulages could not do and – to point to the following chapters – that maps and virus pictures equally failed to convey.

Photographs can never sufficiently define their own content. Photographs of AIDS, particularly medical photographs of AIDS, are no exception to this. As far as a photograph might be trimmed, cropped, tethered to captions and structured through semantic frameworks like an atlas or a medical AIDS briefing, they still fail to arrest a purified vision of the disease to make it a static representation of itself. If we approach such photographs from the strict perspective of their contribution to the endeavor of making AIDS an object of scientific knowledge, they appear to be an extraordinarily weak medium. If a photograph's function were to be defined by its capacity to demonstrate AIDS in an abstracted, generic shape and form, its failure is imminent. But in the case of AIDS, photography was used as a visualization for an emerging epidemic in the 1980s, for its capacity to maintain a presence of disease morphology within the same frame as the presence of social identities was indeed a strong, if not necessary, faculty.

AIDS photography shared this feature within and beyond the realm of a medical atlas. Challenges to medicalization in artistic pictures and sexualization in medical frames both forge a tightly knit connection between what is anticipated as healthy, innocent and inconspicuous, with what appear diseased, disintegrated, disfigured and even as signs of impending death. The history of AIDS photography resembles and reinstates the "epidemic of signification," as the medium could not resolve the ambiguities, uncertainties and unusualness of the emerging epidemic. On the contrary, as Farthing's atlas in particular shows, the long series of photographs made AIDS visible precisely as a syndrome of unusually strong appearances, uncertain symptoms and uncommon patterns of well-known infections in new constellations. If we invoke Preda, this is where the photographs take part in classificatory practices, where the emphasis of unusual appearance sets the groundwork for a new underlying condition, that can be seen as the "unusual usual."[147] A clinical photograph focuses on the recognition of the shape and appearance of signs, but the series of photographs in an AIDS atlas also carried a story in the background, concerned with the presentation of a social denominator, a new habitat in which the unusualness of opportunistic infection became visible.

Precisely this residue of patients' lives, experiences and stories, also aroused suspicion toward the photographic medium. Often perceived as a portrayal of the patient rather than the disease, photography had a tradition of individualizing, of enriching abstracted definitions of specific disease entities. A revised history of medical photography places this visualization practice at the center of this unresolved tension about what medical imagery should seek to do. Photography appears as a practice equally concerned with intelligible, well-established knowledge formations and the appearances of the spectacular and unseen notion of previously unknown diseases. This is the unique value of clinical photography that enabled a translation of AIDS and its "epidemic of signification" into a clinical picture.

Returning to Canguilhem, photography seems to exhibit a strong relationship to thinking about disease as a form of excess, as a picture of an imbalance, a disposition and a dysfunction. Photographs configured an embodiment of AIDS, which cannot be detached from the body in which the condition appeared. An unusual KS, an uncommon rash or a significantly strong outbreak of shingles inherited their unusualness through the depicted affection and embodied experience. In this way, photographs frame the first chapter of AIDS history as the "politics of lifestyle" Epstein discussed, in which Oppenheimer identified the significance of multifactorial models, and where Yingling saw the person with AIDS being made unseen through layers of medical framings.

---

[147] Preda, *AIDS, Rhetoric, and Medical Knowledge*, 61.

Photographs sought an understanding of the relation between communities, practices and the epidemic's distribution.

When Friedman-Kien set out his first atlas in 1989, this first chapter of AIDS history was already ending. As he pointed out himself, the atlas was published at a time when AIDS was on the cusp of becoming a global pandemic with widespread distribution among the general society. Treatment options were not yet available, and the mortality rate was rising at a seemingly unstoppable pace. Aware of this globalization of the epidemic, Friedman-Kien's application of photography was intended to transfer the remaining epidemiological puzzle piece into the next chapter of AIDS. The prevalence of AIDS-related epidemic KS among homosexual men was so striking to him that he coined a new class of KS. Where the defining feature of this new class was the social profile of KS in cases of AIDS, photography again was employed to chart out the landscape of this classification practice, visualizing the epidemiological connection between the morphology of KS lesions and the "sociology" of young, gay men. It took until 1994 to resolve this epidemiological puzzle, when Yuan Chang and others would publish a paper that suggested a significant association between KS prevalence and a new herpes virus, with a widespread circulation in gay communities. The presence of the virus might have contributed to the unusual high occurrence of KS in this population.[148] At the same time, the prevalence of KS among gay men had diminished and was also becoming a picture of the past.

The photographs in Friedman-Kien's second edition from 1996 – although some were identical to those used in the first edition– were put to a different purpose. The atlas rationale was now dedicated to diseases that appear in patients with HIV infections, integrating "a vast amount of new information about HIV-related disease that has been elucidated since the first edition," claim the editors.[149] In this extended, actualized edition, photographs ceased fully to demonstrate an uncertain relation between the syndrome and its human carriers, and no longer were they framed to present the unusualness of the appearance of diseases in specific social settings. Instead the photographs assembled and collected the visible effects of an HIV infection. The clinical gaze that was applied in this second publication of Friedman-Kien did no longer interrogate the very nature of the relationship between the affected

---

[148] Yuan Chang et al., "Identification of Herpesvirus-Like DNA Sequences in AIDS-Associated Kaposi's Sarcoma," *Science* 266 (1994), 1865–9, doi:10.1126/science.7997879.

[149] Alvin E. Friedman-Kien and Clay J. Cockerell, eds., *Color Atlas of AIDS* (Philadelphia: W. B. Saunders, 1996), xi.

patient and their lifestyle and practices but was immediately pointed toward the depth of the syndrome's viral etiology. By 1996, the photograph of bodily symptoms had become a trace of a viral activity, as the syndrome was no longer seen as the quantitative extension of lifestyle and sexual identity, but as the qualitative opponent to life.

Accordingly, the atlas was now filled with photographs of fewer opportunistic infections. Although KS was still a prominent disease, it was demoted to be just one of a variety. Throughout the chapters, patients did not remain anonymous and the majority of photographs are attached to short captions providing information on the visualized cases. The photographs tend to be embedded in additional visual information, such as tissue sections, pictures of histological analysis and models of HIV mechanics. The atlas editors conceded the transformation partly to "changes in the epidemiology, biology, and natural history of the disease,"[150] and partly to intervention of anti-retroviral therapies. Relieved from the original purpose of charting the social conditions of KS appearance, the photographs of the 1996 atlas now appear like a stable catalog of visible traces of an HIV infection.

Photographs persisted in the atlas until 2008, but their function changed to become a medium of surplus illustration. They also acquired a new function as an archive of how AIDS used to look like when its outbreak had not been under control. Photographs increasingly took on the function of demonstrating the spectacle of AIDS as it did – and later, not anymore – appear to the eyes of doctors. The increasing detachment of the syndrome from its embodied appearances – and accordingly the decreasing significance of photography – can best be understood when looking at the final atlas series published by Donna Mildvan from 1995 to 2008. Already in its first edition – as part of the overarching *vademecum* on infectious diseases – other visual representations like diagrams of HIV dominate the overall impression given of AIDS. The atlas carves out a different rationale to either Farthing's or Friedman-Kien's and is mostly concerned with the functionality of the virus and its transmission as well as with various underlying assumptions of possible treatments. In short, the atlas approaches the syndrome from the disciplinary perspective of infectious diseases, focused on the infectious agent and the means of its spread. But as indicated in the atlas's introduction by the series editor, Gerald L. Mandell, "[D]iagnosis and management of patients with infectious diseases are based in large part on visual clues." This "modern, complete collection" of images also forcefully reminds the

---

[150] Ibid., x.

profession, just as Friedman-Kien did, that diseases in AIDS often appear "unique" and "atypical."[151]

Between numerous diagrams and maps, photographs seem only of limited interest to Mildvan and her colleagues. Throughout the detailed and complex atlas some photographs can be found in chapters except the one dedicated to "cutaneous manifestations." A few photographs are used to show characteristic rashes in early stages of HIV infections to draw the reader's attention to the expected "spectrum of HIV disease."[152] Every photograph is accompanied by a detailed discussion of the disease it visualized, while not a single case is mentioned. The sexual identities of most patients remain unknown and the majority of caption end with a description of the typical morphology of the illustrated disease in cases of AIDS or HIV infection. But clinical photographs also become scattered along the sections on AIDS and HIV in women and on pediatric AIDS. Here, the pictures follow the general purpose of the sections to raise awareness to the specific appearances of AIDS in these demographics. But throughout the atlas, photographs remain sidelined for most sections, serving in an illustrative function as photographs did for Lesser and Bramwell. They demonstrated the most typical characteristics of understood and well-enough classified set of disease entities, whose appearance were typical for cases of AIDS.

Beyond the framework of the atlas, AIDS photography also drastically changed in the early 1990s. The image of AIDS as disfigurement found its probably last public scandal in the Benetton Campaign.[153] After that, pictures of bodies overwhelmed by the stigma of disease became pictures of the recent past. Photographing the person with AIDS became increasingly bound to endeavors of visualizing hope or of crafting new images of innocent victims – most prominently in photographs of HIV positive mothers and their children. These introduced the body with HIV into the world of marketing. As Rodney Jones has argued, pictures of healthy and fit bodies with HIV addressed an "idealized 'self' – healthy, empowered and possessing options."[154] With the growing availability of anti-retroviral treatment, photography of people with HIV infections

---

[151] Donna Mildvan, ed., *AIDS*. Vol. 1. Atlas of Infectious Diseases (Philadelphia: Current Medicine, 195), v.

[152] Ibid., 1:4.7.

[153] Les Back and Vibeke Quaade, "Dream Utopias, Nightmare Realities: Imaging Race and Culture within the World of Benetton Advertising," *Third Text* 7, no. 22 (1993), 65–80; Henry A. Giroux, "Consuming Social Change: The 'United Colors of Benetton,'" *Cultural Critique* no. 26 (1993), 5–32.

[154] Rodney H. Jones, "Marketing the Damaged Self: The Construction of Identity in Advertisements Directed towards People with HIV/AIDS," *Journal of Sociolinguistics* 1, no. 3 (1997), 399, doi:10.1111/1467-9481.00022.

became invested in picturing healthy, normal and capable persons, with bodies that have "HIV under control." According to Campbell, photography too had lost its medicalizing capacities in the visual economy of AIDS at the end of the twentieth century; a statement that holds true if we maintain fixed with the American and European body.

Insisting on this claim risks a general assessment of the history of photography of AIDS that would continue an indifference to the rapidly changing geography of the epidemic by the end of the 1980s into the 1990s. A photographic representation of AIDS embodied through a predominantly North American risk group became obscure when the global picture of the epidemic emerged. Prevalence rates among social groups varied drastically from location to location, but the continued absence of successful treatment options until 1995 meant that interventions into social behavior were the most effective means of global health interventions.

AIDS photography accordingly diversified to become a practice as complex and manifold as the epidemic.[155] A pamphlet from 1994, published by the WHO just a year before HAART was announced at the Vancouver AIDS conference, aimed to draw together the new "images of the epidemic."[156] Hundreds of photographs, some in color, aim to show a range of societies, cultures, communities, social practices and fabrics around the world – from prostitution in Thailand, poverty in Brazil, farming families in Tanzania to drug use in Brooklyn. AIDS, the pictures tell, appears everywhere in different conditions, resembling the classic paradigm of global health in which the correlation between resource scarcity, absent primary healthcare and disease prevalence became the frame through which AIDS was visualized. Not a single photograph in the pamphlet shows recognizable signs of disease, indeed most pictures are not even intended to visualize cases but rather draw attention to possible occurrences in estimated populations at risk. This official image of the worldwide crisis of AIDS defined and framed much of the new attitude to the epidemic. Maps and visualizations of HIV show AIDS, its character and spread, while photographs served as pictures of risk, measurements of affect and vulnerability and portraits of the lives threatened by a virus.

---

[155] Ruth J. Prince, "The Diseased Body and the Global Subject: The Circulation and Consumption of an Iconic AIDS Photograph in East Africa," *Visual Anthropology* 29, no. 2 (2016), 159–86, doi:10.1080/08949468.2016.1131517; Julie Livingston, "AIDS as Chronic Illness: Epidemiological Transition and Health Care in South-Eastern Botswana," *African Journal of AIDS Research* 3, no. 1 (2004), 15–22; Julie Livingston, "Figuring the Tumor in Botswana," *Raritan* 34, no. 1 (2014), 10–24.

[156] World Health Organization, *AIDS: Images of the Epidemic* (Geneva: World Health Organization, 1994).

2   Seeing Spaces of AIDS

Maps begin to make sense after the clinical photographer's work is done. Normally, maps move into focus when cases have been diagnosed and verified and a clinical authority is reinstated. Mapmaking means to count cases and to place them into a spatial and temporal order to visualize the disease's location, to ask why cases have appeared in these places and not in others and to conclude, if the emerging pattern can tell us anything, on what this disease *is*. Through photographs, AIDS had become readable as a pattern of discrete infections, symptoms, characteristic signs and visceral impressions on bodies of particular persons, defined as a population at risk. Maps were made to step back from this close clinical perspective and its arbitrary relationship with the individual body. As a view from above, maps resolve momentous encounters with the disease on the ground into a pattern, creating a two-dimensional representation of space and time. Maps do not capture disease: They are a genre of abstraction and imply a theoretical representation of the relationship between disease and its place. They visualize ranges of cases arranged in an order due to their spatial and temporal occurrence to reveal the shape of AIDS as an epidemic.

Infectious diseases become epidemics through scale. The AIDS epidemic was visualized through spatial perspectives from urban to national, from regional to global configurations. To think through the horizontal relationships between disparate local outbreaks, or to conceptualize hierarchies between the experience of "local pain" and the politics of "global prescriptions" are challenges that AIDS provoked on a daily basis.[1] Many metaphors have structured geographical scholarship on the global history of AIDS, reaching from "levels" to "networks" to "assemblages," each of which insinuated an angle to think through the global governance

---

[1] Catherine Campbell, Flora Cornish, and Morten Skovdal, "Local Pain, Global Prescriptions? Using Scale to Analyse the Globalisation of the HIV/AIDS Response," *Health and Place* 18, no. 3 (May 2012), 447–52, doi:10.1016/j.healthplace.2011.10.006.

of AIDS, the transnational AIDS industry or international networks of activism.[2] And last but not least, the characteristic tensions that AIDS poses to local and global perspective have carved out much of the framework of contemporary global health.[3]

In this chapter I will step back from arguments about the relative success and failure of the world's response to the global AIDS crisis and engage instead with maps as instruments that shaped the forms and configurations through which this global crisis has been made visible. Moreover, this begs the question if maps could and should be considered as pictures at all? Maps, I argue, played an essential role in changing the picture of AIDS in the late 1980s. They resolved the syndrome's exclusive association with risk groups and bodily identities to enable a seeing of AIDS in space, scaling up the epidemic from the uniformity of an urban niche to a complex pattern of global diversity.

The individual case, which had been the primary concern of clinical photographers, was flattened down in maps to become a single datapoint in a range of spatially located incidences. The patient became a public health event expected to affect communities, nations and global orders beyond any previous estimations.[4] From here onward, what mattered was not so much the shape and specific configuration of a clinical diagnosis but the number of cases, their spread and the social and cultural structure of their distribution. Nicholas King described this as "scale politics of emerging diseases" to draw attention to the "scalar narratives," in which an epidemic like AIDS appears as an ever-emerging process, overcoming early assumptions, containing of national borders, exceeding known spaces and providing place after place to be mapped and thus better understood.[5]

Districts of AIDS were identified early on in San Francisco, Los Angeles and New York, from which the epidemic was understood to

---

[2] Vinh-Kim Nguyen, "Antiretroviral Globalism, Biopolitics, and Therapeutic Citizenship," in *Global Assemblages*, ed. Aihwa Ong and Stephen J. Collier (London: Blackwell Publishing, 2007), 124–44, doi:10.1002/9780470696569; Mandisa Mbali, *South African AIDS Activism and Global Health Politics* (Basingstoke, UK: Palgrave Macmillan, 2013); Hakan Seckinelgin, "The Global Governance of Success in HIV/AIDS Policy: Emergency Action, Everyday Lives and Sen's Capabilities," *Health and Place* 18, no. 3 (May 2012), 453–60, doi:10.1016/j.healthplace.2011.09.014.
[3] Paul Farmer et al., eds., *Reimagining Global Health* (Berkeley: University of California Press, 2013); Allan M. Brandt, "How AIDS Invented Global Health," *New England Journal of Medicine* 368, no. 23 (June 6, 2013), 2149–52, doi:10.1056/NEJMp1305297.
[4] Tom Koch, *Disease Maps: Epidemics on the Ground* (Chicago: University of Chicago Press, 2011), 7.
[5] Nicholas B. King, "The Scale Politics of Emerging Disease," *Osiris* 19 (2004), 62–76.

have spread across the American continent.[6] But the CDC extended the risk group definition in 1983 to include the 4Hs: homosexuals, Haitians, heroin Users and hemophiliacs.[7] This let a picture of the epidemic's possible extension emerge that photographs simply failed to capture. The visualization of AIDS moved away from the patient and depictions of his or her symptoms to favor a cartography of the epidemic's spaces. With this change in media from photographs to maps, the confined space of the physiological body of patients was exchanged for the limitless spatial coordinates of cities, countries and the international landscape of global health.[8] With the mapping of spaces of AIDS, the bodies affected by the immunodeficiency syndrome fell out of focus.

Maps and practices of mapping have been discussed widely in the history of science and medicine in the last 50 years. As Jacques Bertin had already summarized in his readings of the *Semiology of Graphics* from the 1960s, the map was disentangled from "the dead image, the illustration" and has become a "living image . . . no longer only the 'representation' of a final simplification, it is a point of departure for the discovery of these simplifications and the means for their justification."[9] In the following years, maps and the technology of mapping developed into a cartographic "science of communication."[10] The map has been thought of as a universal metaphor for cognition, thinking, systematizing and observing anything spatial or structured in almost every discipline. Other authors emphasized the analytical capacities of mapping practices and their association with mathematical models, which lead to a tendency to formalize accounts of reality into the simplified doubles of simulacra.[11]

---

[6] Nina Siu-Ngan Lam, Ming Fan, and Kam-biu Liu, "Spatial-Temporal Spread of the AIDS Epidemic, 1982–1990: A Correlogram Analysis of Four Regions of the United States," *Geographical Analysis* 28, no. 2 (1996), 93–107, doi:10.1111/j.1538-4632.1996.tb00923.x.

[7] "Current Trends: Prevention of Acquired Immune Deficiency Syndrome (AIDS): Report of Inter-Agency Recommendations," *MMWR: Morbidity and Mortality Weekly Report* 32, no. 8 (April 3, 1983), 101–3.

[8] Foucault has described this exchange between the spatial coordinates of the body and geographical coordinates as different modes of spatializing or embodying a disease. But the notion of the epidemic gave also birth to a "historical and geographical consciousness of disease." Michel Foucault, *The Birth of the Clinic: An Archaeology of Medical Perception* (New York: Pantheon Books, 1973), 9, 24.

[9] Jacques Bertin, *Semiology of Graphics: Diagrams, Networks, Maps*, trans. William J. Berg (Redlands, CA: ESRI Press, 2011), 17.

[10] Christopher Board, "Cartographic Communication," *Cartographica: The International Journal for Geographic Information and Geovisualization* 18, no. 2 (1972), 42–78; Waldo R. Tobler, "Analytical Cartography," *The American Cartographer* 3, no. 1 (1976), 21–31.

[11] Joel L. Morrison, "The Science of Cartography and Its Essential Processes," *Cartographica: The International Journal for Geographic Information and Geovisualization* 14, no. 1 (1977), 58–71.

In the 1980s, at the time AIDS appeared, mapping and cartography were attracting growing interest as powerful rhetorical instruments, which opened analysis beyond a normative model of cartography. John B. Harley challenged historians to separate their analysis of maps from the narrative claims cartographers held on the products of their own craft.

Once critical analysis moved beyond the idea of the map as an "objective" or "scientific" account of reality, Harley points to two distinct sets of rules that dominated the Western history of cartography.[12] Technical methodologies of data visualization and design as well as questions of accuracy governed the production of maps. A scientific epistemology guided map makers to arrive at correct relational models, translating spatial coordinates into appropriate representation. Only through observation and measurement could cartographic truth be acquired. A second set of rules, Harley argues, structured the cultural production of the map. This is where values, politics and ethics find their way into the production of maps, although often opaque or hidden in the cartographer's intention to produce an objective account of reality. Accordingly, Harley asked how historians of maps could depart from reading maps in the way cartographers intended them to be read, to engage instead with the invisible ingredients and the unseen silence in the visualization of a map.[13] In this sense, I ask how maps were invested in a true visualization of the AIDS epidemic and how this mode of visualization enabled certain ways of seeing the epidemic, attached to specific values and ethics, while rendering others unseen.

One of the two maps printed in the first AIDS atlas published by Farthing in 1986 is concerned with the global transmission routes of the epidemic (Fig. 2.1). A black-and-white background with outlined contours of the world's continents is centered on the Atlantic Ocean and visualizes the "probable origin" through routes of transmission between the continents. The map uses colorful arrows to indicate the supposed direction of spread. The title announces this despite the tentative caption to be a representation of "the AIDS epidemic," which presents the map's content as a model of the historical and global shape of AIDS. Both its particular cartographical argument as well as its graphical implementation acts as an exemplary predecessor to many similar mappings of AIDS that appeared in the years after the atlas was published.

---

[12] John Brian Harley, "Deconstructing the Map," *Cartographica: The International Journal for Geographic Information and Geovisualization* 26, no. 2 (1989), 4.

[13] John Brian Harley, *The New Nature of Maps: Essays in the History of Cartography* (Baltimore: Johns Hopkins University Press, 2002), 12.

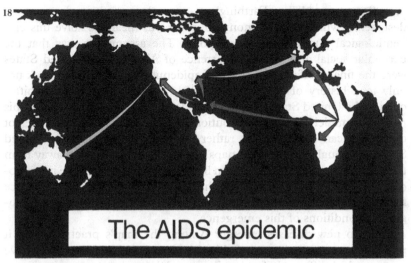

18 Probable origin and spread of the AIDS
virus – worldwide.

Fig. 2.1 A map visualizing the AIDS epidemic and indicating a
probable origin and spread. It presents one of the first consistent models
of AIDS' original distribution, often called the Gallo Model, which
aimed to align the occurrence of AIDS in the United States with earlier
cases on Haiti and Central Africa.
Source: Charles F. Farthing, Simon E. Brown, Richard C. D. Staughton,
Jeffrey J. Cream, and Mark Mühlemann, eds., A Colour Atlas of AIDS: Acquired
Immunodeficiency Syndrome (London: Wolfe Medical Publications, 1986), p. 14.
Permission granted by Elsevier.

While Farthing's map seems to imply a general argument about the
epidemic's global distribution, by 1986 what would become the global
expanse of the epidemic was not widely acknowledged. As discussed
previously, photographs dominated in this first atlas as means to demonstrate what AIDS was. As only one of two maps in Farthing's atlas, this
figure's main purpose was to resolve a very specific problem of AIDS
between 1983 and 1986. The occurrence and initial classification of
AIDS through the rationale of risk groups, most notably the 4H, was
problematic for attempts to align the epidemic profile with the concept of
a causal viral agent. Since 1983 such a virus was the widely accepted
mode of transmission for AIDS, but a viral infection should have
achieved a larger distribution and a very different epidemiological pattern. Models were required that had the power to align a viral etiology
with the emergence of the particular social pattern associated with AIDS

in its first years.[14] When Farthing's map was drawn – the author and the designer of which remain anonymous – it was meant to solve this epidemiological puzzle from its endpoint. The assumption was that the particular social and spatial occurrence of AIDS in the United States were the final footfalls in a chain of epidemic events that lead back not only to a history of AIDS before 1981, but also to original habitats outside the United States. In other words, the origin of the narrative this particular model of AIDS distribution suggested was not a random spot on the African continent but rather the point of arrival in the United States. Although the genre of maps marked a shift in interest away from the body of person's suffering from illnesses associated with the immuno-deficiency syndrome, its cartographic isolation of geographic incidence focused on the same populations and asked for the historical and geographic conditions of this emergence.

How do new diseases emerge? Among the map's practical uses, it provided some commentary on this old, yet pressing question. How have maps worked differently from written models on the communication of unknown origins and spatial extension? Why do we need maps, and what kind of visualization do they produce that can assist our understanding, analysis and ultimately our containment of epidemic threats? Furthermore, how and to what end do spatial and temporal dimensions, on which diseases are plotted, become significant through maps? How were these visual arguments about space then understood and applied in frameworks of local public health strategies, national AIDS politics and global health institutions such as the WHO? In different forms, at different times and different places, maps were used to problematize AIDS within different spatial, ecological, historical and etiological frameworks. The resolution that maps provided to preexisting ways of seeing AIDS, increased diversity, extended variability and communicated a lasting anxiety that accompanied the globalization of AIDS.

Many historical traditions of mapping diseases in space were revived to make the global vision of AIDS. Ackerknecht considered geographical thinking to be essential in the genesis of a modern disease concept in the nineteenth century.[15] Separating, clustering and mapping diseases helped crafting the specific entities of cholera, typhus, typhoid fever, bubonic plague and many more. This practice was showcased in the

---

[14] Gerald M. Oppenheimer, "In the Eye of the Storm: The Epidemiological Construction of AIDS," in *AIDS: The Burdens of History*, ed. Elizabeth Fee and Daniel M. Fox (Berkeley: University of California Press, 1988), 267–300.
[15] Erwin H. Ackerknecht, *Geschichte und Geographie der wichtigsten Krankheiten* (Stuttgart: Enke, 1963).

mid-nineteenth-century diagrams of John Snow's Broad Street pump affair in London and culminated in August Hirsch's extensive work on the historical geography of diseases.[16] Frank Barrett has shown that the methodological underpinnings of medical geography made it indispensable for the growing significance of scientific methods in medical thinking. Beyond the nineteenth century, this legacy continued to structure thinking on infectious diseases that was not segregated from bacteriological models but evolved tangentially to the new laboratory sciences.[17] Medical geography found its destination in the birth of modern tropical medicine. Deeply implicated in colonial and postcolonial frameworks, here the mapped ecology of certain diseases became the most important way of understanding the increasing complexities of yellow fever, malaria and sleeping sickness.[18] It was Jacques May who proposed in the 1950s that "many secrets of nature" could have been revealed if diseases had been accurately mapped throughout history.[19]

Tom Koch has provided the most extensive and ambitious work on the history of mapping diseases to date. Placing a disease on the ground, embedding a disease in its pathways through social, natural and geological spaces, Koch argues, has enabled productive methods for combining and assembling data, theories and models to arrive at pictures of diseases. These maps seek to answer the three most essential question of modern epidemiology: Where did this disease come from? How is it distributed? What is it?[20] But maps can hardly be approached as representations of the disease, Koch warns us. The map has traditionally been a thinking device and a means of experimental combination and thus resembles the epistemic structure of a laboratory rather than the presentation of final outcomes and results. Maps create the context in which proposals can be tested, or rather, "mapping is a method of assemblage

[16] John Snow, *On the Mode of Communication of Cholera* (London: John Churchill, 1855); August Hirsch, *Handbook of Geographical and Historical Pathology* (London: New Sydenham Society, 1883); Kari S. McLeod, "Our Sense of Snow: The Myth of John Snow in Medical Geography," *Social Science and Medicine* 50, no. 7 (2000), 923–35.

[17] Frank A. Barrett, *Disease and Geography: The History of an Idea*. Vol. 23 (York: York University Press, 2000).

[18] World Health Organization, "Geographical Reconnaissance for Malaria Eradication Programmes" (Geneva: World Health Organization, 1965), www.who.int/iris/handle/10665/70045; François Delaporte, *The History of Yellow Fever: An Essay on the Birth of Tropical Medicine* (Cambridge, MA: MIT Press, 1991); Maryinez Lyons, *The Colonial Disease: A Social History of Sleeping Sickness in Northern Zaire, 1900–1940* (Cambridge: Cambridge University Press, 2002).

[19] Jacques Meyer May, *The Ecology of Human Disease* (New York: MD Publications, 1958), 25.

[20] Koch, *Disease Maps: Epidemics on the Ground*, 25.

within which ideas are constituted and then argued about specific experiences."[21] Maps, Koch concludes, craft the conditions for scientific approaches to epidemics. Maps should be approached as a "making of" arguments about diseases and, hence, are well-suited to epidemiology.

Following Koch's journey through centuries of disease geography, the history of epidemic mapping can be extended into the emergence of digital methods for disease mapping, such as geographic information systems (GIS).[22] AIDS was the testing ground for many new technical procedures. It was seen by many geographers as an ideal field to approach large datasets with GIS methods. The history of AIDS's transformation into a global phenomenon is as much characterized by inventive new mapping technologies, as it is shaped by a revision of what was assumed to be the place of AIDS. It can seem as if the fast tempo with which the epidemic transformed in its approach to a second decade forced the development of new mapping technologies to keep up.[23] Quantitative approaches to the epidemic were published to find logical and affect-free answers to the puzzling conditions under which the epidemic had left its original territory, its district and space in the gay communities and inner-city pockets of poverty.[24] Mapping AIDS would not only provide a broader vision of a disease distributed globally, but also of an infectious epidemic overcoming national, continental, social as well as – once again – epistemic borders.

With regard to the extensive and complex set of forms, genres, aesthetics and styles applied to mapping AIDS, this chapter focuses on three distinctive ways in which maps have shaped the history of AIDS. First, the chapter will open with an interrogation of the conditions under which maps became necessary in the first place. What remained initially unseen that maps could turn into visible information? And then, what was made unseen in the transformation of visualization styles and scales from clinical photographs to maps? Second, this chapter shows how the history of maps characterizes a history of constantly fleeing spatial certainties. With every map, with every new way of charting the territory of AIDS – the gay district, the urban environment, the metropolitan areas, the national states, the Western world and finally the globe – the story of

---

[21] Ibid., 13.

[22] J. Terry Coppock and David W. Rhind, "The History of GIS," *Geographical Information Systems: Principles and Applications* 1, no. 1 (1991), 21–43.

[23] Tom Koch, *Cartographies of Disease: Maps, Mapping, and Medicine* (Redlands, CA: ESRI Press, 2005), 271 ff.

[24] Ron Brookmeyer and Mitchell H. Gail, *AIDS Epidemiology: A Quantitative Approach* (Oxford: Oxford University Press, 1994); W. Y. Tan, *Stochastic Modeling of AIDS Epidemiology and HIV Pathogenesis* (London: World Scientific, 2000).

mapping AIDS is a history of spaces and coordinates that have at some point left the picture. Third, the chapter will look to the newly emerging home of the epidemic, as AIDS became a disease of the global south. It became an epidemic of poverty, neglect and Western ignorance. Maps contributed to crafting AIDS into a new paradigm of thinking and practicing global health policy, where the key challenges were scarcity, education and – later – as TAC, the South African Treatment Action Campaign amplified an old activist's slogan, to get "drugs into bodies."[25] As Didier Fassin said so well, the question was how maps contributed to a widespread "political anesthesia,"[26] which characterized many years of the West's attitude to AIDS in Africa.

As AIDS became global, photographs of patients certainly did not disappear. But their meaning drastically changed once the genre had lost its monopoly as a representation of the epidemic. In some countries such as Brazil, photography inherited a critical vision, amplified by anthropological research but never fully separated from its clinical and medical heritage.[27] In Botswana, photographic captions of AIDS became personalized, were integrated into the scarcity of basic medical resources and used sometimes as a last resort to organize the individual deidentification with the horrible realities of disease.[28] But medical photographs also came to serve in East African public health campaigns, which favored the before-and-after cut-up as incentives for taking up treatment.[29] As already indicated with the WHO's image of AIDS, photography became crudely ethnographic and an instrument to enhance the perception of AIDS's diverse global appearance. Photographs depicted radically discrete ecologies, social and cultural environments in which AIDS appeared, working in opposition to maps designed to join the dots.[30]

In the AIDS atlas, the epidemiological design of AIDS was delegated exclusively to maps. In the first series, Farthing's 1986 and 1988 edition's question of both geographical and biological origin and causation

---

[25] Mbali, *South African AIDS Activism and Global Health Politics*, 184 ff.
[26] Didier Fassin, *When Bodies Remember: Experiences and Politics of AIDS in South Africa* (Berkeley: University of California Press, 2007).
[27] João Guilherme Biehl, *Will to Live: AIDS Therapies and the Politics of Survival* (Princeton, NJ: Princeton University Press, 2007).
[28] Julie Livingston, *Improvising Medicine: An African Oncology Ward in an Emerging Cancer Epidemic* (Durham, NC: Duke University Press, 2012); Julie Livingston, "Figuring the Tumor in Botswana," *Raritan* 34, no. 1 (2014), 10–24.
[29] Ruth J. Prince, "The Diseased Body and the Global Subject: The Circulation and Consumption of an Iconic AIDS Photograph in East Africa," *Visual Anthropology* 29, no. 2 (2016), 159–86, doi:10.1080/08949468.2016.1131517.
[30] World Health Organization, *AIDS: Images of the Epidemic* (Geneva: World Health Organization, 1994).

were key to the unknown mapmakers as well as to the atlas editors. Geographical visualization was combined with diagrams of the phylogenetic heritage of the virus.[31] Spatial patterns seemed to provide the missing link in the story of how the virus emerged out of a long-standing genealogy of existing and known viruses. The epidemiological chapter in Farthing's atlases used maps in this way to visualize regions susceptible to the evolutionary excess in which the virus appeared. The two printed maps in each edition drew attention to different host species that were suspected for enabling transmission, yet it remained a mystery how the virus seemingly jumped from an isolated region in Central Africa to the continent, and how this then caused a pandemic.

The KS-focused atlases of Friedman-Kien did not include any maps. Although his argument relied on various geographies of KS, maps seem to have been insignificant to his nosological claims. But with the publication of Mildvan's first atlas in 1995, the map became a crucial and highly professionalized tool to argue for historical developments, as much as to emphasize prognostic claims about the "future epidemic."[32] As visualizations of statistical data of the successive distribution in the United States, or as representations of hypothetical models relating AIDS to social patterns of gender, drug usage or income, the five (in 1995) to eight (2008) maps throughout Mildvan's atlas series are a key medium to relate what was known about the biological nature of AIDS with its social, cultural and spatial determinants. In the last issue from 2008, AIDS is fully recognized as a global issue, which is reflected by the framing of the atlas as an *International Atlas*, constituted through a variety of world maps plotting HIV and its effects on the background of global health.[33]

The main concern to atlas editors as they integrated and discussed the maps was the social and cultural diversity that appeared once AIDS was visualized through geographical filters. Why did AIDS appear in many of the Western countries as a male homosexual-transmitted disease, while its distribution on the African continent seemed to be overwhelmingly heterosexual? What was driving an almost exclusively male infection rate in United States and Europe, while it appeared predominantly female in other areas? Why was transmission from mothers to children such a problem in countries of the Southern Hemisphere, while it seemed a

[31] Charles F. Farthing et al., eds., *A Colour Atlas of AIDS (Acquired Immunodeficiency Syndrome)* (London: Wolfe Medical Publications, 1986), 6 f.; Charles F. Farthing, ed., *A Color Atlas of AIDS* (Chicago: Year Book Medical Publishers, 1988), 17 ff.

[32] Donna Mildvan, ed., *AIDS*. Vol. 1. Atlas of Infectious Diseases (Philadelphia: Current Medicine, 1995).

[33] Donna Mildvan, ed., *International Atlas of AIDS*, 4th ed. (Philadelphia: Springer, 2008).

moderate issue in the Northern Hemisphere? Maps were concerned with questions that challenged a unified idea, a homogenous concept and an all-encompassing picture of AIDS because they presented significant local differences.

As geographers know all too well, maps are essential to turn a space into a place, to render a nondescript set of coordinates into a lived, meaningful and visible entity.[34] Maps constitute places, but a place is rarely understood to be characterized as a set of static qualities, rather a locale in flux. It is mobility that makes space and place interesting in the study of phenomena such as diseases. A disease's arrival and its circulation within confined spaces, as well as its departure, challenge geographers to map a static picture of a constantly moving, evasive and fluid process. Through a map, particular qualities of space are interrogated as a means of understanding why an epidemic appeared in that specific mapped place. The map seems to ask its readers what allowed the epidemic to thrive in this place, and what can be learned from these particularities to contain further distribution. Maps draw theories, data, visions and histories together through intensely versatile diagrammatic techniques.[35] As an effect, maps present themselves as "sampling devices" of plagued places. But where Rosenberg saw the epidemic as a device to unpack social, cultural and political histories, the map offers an instrument of linkage between the conditions of a place that become visible through the lens of the mapped epidemic, while the epidemic is mapped through the lens of these local conditions.[36]

Losing the AIDS Space

By 1986, when Farthing included the map resembling Gallo's model, the global dimension of AIDS and the syndrome's occurrences in European, Latin American and African countries were verified and officially acknowledged by public health institutions around the world. But the image of the epidemic as a global phenomenon did not change as quickly as its trajectory took on speed in reaching new locations, addressing new patterns of distribution and posing new challenges to its containment. A crescendoing chorus of voices who raised their concern throughout the

[34] See, e.g., Edward Casey, *The Fate of Place: A Philosophical History* (Berkeley: University of California Press, 1997).
[35] Christina Ljungberg, "The Diagrammatic Nature of Maps," in *Thinking with Diagrams: The Semiotic Basis of Human Cognition*. Vol. 17, ed. Christina Ljungberg and Sybille Krämer (Berlin: De Gruyter, 2016).
[36] Charles E. Rosenberg, "What Is an Epidemic? AIDS in Historical Perspective," in *Living with AIDS*, ed. Stephen R. Graubard (Cambridge, MA: MIT Press, 1989), 1–17.

1980s about the overly narrow geographical perspectives on the distribution of AIDS slowly changed the popular perception of AIDS into a global disease. In many cases, maps were an essential and effective tool in bringing about this new view of AIDS as a crisis without borders.

Among the chorus were global health advocates like Jonathan Mann, who was recruited by the director of the CDC's AIDS program in 1984 to join one of the earliest programs established to grapple with the scope of the AIDS epidemic in Africa.[37] Project SIDA was located in Kinshasa, Zaire (today's Democratic Republic of Congo), operated from the Mama Yemo hospital and worked as cooperation of the CDC with the National Institute of Allergy and Infectious Diseases (NIAID) and the Belgium Institute for Tropical Medicine. The group was headed by Peter Piot, who would later become the first director of Joint United Nations Programme on HIV/AIDS (UNAIDS).[38] Projet SIDA was described as the earliest systematic attempt to answer fundamental epidemiological questions about AIDS beyond the North American and European soil.[39] As Jon Cohen recalls, the project found its own purpose and, more crucially, funding when the first plausible infectious chain was proposed that would connect cases in Zaire with cases in New York and in Los Angeles.[40]

Peter Piot had seen patients with clinical signs resembling a pattern of AIDS in his previous research in Zaire and had tried since 1983 to find the money for further investigations to prove his suspicions that AIDS was rampant on the African continent. Thomas Quinn and Richard Krause from the NIAID had also in 1983 worked in Haiti to investigate claims of a Haitian vector of the epidemic. On the island, they had learned about large groups of Haitians who had worked in Zaire after its independence was wrestled from Belgium but were forced to return to Haiti in the late 1970s. Once the details of this migration pattern emerged, a possible trajectory seem to be found and much of the CDC's interest in Zaire was guided by finding out where the disease's might had come from.[41] As Mann was sent by the CDC to head a small research

---

[37] Elizabeth Fee and Manon Parry, "Jonathan Mann, HIV/AIDS, and Human Rights," *Journal of Public Health Policy* 29, no. 1 (2008), 57.

[38] Piot was later known for his ground-breaking research on Ebola and since 2010 is the director of the London School of Hygiene and Tropical Medicine.

[39] Jon Cohen, "The Rise and Fall of Projet SIDA," *Science* 278, no. 5343 (November 28, 1997), 1565–8, doi:10.1126/science.278.5343.1565.

[40] Jon Cohen, *Shots in the Dark: The Wayward Search for an AIDS Vaccine* (London: Norton, 2001).

[41] Richard A. McKay, "'Patient Zero': The Absence of a Patient's View of the Early North American AIDS Epidemic," *Bulletin of the History of Medicine* 88, no. 1 (2014), 161–94, doi:10.1353/bhm.2014.0005.

team accompanied by two physicians from Zaire, Bosenga Ngali and Eugene Nzila, they quickly arrived at the essential conclusion that the transmission occurred predominantly through heterosexual intercourse. Attempts to publish these findings failed initially, as the historian Elizabeth Fee reports, when their paper was rejected by the *New England Journal of Medicine*.[42] The growing presence of AIDS in Africa and the possibility of heterosexual transmission was widely refuted by peer reviewers and by many attendants of the first international AIDS conference. After Piot and colleagues experienced rejection from a dozen further journals their findings were finally published in 1984 by *The Lancet*.[43]

It took until roughly 1987 for a larger American and European public to wake up to the looming reality of an epidemic reaching far beyond its assumed urban pockets of sexual deviance. One condition for this acceptance of AIDS's global dissemination was its framing as a disease that posed a threat to the general public. The AIDS report of the American Surgeon General, published in 1986,[44] articulated a drastic warning of impending epidemic catastrophe that could affect anyone, anywhere. The old image of AIDS as a disease of "AIDS victims" who were inherently different and geographically separated in urban enclaves was challenged. As the *Scientific American* wrote, "[T]hat security blanket has now been stripped away."[45] The overt identification of AIDS with other bodies in their supposedly closed communities posed now an increased risk, rather than any form of containment. Considering this, doctors such as Abraham Verghese, a general practitioner from rural Tennessee, understood the need to map the epidemic's arrival in the hinterland.[46] Geographers like Peter Gould described the creeping advance of the epidemic over the American landscape.[47] Countless

---

[42] Fee and Parry, "Jonathan Mann, HIV/AIDS, and Human Rights," 55.

[43] P. Piot et al., "Acquired Immunodeficiency Syndrome in a Heterosexual Population in Zaire," *Lancet*, 2, no. 8394 (1984), 65–9; Jonathan M. Mann et al., "Surveillance for AIDS in a Central African City: Kinshasa, Zaire," *JAMA* 255, no. 23 (1986), 3255–9, doi:10.1001/jama.1986.03370230061031.

[44] Koop C. Everett, *Surgeon General's Report on Acquired Immune Deficiency Syndrome* (Washington, DC: US Public Health Service, 1986).

[45] 1987 *Scientific American*, quoted in Paula A. Treichler, "AIDS, Homophobia, and Biomedical Discourse: An Epidemic of Signification," in *AIDS, Cultural Analysis, Cultural Activism*, ed. Douglas Crimp (Cambridge, MA: MIT Press, 1988), 66.

[46] Abraham Verghese, *My Own Country: A Doctor's Story* (New York: Vintage Books, 1994).

[47] Peter Gould, *The Slow Plague: A Geography of the AIDS Pandemic* (Oxford: Blackwell Publishers, 1993).

authors acknowledged what appeared to be a new outlook: AIDS was becoming a pandemic.[48]

The most striking argument for the grander scale of an epidemic that transgressed local, regional and national boundaries was to prove its original global history. The first model, which narrated how AIDS arrived in the United States, served as a paradigm for the atlas visualization previously mentioned (Fig. 2.1) and became popular as the "Gallo-Model" with the publication of a series of articles in the *Scientific American*.[49] The publications were authored by microbiologist Robert Gallo, who presented his model to a wider public in his quest to demonstrate the validity of his hypothesis for a retroviral cause of AIDS.[50] His model of original distribution connected the local appearance of AIDS in specific subpopulations in the United States with a retroviral agent of probable zoonotic ancestry from Central Africa. He linked the parameter under which the epidemic was first recognized in homosexual urban communities with a plausible model of original distribution, and the model also importantly crafted an argument to emphasize the sexual transmission of AIDS. The model and the map (Fig. 2.1) were used as evidence that the scale of AIDS was indeed driven by a single viral agent, even if it was believed to be a notably inefficient kind of virus.

The map and the underlying model resonated with a long-standing problem in epidemiology. Maps rarely visualize certainty about a disease's occurrence and ecology, but rather interrogate the conditions under which existing knowledge can be aligned with plausible hypotheses. In the discipline of geography maps are normally understood to be instruments that enable and encourage controversy rather than aspire to define fact or invest in unshakeable propositions. Gallo discussed four different possible explanatory models for the newly emerging epidemic, each of which would have aligned with the cartographic picture of the epidemic deriving from his model. (A) The appearance of AIDS could be attributed to an old, but not yet isolated disease. As its appearance was

---

[48] Cindy Patton, *Globalizing AIDS* (Minneapolis: University of Minnesota Press, 2002); Cristiana Bastos, *Global Responses to AIDS: Science in Emergency* (Bloomington: Indiana University Press, 1999); Johanna Tayloe Crane, *Scrambling for Africa: AIDS, Expertise, and the Rise of American Global Health Science* (Ithaca, NY: Cornell University Press, 2013).

[49] For a discussion and critical reading of the Gallo model in geography see: Matthew Smallman-Raynor, Andrew Cliff, and Peter Haggett, eds., *London International Atlas of AIDS* (Oxford and Cambridge: Blackwell Publishers, 1992), 141.

[50] Robert Gallo, "The First Human Retrovirus," *Scientific American* 255, no. 6, December (1986), 88–99; Robert Gallo, "The AIDS Virus," *Scientific American* 256, no. 1 (1987), 46–57; Robert Gallo, *Virus Hunting: AIDS, Cancer, and the Human Retrovirus* (New York: Basic Books, 1991).

characterized by the aggregation of known diseases, it might have gone unseen for an unknown amount of time. For Gallo, the absence of traces of the virus in human blood samples before the 1960s was evidence enough to eliminate this option. (B) The virus could be understood as a mutated version of a well-distributed nonpathogenic virus, a theory that he could have proven by analyzing antibodies in stored blood samples. (C) The zoonotic explanation was a crucial element to Gallo, as the virus appeared as a mutated version of a virus found in African Green Monkey. But most crucially, Gallo argued that (D) the "recent spread of the virus from an isolated group [was] due to social change."[51]

The Gallo-Model is central to the history of geographic visualizations of AIDS. Maps like the one in the 1986 atlas must be understood as simplifications of the model, reducing it to scant visual information only. Gallo did not use maps to visualize his assumptions in his contributions to the *Scientific American*, but instead adopted the initial assumptions raised by Mann, Krause and others about the Zaire-Haiti-US connection to advance the argument on probable points of origin and pathways for the distribution of HTLV-III/HIV-1.[52] Gallo claimed that STLV-III, a virus prevalent in the African green monkey, developed into HTLV-III/HIV-1 through a series of mutations (HTLV-IV and HIV-2). He believed these variants of the virus circulated throughout the 1960s and 1970s, barely recognized in some Central African countries. Retrospective blood analysis suggested that this region was the most likely origin, as by 1986 comparable viruses had not been found in other countries. The open question Gallo posed in 1986 included how exactly the virus had become the deadly variant HIV-1, how this particular virus left the African continent and how the former endemic situation in Africa turned into an epidemic.

The three geographers Smallman-Raynor, Haggett and Cliff based in Cambridge, the United Kingdom, published in 1992 *The London International Atlas of AIDS*, which was the result of extensive studies conducted both locally and globally over the course of the late 1980s. Smallman-Raynor and his colleagues discussed Gallo's model as one of the first valid proposals of original distribution and drew an annotated

[51] Robert Gallo, "HIV-The Cause of AIDS: An Overview on Its Biology, Mechanisms of Disease Induction, and Our Attempts to Control It," *Journal of Acquired Immune Deficiency Syndromes* 1, no. 6 (1988), 529.

[52] While Gallo believed that HTLV-III was the original AIDS virus, which he therefore called HIV-1, his claims were later refuted by Barre-Sinnousi and other virologists. See Chapter 3 and Epstein on the details of the historical virus dispute. Steven Epstein, *Impure Science: AIDS, Activism, and the Politics of Knowledge* (Berkeley: University of California Press, 1996), 79 ff.

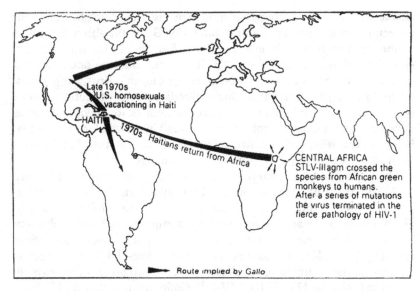

Fig. 2.2 Map of the original route implied by Robert Gallo from the
London International Atlas of AIDS. Annotated with additional details
of Gallo's model, the geographers discuss the validity of the model
and point to its already outdated assumptions in 1992.
Source: Matthew Smallman-Raynor, Andrew Cliff, and Peter Haggett, eds.,
London International Atlas of AIDS (Oxford and Cambridge: Blackwell
Publishers, 1992), p. 144. Permission granted by Wiley.

version for their atlas (Fig. 2.2). As the geographers pointed out, Gallo's
model was not cemented in data but can best be understood as a thought
experiment to align the very short history of AIDS at the beginning of the
1980s with the emerging hypothesis of a causal retrovirus.[53] The hypothesis connected the occurrence of AIDS-related diseases in specific populations to the social change that led the virus to spread "from an isolated
group in East Africa."[54] Mass migration between Zaire and Haiti might
have caused the virus to cross the Atlantic, and as Haiti was perceived by
Gallo as a favored holiday resort for metropolitan American homosexual
men, it seemed plausible that the virus found its entry point to the United
States here.[55] But Gallo's model fell from favor due to questionable

---

[53] Smallman-Raynor et al., *London International Atlas of AIDS*, 141.
[54] Gallo, "The First Human Retrovirus," 92.
[55] Haiti was suspected throughout history to have harbored many diseases, such as
syphilis, cholera and yellow fever. See, e.g., R. C. Holcomb, *Who Gave the World
Syphilis? The Haitian Myth.* Vol. 01270. Harvard Medicine Preservation Microfilm
Project (New York: Froben Press, 1937).

accuracy as data and theories about the origins of AIDS became more complex.[56] But as the map in the 1986 atlas demonstrates, it was one of the first consistent models that crafted a vision of a history and geography of the epidemic before AIDS history officially began in 1981.

Diagrams of the Topography of Outbreaks

Already in 1983, when the CDC published a paper that indicated increased risk of contracting AIDS among homosexual men, heroin drug users, hemophiliacs and Haitians, the "geographical question" could no longer be ignored. Only the first three groups of the 4Hs supported a case for locally limited distribution. Cases among Haitians were scattered across the United States, almost none of which were reported to be homosexual or directly implicated in drug use. These "anomalous many" presented the scientists with a puzzle.[57] Some argued that the unusual social pattern undermined the validity of a viral cause altogether, while others, like Gallo, used the distribution pattern to turn geographical aspects into supporting evidence of specific viral candidates.[58] Etiology and ecology, theory about the syndrome's cause and theory about the local conditions that contribute to significant local prevalence needed alignment.

By 1989 it seemed like common sense that "individuals with HIV-1 infection in different transmission categories, geographic locations, or ethnic groups have demonstrated distinctive patterns of occurrence and manifestations of AIDS."[59] But old assumptions about where AIDS would be, how it was transmitted and who was at risk persisted long into the 1980s and proved difficult to resolve. Spaces like the rural hinterland lost their imagined immunity and as clear boundaries between the "implicated and the immune"[60] began to falter, representations of the spatial structure of the epidemic's transition became a key instrument in proving old assumptions wrong and making previous pictures of AIDS

---

[56] M. Deschamps, "AIDS in the Caribbean," *Archives of AIDS Research* 2 (1988), 51–6.

[57] Epstein, *Impure Science*, 56.

[58] J. Sonnabend, S. S. Witkin, and D. T. Purtilo, "Acquired Immunodeficiency Syndrome, Opportunistic Infections, and Malignancies in Male Homosexuals: A Hypothesis of Etiologic Factors in Pathogenesis," *JAMA* 249, no. 17 (1983), 2370–4, doi:10.1001/jama.1983.03330410056028; Anthony S. Fauci, "25 Years of HIV," *Nature* 453, no. 7193 (2008), 289–90, doi:10.1038/453289a.

[59] Richard A. Kaslow and Donald P. Francis, eds., *The Epidemiology of AIDS: Expression, Occurrence, and Control of Human Immunodeficiency Virus Type 1 Infection* (New York: Oxford University Press, 1989), 90.

[60] Richard Goldstein, "The Implicated and the Immune: Cultural Responses to AIDS," *The Milbank Quarterly* 68 (1990), 295–319, doi:10.2307/3350055.

unseen. Maps approached the new puzzle of ever-increasing variance in occurrence patterns and – crucially –warned of expected distribution into the general population.

Indeed, one of the first local spatial models of AIDS was called the "San Francisco model" and published in a 1983 issue of *The Lancet*. The authors combined incidence rates, clinical reports and rather fixed assertions about the homosexual geography of districts within the city, to argue for an overriding sexual transmission of the disease, driven by geographical proximity.[61] A shared lifestyle, the authors claim, was indicative that social proximity was a condition for the distribution of AIDS, so that social practices became a geographic risk. As Preda argues, these associations of spaces, which had been associated with particular risk behavior, exaggerated the importance of risk groups in a geographic narrative, in which the classification of social groups according to risk zones and transmission categories along spatial determinants cemented their association with AIDS.[62]

Following the trend of how, why and when AIDS had left the place assumed to be its original environment, the authors of the 1992 *The London International Atlas of AIDS* produced a detailed spatio-temporal analysis of San Francisco. They demonstrate the patterns of distribution within the city's boundaries and question existing assumptions and framings about the epidemic's supposed natural spaces, such as presented in the 1983 paper. Geographical reasoning, the art of linking different variables within a confined environment, was pursued and praised by these authors as a method of critical inquiry, which should improve strategies of intervention and prevention in a field marked by a rapid pace of transformation.[63]

For their study, a sequence of six maps of San Francisco was plotted onto one page of the geographical atlas (Fig. 2.3). The upper row relates the point datasets of approximately 7,000 AIDS cases to the standardized morbidity rate (SMR) of San Francisco. The size of the points denotes the number of cases, while the shading is used to visualize the SMR. The three principal transmission categories of homosexuals, homosexual

[61] Andrew R. Moss et al., "AIDS in the 'Gay' Areas of San Francisco," *The Lancet* 321, no. 8330 (1983), 923–4, doi:10.1016/S0140-6736(83)91346-6. Also See Richard A. McKay, *Patient Zero and the Making of the AIDS Epidemic* (Chicago: University of Chicago Press, 2017).

[62] Alex Preda, *AIDS, Rhetoric, and Medical Knowledge* (Cambridge: Cambridge University Press, 2005), 191. Furthermore, Preda argues that these practices were indicative of a combination of contagious and infectious models of how AIDS was transmitted.

[63] Smallman-Raynor et al., *London International Atlas of AIDS*; Andrew D. Cliff, *Atlas of Disease Distributions: Analytic Approaches to Epidemiological Data* (Oxford: Basil Blackwell, 1988), 12 ff.

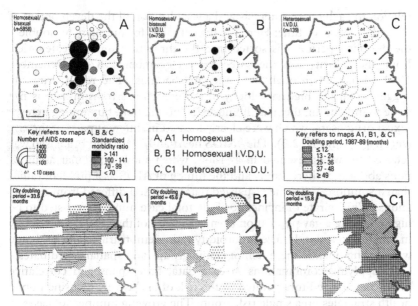

Fig. 2.3 Six maps of local patterns of AIDS distribution in San
Francisco in Smallman-Raynor's geographical atlas from 1992. The
editors used different models and different methods of visualizing to
demonstrate the dangerously flawed assumption of an exclusively
homosexually driven epidemic. As these maps show, a significant
increase of cases can be observed in heterosexual transmission beyond
the geographic confines of traditionally gay districts.
Source: Matthew Smallman-Raynor, Andrew Cliff, and Peter Haggett, eds.,
London International Atlas of AIDS (Oxford and Cambridge: Blackwell
Publishers, 1992), p. 214. Permission granted by Wiley.

intravenous drug users and heterosexual intravenous drug users are used
to compare three different visions of total AIDS mortality in the same
district. Almost 87 percent of registered cases before 1989 are shown to
be due to homosexual transmission. These cases are pinned to the
traditionally gay districts of San Francisco, the Castro, Upper Market,
Noe Valley and Diamond Heights. With lower total numbers, the distribution of heterosexual transmission and drug-related transmission seem,
on first sight, to resemble the same spatial pattern.

The bottom row of the map adds a visualization of *interval* to the ratio
graph mentioned previously.[64] Where ratio graphs plot datapoints in

---

[64] The characteristics of mapping data can be divided formally into four different scales:
nominal, ordinal, interval and ratio. While the nominal scale presents the weakest form

relation to each other, intervals add a visualization of the development of these datasets over time: Here the time it takes for numbers to double – the doubling period – is sorted into the three transmission categories. Epidemic velocity was measured from December 1987 to December 1989, visualized through five different shadings. The result primarily suggests that the highest velocity of the epidemic's transmission is not to be found among the male homosexual population, but among hetero-sexual drug users, which were clearly located in different parts of the city (see map C1 in Fig. 2.3). The "AIDS heartland,"[65] as San Francisco was referred to, was presented in a vision, which showed popular assumptions about the whereabouts and the timing of AIDS as a problem rather than a solution. What the visualized data disclosed differed from expectations. While a rate of incidence of the total case number persisted to be higher among a gay population even at the end of the 1980s, the velocity in relation to a standardized morbidity ratio demonstrated the epidemic was soaring outside these demographic groups and spatial coordinates.

By applying combinations of case data, time spans and correlative SMR, the atlas editors pointed to the risk of exclusively focusing public health strategies on a single risk group. The growing numbers of cases in other subpopulations had fallen outside of the spotlight. The underlying trends and velocities were made visible by turning the geographic per-spective from a *ratio* into an *interval*: While the first row suggests a common and all too familiar spatial structure in which AIDS is found where it was expected to be found – roughly the Castro – it is only in the interval that the displacement of the epidemic, its threat beyond assumed spaces, became visible and vivid.

Similar models were created for New York and other "Metropolitan-Level Epidemics" of AIDS in and outside the United States.[66] To demonstrate the necessary widening, restructuring and reconsideration of who were at risk, maps provided a new, spatial framing that pointed beyond identities and familiar lifestyle practices. To include risk for nonwhite populations, to draw attention to developing patterns within the urban space and to raise awareness to the growing historicity of clear-cut assumptions about AIDS districts is, what Smallman-Raynor, Cliff and Haggett considered the particular capacity of their geographic visual commentary on the epidemic. After all, they concluded this section of the

---

in which numbers and symbols are equivalent with cases of a specific disease, ordinal scales present a form of ranking, in which different sizes, masses and disease burdens can be visualized in relation to one another. Ratio and interval scales present data in equivalence, in rank and in the ration between intervals. See Cliff, *Atlas of Disease Distributions*, 13.

[65] Smallman-Raynor et al., *London International Atlas of AIDS*, 215.   [66] Ibid., 227 ff.

atlas with a warning to white, heterosexual populations about the very categories in which AIDS incidence was originally registered, counted and plotted. "If the epidemic continues to burgeon," they forecast, "such sharp contrasts may disappear as HIV becomes more widely dispersed in the heterosexual population."[67]

The way AIDS was visualized in these accounts of the urban space was independent of individual symptoms but relied on the formalization of patterns. Historically, epidemiology has been described as the substantial driver for disease entities to be defined as unambiguous as possible because only the well-defined class allows for counting, calculation and depiction.[68] To arrive at a characteristic spatial pattern of scattered incidents, the events of infection and the moments of succumbing to illness on the "epidemic streets"[69] require classification, abstraction and simplification. Catherine Waldby has discussed this transformation of AIDS-related disease events among individuals into spatial temporal pattern as a compression of complex, far-flung and heterogeneous processes. The huge variety of stories, experiences and encounters of each AIDS outbreak is reduced to a simple numeric expression. To enable the biopolitical-surveying eye of epidemiology, Waldby continues, the map needed to become a technology that diagnosed the epidemic within the fabric of the population. "Epidemiology is the science of the repetition of disease in the population, but in the analysis of such repetitions it also seeks to generate a higher order system of explanation than that of clinical medicine,"[70] she explains. Waldby's conclusion suggests this higher order is to be found in epidemiology's fixation on the risk group of gay men. Combining the sexualized population with the diseased population thus established a biopolitical order in which maps and geographical technologies became instruments to make those populations visible; to make communities seen in which the infectious risk was supposedly harbored from where AIDS might spread and threaten the healthy majority of the US population. But maps are more versatile than this, as the example of San Francisco shows. They indeed work as powerful visualizations of populations whose very shape was crafted in the eye of epidemiological consideration of their relationship to a disease,

[67] Ibid., 231.
[68] J. Rosser Matthews, *Quantification and the Quest for Medical Certainty* (Princeton, NJ: Princeton University Press, 1995); Ian Hacking, *The Taming of Chance* (Cambridge: Cambridge University Press, 1990).
[69] Anne Hardy, *The Epidemic Streets: Infectious Disease and the Rise of Preventive Medicine, 1856–1900* (Oxford: Clarendon Press, 1993).
[70] Catherine Waldby, *AIDS and the Body Politic: Biomedicine and Sexual Difference* (London: Routledge, 1996), 92.

but maps can also unfold a powerful intervention in established and sometimes epidemiologically concerning assumptions. To overcome the idea of an AIDS heartland meant to leave the impression of a space of containment behind.

Mappings like the ones previously shown sit comfortably in the long history of mapping disease within the urban environment.[71] The most prominent example is clearly to be found in the history of cholera in London in the mid-nineteenth century. After the outbreak of 1849 killed more than 62,000 inhabitants, controversy about the means of distribution achieved new urgency. The majority of medical experts at that time stuck to their conviction that cholera was caused by bad air, inherently connected to filth and waste, and thus cholera was a disease characterized by poverty. As low standards of living were predominantly found in districts close to the Thames, the wealthier parts of London were seen by comparison as safe spaces. Many of what we would call epidemiological arguments today, were in the mid-nineteenth century based on spatial coordinates. It was not only the famed John Snow who tried to convince the community of his hypothesis with the visual support of maps (Fig. 2.4). While Snow's opponent Edmund Cooper deployed maps to suggest a connection between foul water exhausts and cholera case density, the Reverend Henry Whitehead agreed with many of Snow's assumptions about the implication of water, but ultimately rejected the idea of a contagious agent.[72] Snow mobilized extensive case data and correlated it with the geographical position of water pumps. Moving beyond a Euclidian proximity and integrating the local features and conditions that structured the social life of inhabitants, Snow's map became the most convincing instrument to argue for a cause for cholera other than poverty and its associated stench.

As Snow described in his own book *On the Mode of Communication of Cholera*, he used the map to reveal geographical patterns that might help to explore the specific cause of London's 1854 epidemic. Snow called

---

[71] See, e.g., Eckstein on an Early Modern practice of urban disease mapping and Monmonier and Koch for the lasting significance of the urban space in public health propaganda. Nicholas A. Eckstein, "Florence on Foot: An Eye-Level Mapping of the Early Modern City in Time of Plague," *Renaissance Studies* 30, no. 2 (2016), 273–97, doi:10.1111/rest.12144; Mark Monmonier, "Maps as Graphic Propaganda for Public Health," in *Imagining Illness: Public Health and Visual Culture*, ed. David Harley Serlin (Minneapolis: University of Minnesota Press, 2010), 108–25; Koch, *Disease Maps: Epidemics on the Ground*, 49 ff.

[72] Koch, *Cartographies of Disease: Maps, Mapping, and Medicine*, 108–11; Tom Koch and Kenneth Denike, "'Crediting His Critics' Concerns: Remaking John Snow's Map of Broad Street Cholera, 1854," *Social Science and Medicine* 69 (2009), 1246–51.

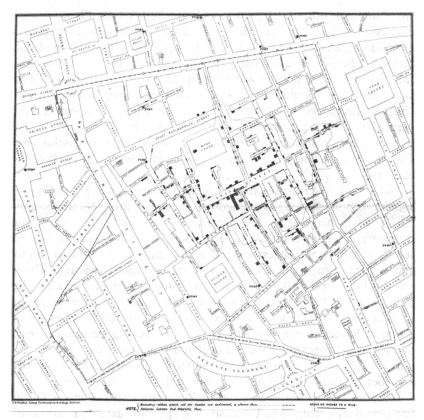

Fig. 2.4 John Snow's famous visualization of cholera in 1854 London.
Through spatial reasoning Snow was able to demonstrate that not
merely geographical incidence but a spatial proximity to the Broad
Street water pump was crucial for cholera to spread. This map stands
as a historical example of how maps can provoke new ways of thinking
about infectious diseases.
Source: John Snow, *On the Mode of Communication of Cholera* (London:
John Churchill, 1855), p. 46. Courtesy of the Wellcome Collection.

this now-famous map a "diagram of the topography of the outbreak."[73]
Cholera death data, collected from the city's registers, were placed in
tables and connected to as many case histories as Snow could find.
Denoted by small squares, deaths are affixed to particular addresses,
where they occurred to reveal a suggestive pattern of distribution in the

[73] Snow, *On the Mode of Communication of Cholera*, 45.

city. "It will be observed," Snow concluded "that the deaths either very much diminished, or ceased altogether, at every point where it becomes decidedly nearer to send to another pump than to the one in Broad Street."[74] Snow's diagrammatic device relied on statistical data that specific contaminated water was to blame for the distribution of cholera and, maybe more importantly, could show that neither bad air nor any kind of effluvia were responsible for the epidemic. The map in this particular case and its framing as part of an ongoing heated controversy plotted a spatial structure of the disease not so much to disclose the disease's locality but to deliver a spatial argument about cholera's etiology.

McLeod argued recently that the spatial structure delivered in Snow's cholera map uses place "as defined and mediated through human activity,"[75] rather than just a geometrical set of coordinates in space. Snow interwove his conviction about contagious substances in water with statistical data from tables, case histories and particular observations about social behavior in the districts with the highest case rate. From the resulting tapestry he made his recommendation of removing the pump handle. This intervention stopped the epidemic's spread. Maps such as Snow's added a radical new level to the spatial visualization of diseases. Rather than assembling cases and revealing density patterns, the map is built around an *ordinal* structure, which puts data and objects into a specific relation on the place charted by the map to argue visually for a better understanding of the nature of the visualized disease.[76]

In both cases – cholera in nineteenth-century London and AIDS in late-twentieth-century San Francisco – maps were used to relate additional data to case statistics to prove or disprove a hypothesis. Both the spatial diagram of Snow and the devices of Smallman-Raynor and colleagues allow for an indefinite number of assumptions, datasets, theories and critical inquiries to be applied to the spatio-temporal structure of an outbreak of a disease. Maps provide convincing visual arguments to overcome previously entrenched way of seeing, understanding and approaching the nature of an epidemic. As Monmonier observed, "[E]ven when authors of disease maps assert an exploratory or scientific intent, their maps and atlases serve to promote a particular viewpoint."[77] After Snow, cholera gradually ceased to be seen as purely a disease of

---

[74] Ibid., 47.   [75] McLeod, "Our Sense of Snow," 926.

[76] Cliff, *Atlas of Disease Distributions*, 13 f.; Tom Koch and Ken Denike, "Essential, Illustrative, or ... Just Propaganda? Rethinking John Snow's Broad Street Map," *Cartographica: The International Journal for Geographic Information and Geovisualization* 45, no. 1 (March 2010), 19–31, doi:10.3138/carto.45.1.19.

[77] Monmonier, "Maps as Graphic Propaganda for Public Health," 109.

filth, stench and, by logical extension, poverty. AIDS, when mapped through models, was also no longer just a disease of homosexual men confined to the territory of certain stigmatized districts.

The Geographical Bloodhound

By 1990, focus in the United States had shifted to locate and visualize the pathways between assumed epicenters of the epidemic's early days and the majority of American society. Maybe the proto-narrative, certainly one of the most repeated stories of how AIDS overcame the walls of urban societies, was given by Abraham Verghese, a writing clinician from Johnston City, Tennessee. He told a captivating and celebrated first-person account of the epidemic's arrival in rural America at the end of its first decade. A key element of his experiences was the fact that most patients who he encountered in the small Johnston City Hospital, in which he worked, seemed to have acquired their infection elsewhere and who had after longer absence only recently returned to their home city. The persistent lack of accessible healthcare and political visibility about AIDS, Verghese assumed, meant some patients had to rely eventually on palliative care from family and friends back at home.[78] Joining the dots between 81 cases in 1989 from around Johnston City, the constellation suggested that most patients probably became infected in one of the urban centers of the United States: New York, San Francisco, Los Angeles or Houston. Furthermore, the small sample of rural AIDS cases Verghese was confronted with seem to fit all too neatly into the cluster of risk groups defined by the CDC in the early 1980s. Verghese drew a map that demonstrated the fate of young, white homosexual men, who had left their hometown to flee homophobia, prejudice and stigmatization, only to return to their families as neither healthcare nor other charitable acknowledgment was provided in the urban centers from where AIDS seemed to stem.[79]

Certainly, this story showed Verghese's sympathy, committed to following the fate of ostracized persons with AIDS who sought shelter and care, but his tale also served as a warning to a complacent public. As AIDS reached the countryside, many new areas, which were considered to be in safe distance, were at heightened risk. Verghese articulated his worry about this newly emerging pattern of the migrating persons with

---

[78] Abraham Verghese, Steven L. Berk, and Felix Sarubbi, "Urbs in Rure: Human Immunodeficiency Virus Infection in Rural Tennessee," *Journal of Infectious Diseases* 160, no. 6 (1989), 1051–5.
[79] Verghese, *My Own Country*.

AIDS, and he and his co-authors concluded that "[u]nfortunately, persons outside the AIDS epicenters less often adopt safer sex and needle practices."[80] Here again, we can see a motive introduced in the chapter on photography: Imagining the person with AIDS as "still sexual" drew attention to new places of distribution and new patterns of emergence in the previously safe hinterland.

Eventually AIDS came to be perceived as a thread to everyone. In the late 1980s AIDS was gradually taking over – or so it seemed – the whole country. This alarming impression led to a high priority of new map making: Models of the progression of AIDS county by county had been in production since the mid-1980s. Clustered visualizations of CDC datasets were presented by Dutt and colleagues, while others exploited the spatial data from the US Department of Defense's screening program for military applicants to argue for spillovers into previous low-prevalence regions.[81] All spatial arguments shared a recurring way of visualizing the progression of AIDS beyond its assumed locales: Typically a map of the United States, plotted in a consecutive series for comparison, shows the epidemic's ratio in shaded patterns, county by county and state by state[82] The geographer Peter Gould wrote that "Anyone, scanning that sequence of maps..., looking at AIDS spreading in Pennsylvania like a photographic plate developing in the darkroom, can see intuitively an enormous amount of spatial-temporal regularity."[83] One such map sequence illustrates the cover of Gould's book contribution to the geography of AIDS, which – reiterating the visual impression of an increasingly deadly density – is entitled "The Slow Plague."[84]

The atlas series published by Mildvan established an even stronger visualization of the "creeping" transition of the epidemic. In the first edition in 1995, the chapter "Epidemiology, Natural History, and Prevention," edited by Sten H. Vermund and D. Peter Drotman, combined a number of tables, bar graphs and statistical plots illustrated with a map

---

[80] Susan E. Cohn et al., "The Geography of AIDS: Patterns of Urban and Rural Migration," *Southern Medical Journal* 87, no. 6 (1994), 604.

[81] Ashok K. Dutt et al., "Geographical Patterns of AIDS in the United States," *Geographical Review* 77, no. 4 (1987), 456–71; Andrew Golub, Wilpen L. Gorr, and Peter R. Gould, "Spatial Diffusion of the HIV/AIDS Epidemic: Modeling Implications and Case Study of AIDS Incidence in Ohio," *Geographical Analysis* 25, no. 2 (1993), 85–100, doi:10.1111/j.1538-4632.1993.tb00282.x; Lam et al., "Spatial-Temporal Spread of the AIDS Epidemic, 1982–1990."

[82] See, e.g., the map sequences in Kaslow and Francis, *The Epidemiology of AIDS*, Brookmeyer and Gail, *AIDS Epidemiology*, Mildvan, *AIDS* and on the cover of Gould, *The Slow Plague*. Until today the style of map is used to visualize the progression of AIDS or respective, HIV, in the United States on CDC websites and elsewhere.

[83] Gould et al., "AIDS: Predicting the Next Map," *Interfaces* 21, no. 3 (1991), 90.

[84] Gould, *The Slow Plague*.

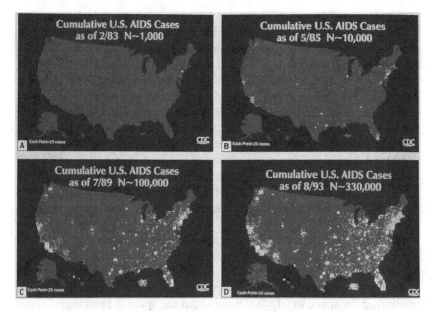

Fig. 2.5 A series of dot maps in the AIDS atlas by Donna Mildvan
from 1995. The serial arrangement suggests a "flooding" of the
United States as the epidemic spills out of the urban epicenters
in which AIDS was assumed to be contained.
Source: Donna Mildvan, ed., *AIDS*. Vol. 1. Atlas of Infectious Diseases
(Philadelphia: Current Medicine, 1995), p. 1.4. Courtesy of the CDC.

sequence on the distribution of AIDS in the United States (Fig. 2.5).[85]
Each white dot on the maps represented 20 cases of AIDS, their increasing density demonstrating the magnitude of the epidemic. Similar to the
maps used by Gould, the series invoked a developing picture of an
epidemic, sweeping from the urban centers to the rest of the country
between 1983 and 1993.

Already by 1990, Gould was not satisfied with the picture of AIDS
proposed in these sequenced maps. These visualizations, he argued,
allowed for complacency regarding the spatial pattern he had observed
and that was not comparable to a slow homogenous spreading. He
developed a competing geographical model that would capture the actual
pathways and complicated spatial-temporal distribution of AIDS. He
developed his model with the ambition of predicting the next outbreak
because he was convinced sequential series of maps could only deliver a

[85] Mildvan, *AIDS*, 1:1.4.

vague picture of threat and in fact could shore up a sense of false security. To make his students at the University of Pennsylvania aware of the real risks about the arrival of the epidemic, he crafted what Koch has called a geographical "bloodhound."[86] The formula laid out a model for rethinking the distribution of AIDS in relation to relative population density. The argument went that AIDS could be differentiated from a contagious disease like plague, for which diffusion follows a gradual distribution over geographical space, reaching village after village as if it were a map of an extending flood. This predominant but misleading image for plague prompted Gould to design the "next map" to give a better, informed account of how the particular disease of AIDS made its way across the United States. His intent was emphatically to scare teenagers and to wake up health practitioners who would not acknowledge their own proximity to the epidemic.[87]

AIDS spread from city to city by slow diffusion to surrounding countryside. To communicate this powerfully in a map, Gould dissolved the geographical distance of the cities affected by AIDS. In doing so he crafted a geographic projection, in which the disease is not plotted in relation to the space in which it moves, but the space is rearranged along the characteristic movements of the epidemic. Taking the example of the US state of Ohio, Gould plotted an "AIDS space"(Fig. 2.6) by moving the urban centers of the state out of their geographic position and grouping them together according to the probability of the preparation for the next infection, the next AIDS event.[88] In this innovative map, Gould had made a mathematical model that correlated the hierarchical spatial transmission of AIDS along the density of population in urban centers. He intended the map to visualize the "step-jump" situation that was to set the diffusion of AIDS apart from the common picture of epidemics as extending flood.[89] Both an instrument for open ended interrogation, and a symptom of the narrowly focused surveillance of AIDS up until that point, Gould's AIDS space became a timely reminder that social and cultural framings of the epidemic had misled both the research community as well as the general public. Thinking AIDS through its spatial pattern was an invitation to unsee the epidemic's limited and epidemiologically dangerous entanglement with homosexual men, heroin users, hemophiliacs and Haitians.

There are many historical cases of how shifting ideas about where a disease is and what it means have enabled a reimagining of what the

---

[86] Koch, *Cartographies of Disease: Maps, Mapping, and Medicine*, 272.
[87] Monmonier, "Maps as Graphic Propaganda for Public Health," 119.
[88] Gould et al., "AIDS: Predicting the Next Map," 87.   [89] Ibid., 89.

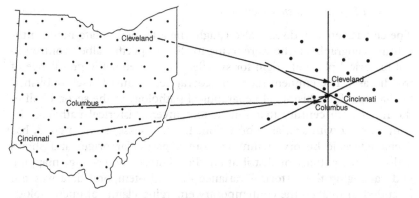

Fig. 2.6 A visualization of the AIDS space as developed by Peter Gould in 1991. To emphasize the epidemic's jumping transmission from city to city he shortened geographical coordinates to rearrange the state of Ohio according to the characteristic movement of the epidemic. *Source:* Peter Gould, J. Kabel, W. Gorr, and A. Golub, "AIDS: Predicting the Next Map," *Interfaces* 21, no. 3 (1991), 80–92, p. 86. Permission granted by the Institute for Operations Research and the Management Sciences.

disease was thought to signify. In the West, tuberculosis was reframed from a disease believed to be intimately attached to poverty and filth, to being seen as a disease more closely associated with migration and social groups outside the scope of medical surveillance.[90] Bubonic plague was known as "yellow peril" when it arrived at the American West Coast in 1899, but health officers and boards were quick to undo the stereotypes as they invoked a sense of false security.[91] But a look at the history of other sexually transmitted diseases brings up an example that proved to be a valuable model through which to understand the AIDS epidemic: syphilis.[92]

---

[90] Janina Kehr, "Blind Spots and Adverse Conditions of Care: Screening Migrants for Tuberculosis in France and Germany," *Sociology of Health and Illness* 34, no. 2 (2012), 251–65, doi:10.1111/j.1467-9566.2011.01415.x; René Dubos and Jean Dubos, *The White Plague: Tuberculosis, Man, and Society*, 3rd ed. (New Brunswick, NJ: Rutgers University Press, 1996); Flurin Condrau, "The Patient's View Meets the Clinical Gaze," *Social History of Medicine* 20, no. 3 (2007), 525–40, doi:10.1093/shm/hkm076.

[91] Nayan Shah, *Contagious Divides: Epidemics and Race in San Francisco's Chinatown* (Berkeley: University of California Press, 2001).

[92] Sander L. Gilman, "AIDS and Syphilis: The Iconography of Disease," in *AIDS, Cultural Analysis, Cultural Activism*, ed. Douglas Crimp (Cambridge, MA: MIT Press, 1988), 87–107; Allan M. Brandt, *No Magic Bullet: A Social History of Venereal Disease in the United States since 1880* (New York: Oxford University Press, 1987); Allan M. Brandt, "The Syphilis Epidemic and Its Relation to AIDS," *Science* 239 (1988), 375–80.

Mapping Endemic Contours

The classic venereal disease also caught the attention of late-nineteenth-century geographers who were trying to align a specific, albeit controversial historical place of origin for syphilis with the endemic prevalence of the disease. The eminent medical geographer August Hirsch published his handbook for historical-geographical pathology in the second half of the nineteenth century that sought to reinvent historical pathology by combining it with spatial information. Every disease, so he argued, has a characteristic history stemming from a particular origin and shows a distinctive pattern of distribution. For Hirsch, describing, mapping and cataloging the historical variance of spatio-temporal data was not intended to weaken the contemporary emerging claims of microbiology and cell pathology, but to accompany their endeavor in forging and unifying disease entities through time and space.[93]

Syphilis became the unofficial poster child of this enterprise toward the end of the nineteenth century. Disagreements about its origin spanned from the idea of an autochthon emergence from sideric influences, to zoonotic transgressions and to the popular idea of an American origin,[94] while Hirsch insisted on the enduring presence of syphilis throughout history. He detailed its overarching presence and indifference to geographic districts as well as mentions a "specific infective substance."[95] Moving away from historic accounts of syphilis as the paradigmatic disease of specific groups and places ("morbus Neapolitans, gallicus, franzos, americanus"), geographers at the turn of the twentieth century tried to establish a new account of the general endemic situation of syphilis. Neither the question of origin nor its classification as a disease of a particular kind of population made sense any longer. Instead, some historians of the disease arrived at the conviction that the history of syphilis resembled the history of mankind. In 1901 Iwan Bloch came to the conclusion that syphilis must be understood as a symptom of the

---

[93] Hirsch, *Handbook of Geographical and Historical Pathology*; Ackerknecht, *Geschichte und Geographie der wichtigsten Krankheiten*, 3; F. A. Barrett, "August Hirsch: As Critic of, and Contributor to Geographical Medicine and Medical Geography," *Medical History Supplement* no. 20 (2000), 98–117. On the significance of historical pathology at the end of the nineteenth century see Johanna Bleker, "Die Idee einer historischen Entwicklung der Krankheiten des Menschengeschlechts und ihre Bedeutung für die empirische Medizin des frühen 19. Jahrhunderts," *Berichte zur Wissenschaftsgeschichte* 8 (1985), 195–204.
[94] Holcomb, *Who Gave the World Syphilis? The Haitian Myth*.
[95] Hirsch, *Handbook of Geographical and Historical Pathology*, II, 84.

development of human civilization and the expansion of human culture.[96] The history of civilization has also been a history of the "syphilization" of the West.[97] Syphilis was seen as a strange object in which the entanglement of cultural history and medical history seems not only accidental, but also a characteristic feature of a modern understanding of this venereal disease that focused now on practices of transmission.[98]

When syphilis lost in the late nineteenth century its image as a foreign illness and became instead a disease of sexual transmission, sexual deviation and sex work, so too did it lose its characteristic geographical patterns, through which it had been perceived for centuries.[99] As the cultural and medical history of syphilis became blended together, syphilis developed yet again into a new disease.[100] In this new figuration, syphilis became essentially endemic, and its vectors were thought too extensive to map through districts or to isolate occurrences that would not eventually resemble the shape of general population density. Rarely a subject in maps of modern medical geography, syphilis became a disease whose pattern would be understood only in close relation to the everyday structures of societies. A recent example is found in Cliff's atlas of epidemic diseases, which emphasizes that syphilis only appears to the eyes of the geographer when an extremely high resolution is applied. Only then, Cliff argues, could the fine-grained prevalence of syphilis in certain lower income populations in the United States be observed at all.[101]

Fears spiked at the end of the 1980s that AIDS distribution might follow the example of syphilis and would eventually become uncharted territory as a widespread endemic crisis. But these fears never played out. AIDS did in fact maintain a quite recognizable social and racial structure throughout the United States until today and never fully dispersed into the general public. Whereas Mildvan with many others were inclined to foreground the map sequence of AIDS slowly covering the landscape of the US territory, she also invested in maps demonstrating the newly emerging patterns of social AIDS distribution in the early 1990s. The

---

[96] Iwan Bloch, *Der Ursprung der Syphilis. Eine Medizinische und Kulturgeschichtliche Untersuchung* (Jena: Fischer, 1901).

[97] Ibid., 6.

[98] Brandt, *No Magic Bullet*; Lutz Sauerteig, *Krankheit, Sexualität, Gesellschaft. Geschlechtskrankheiten und Gesundheitspolitik in Deutschland im 19. und frühen 20. Jahrhundert* (Stuttgart: Steiner, 1999).

[99] Claude Quétel, *History of Syphilis* (Cambridge: Polity Press, 1990).

[100] On the changing nature of syphilis and for a reflection of the styles of thought associated with the disease, see: Ludwik Fleck, *Genesis and Development of a Scientific Fact* (Chicago: University of Chicago Press, 1981).

[101] Andrew D. Cliff, *World Atlas of Epidemic Diseases* (London: Arnold, 2004), 4.2.

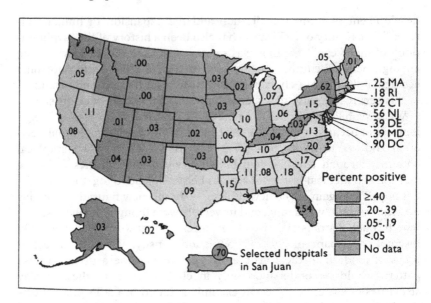

Fig. 2.7 A map of HIV rates among childbearing women in the United States in Mildvan's AIDS atlas from 1995. The increasing diversification of the epidemic's social profile was emphasized through maps, which could visualize the presence of the epidemic in almost every US state and yielded an informative pattern of high prevalence. *Source:* Donna Mildvan, ed., *AIDS*. Vol. 1. Atlas of Infectious Diseases (Philadelphia: Current Medicine, 1995), p. 1.5. Courtesy of the CDC.

overall impression of a "slow plague" in Mildvan's atlas was contextualized on subsequent pages with extensive information about what in 1995 was yet another newly emerging social structure of the epidemic. Previously overlooked, the "minority composition of AIDS cases"[102] was now incorporated into a geographic picture that still characterizes AIDS distribution in the United States today.

One example is given in this map (Fig. 2.7) that appeared in tweaked versions throughout Mildvan's atlas series, which detailed the HIV seroprevalence among "childbearing women." Like others of its kind, it demonstrated the sweeping distribution of heterosexual infections far beyond the original urban centers of the epidemic, with particular emphasis of a rate above 4/1000 in 1991 in Florida and Puerto Rico.[103] Charting AIDS along the disadvantaged groups of society through several graphs suggested a disproportionate number of African American

---

[102] Mildvan, *AIDS*, 1:1.5   [103] Ibid.

and Latin cases, representing 45 percent of new infection rates. Both groups exceeded their statistical relativity to the general public by 200 percent.[104] Furthermore, the atlas editors invested considerable attention to positioning pregnant women in the epidemic. An increasing number of new infections among women – from 8 percent in 1985 to 14 percent in 1992 – correlated, as the maps demonstrated, with the increasing number of infected pregnant women. This suggested that the total number of new infections had left the niche of drug use behind and were now increasingly occurring through heterosexual transmission. A developing dot map as well as the ratio-visualizations of minority composition worked by visualizing unseen and largely invisible domains of the epidemic in its second decade. Especially African American clusters of cases had long remained invisible in the spatial narratives of the epidemic, as they were either counted among drug user incidence or simply overlooked. A lack of surveillance, a lack in good classification, led to a persistent gap in public health campaigns, which might in turn have contributed to a false sense of immunity among African Americans, as described by Cathy Cohen.[105] The map's purpose in Mildvan's atlas lies too in the forceful demonstration of a changing picture in which previous perceptions and strategies of containment, like the urban center, the 4Hs and the perception of an immunity of the national body are systematically made unseen.

However, by the end of 1991 the United States still had more than half of the world's reported cases of AIDS.[106] At the beginning of the epidemic's second decade, geographers like Gould engaged largely in a reconstruction of how this catastrophe had happened and tackled the conditions under which it went unseen for too long. Gould attributed the new "explosive nature of the beast"[107] to a "stinging indictment of arrogant professional blindness and unconscionable neglect," which had characterized both political and medical receptions of the epidemic in its first years.[108]

The geographers Gary Shannon and Gerald Pyle insisted in their critical contribution from 1989 on the diffusion pattern of AIDS that the perception of homosexual men as a single risk group and isolated geographic arena for the disease had always been an epidemiological

---

[104] Ibid.
[105] Preda, *AIDS, Rhetoric, and Medical Knowledge*, 199; Cathy J. Cohen, *The Boundaries of Blackness: AIDS and the Breakdown of Black Politics* (Chicago: University of Chicago Press, 1999).
[106] Center for Disease Control, "HIV Surveillance – United States, 1981–2008," *Morbidity and Mortality Weekly Report* 60, no. 21 (2011), 689–93.
[107] Gould, *The Slow Plague*, 114.   [108] Ibid., 122.

oversight. It did not even resemble the reality of AIDS when it was first identified.[109] Both authors conceded that the social structure and distribution of the epidemic in the United States have followed largely different patterns than originally suspected, to finally point to the other, largely invisible aspect of the epidemic's geography: its international impact. To integrate a global vision, substantial geographical differences in the diffusion of infected populations and of diseases and infections associated with the immune deficiency became starkly clear. Based largely on research carried out by Jonathan Mann at the WHO, the geographers conclude their spatial argument that the "importance of spatially variable behavior, social and environmental factors" suggested the crucial significance of socioecological models of disease in the future perception of what was already a globalized picture of AIDS.[110]

In the United States, not only did the epidemic leave its assumed urban foci behind, its socioecological shape shifted slowly into a disease of poverty, fueled by lack of access to healthcare. What was originally perceived as an isolated incident, politically neglected by the Reagan administration, transformed substantially, as AIDS had become an "American Epidemic." Maps facilitated the departure from what could be called a "single cause, single location" model, in which the threat of AIDS was contained through the risk group in which it first appeared.[111] Instead, maps showed AIDS to affect different communities in different places in different ways, an insight gained through and reliant on intricate visualizations of space to enable perceptions of the disease in its unselective and almost arbitrary nature. Maps were rather practical instruments of forging a new medical and geographical understanding, which served as a cornerstone in epidemiological perception, signaling both a practice of surveillance as well as a clear intention to understand AIDS through its spatial coordinates rather than its individual bodies and their symptoms.

Globalizing the Pandemic

The map of the AIDS epidemic printed in the first AIDS atlas of 1986, loosely based on the Gallo model of original distribution, captured

[109] Gary W. Shannon and Gerald F. Pyle, "The Origin and Diffusion of AIDS: A View from Medical Geography," *Annals of the Association of American Geographers* 79, no. 1 (1989), 1.

[110] Ibid., 2; Jonathan M. Mann, "The Global AIDS Situation," *World Health* (Geneva: World Health Organization, 1987), www.who.int/iris/handle/10665/53236; Mann et al., "Surveillance for AIDS in a Central African City."

[111] Bastos, *Global Responses to AIDS*, 56.

probably the earliest way in which a global history of AIDS was understood. As discussed previously, the map offered an argument on plausible explanations of how AIDS arrived to the American research community and suggested an explanatory framework for AIDS's arrival in the United States. In other words, maps of the original global distribution masked ideas of an American origin of AIDS and helped to make the entanglement of AIDS and the United States unseen.

This leaves us with the dilemma of two kinds of origin of the epidemic: on the one hand, a narrative origin in the United States in 1981 and, on the other hand, the narrative of a natural origin, vaguely tied to the beginning of the twentieth century in Central Africa. Do we attribute a notion of origin to the longer natural history, which has been reconstructed ever since comparable cases in Zaire appeared? Or is the origin of AIDS to be found in the place where it was first recognized, named and framed into the epidemic that it then became? The epidemic's "cognitive birth" in the United States marked the analysis of the epidemic, as Christiana Bastos argued, whereas "a search for its origins helped make it visible everywhere."[112] While it is important to acknowledge that AIDS affected hundreds of thousands of people before it was originally conceived of as AIDS, these cases will inevitably remain part of a history of an epidemic that was not yet AIDS. Its official birth in 1981 United States delivered the conditional framework through which a cultural, a social, a medical and even the natural history of the epidemic was perceived. From here, the global prehistory of AIDS was crafted, and it is from this same point of origin that the globalization of the epidemic was thought through in the late 1980s. While it is tempting to assign phylogenetic trees identified in traces of HIV in historic blood samples, a trumping truth in determining an original, authentic historical and global picture of the epidemic, we will not ever arrive at a purified natural history of the disease in which a geographic and historic origin reveals itself as sufficient to render the social and cultural history of AIDS and its American origin, unseen.

The history of the globalization of AIDS thus departs from a history that began in 1981 United States. "Without a doubt," Cindy Patton writes in her account of the globalization of AIDS, "the United States had a crucial role in setting global trends in thinking about and handling AIDS, but the international and transnational formulations of the epidemic have also shaped the way the United States can represent its place to itself."[113] This transition, Patton argues, was marked by contradicting

---

[112] Ibid., 57.   [113] Patton, *Globalizing AIDS*, 26.

thought styles as different geographic approaches and different medical understandings collided. But beyond this complicated setting, Patton also notes the challenge of making an epidemic global that had originally been American. As a constant exchange of expertise between scales of local places, national politics and international organizations became the *modus operandi*, the crucial question was to what end practices of containment from the United States could ever be applied to the newly emerging foci of crisis in Africa.[114]

For Bastos, the globalization of AIDS was not only marked by different approaches to dealing with the epidemic but happened in a period of AIDS history characterized by the persistent absence of cure or any successful medical interventions. The crucial years between 1986 and 1995 saw the advent of a global pandemic as well as the incapacity of biomedicine to deliver convincing and unified means of intervention. The science of AIDS, already a rapidly advancing specialty, appeared to be in a state of emergency, with "each statement turning out to be as fragile as the one it replaced."[115]

While this period began with a broad agreement on HIV as causal agent, it also began with the first international conference on AIDS.[116] This meeting left an impression of the epidemic's overwhelming global dimensions. The WHO AIDS program – one of the later outcomes of the conference – Bastos argues, emphasized prevention, education and social issues such as political change, empowerment of minorities, justice in gender relations, sex work, drug politics and controlling blood products to effectively prioritize social dimensions over medical solutions in the global response to AIDS: "The absence of a unified and strong response on the part of science had as a counterpart the development of a multifocal panoply of responses."[117] As the AIDS crisis became global, the absence of unified medical strategies was utilized to mobilize a response deeply rooted in the program of social medicine.[118]

The WHO initially considered AIDS to be largely an American disease and problem and only launched a new, global strategy once the minister of health of Uganda had reported on the drastic AIDS crisis developing in Central Africa at the World Health Assembly in 1986. Jonathan Mann was approached a couple of months later to become the director of the

---

[114] Ibid., xx.   [115] Bastos, *Global Responses to AIDS*, 16.

[116] Gary R. Noble, "International Conference on Acquired Immunodeficiency Syndrome: 14–17 April 1985, Atlanta, Georgia," *Annals of Internal Medicine* 103, no. 5 (November 1, 1985), 653, doi:10.7326/0003-4819-103-5-653.

[117] Bastos, *Global Responses to AIDS*, 9.

[118] Elizabeth Fee and Daniel M. Fox, eds., *AIDS: The Burdens of History* (Berkeley: University of California Press, 1988).

new Global Program on AIDS.[119] Equipped with an impressive budget, Mann set out to design a global health policy that attempted to meet the epidemic on as many diverse grounds as possible, while keeping human rights its guiding political focus. As Fee quotes from WHO meeting records, Mann was committed to define AIDS as three discrete epidemics. Each of the three had distinct features requiring a specific resolution. AIDS was thus understood to be (1) an infection, (2) an epidemic of devastating illness and (3) a social, cultural and political epidemic that required a depoliticized approach and a strict focus on the distinct but limited transmission routes of HIV in affected countries.[120]

Mann's mission was to change a resilient paradigm of public health policy by fighting for a global acknowledgment of the unique appearance of AIDS and its many national crises. A concern for individual rights, stigmatization and strategies to overcome the image of AIDS as a disease of homosexual transmission led the WHO to argue strictly against coercive measures. The notion of forcing people into regimes of assumed healthy behaviors was unacceptable. As Allan Brandt notes 2013:

Most notably, the AIDS epidemic has provided the foundation for a revolution that upended traditional approaches to "international health," replacing them with innovative global approaches to disease. Indeed, the HIV epidemic and the responses it generated have been crucial forces in "inventing" the new "global health."[121]

Accordingly, the new policy was driven by calls for transparency, for inclusion of civil society groups and activism on both national and international scales and to develop a policy of nondiscrimination within the WHO. It was thanks to their strong position that the intentions of some nations to restrict traveling were halted.[122] Mann's leadership of the AIDS program at the WHO established a lasting public health paradigm of nondiscrimination. The protection of individual rights was considered essential "as the stigma of the disease threatened to drive infected persons to conceal their status."[123]

Mann's pragmatic approach needed new instruments for mapping, surveillance and containment on the ground. WHO's malaria and smallpox campaigns of the 1950s and 1960s were characterized by large-scale mappings of communities, villages, social structures and cultural

---

[119] Fee and Parry, "Jonathan Mann, HIV/AIDS, and Human Rights," 59.
[120] Ibid., 61.   [121] Brandt, "How AIDS Invented Global Health," 2149.
[122] Jonathan M. Mann, D. Tarantola, and Thomas W. Netter, *AIDS in the World* (Cambridge, MA: Harvard University Press, 1992).
[123] Fee and Parry, "Jonathan Mann, HIV/AIDS, and Human Rights," 62.

boundaries to vaccination programs.[124] But a fine-grained geographical visualization of HIV-positive populations to determine risk and to enable focused interventions violated the principles of protecting individual rights and nondiscrimination of HIV positive persons. Geographic reconnaissance, with the systematic mapping of social communities in their spatial and temporal distribution among specified risk areas was not an option. The anthropologist Robert Thornton has shown that in place of these old techniques a new kind of mapping was introduced to solve the unprecedented epidemiological puzzles of AIDS.[125]

A strategy emerged that adopted some of the methods developed by Gould and others, in which the mapping of an AIDS space focused on the visualization of network structures disconnected from spatial coordinates. These mappings were concerned with the social network structures in which HIV was sexually transmitted. But what had been originally a strategy of charting the sexual life of a specific population in 1984 San Francisco, who were perceived of sharing a common lifestyle and specific districts, the same practice now was applied to fragments of the general population. In San Francisco, Auerbach and his colleagues had begun in 1984 to map the homosexual networks around their patients to arrive at visual clusters of infection.[126] But while old patterns were never fully disconnected from attempts to identify index patients, or indeed to find "patient zero," new methods of visualizing sexual networks emphasized the complexity of a relation between HIV transmission and sexual behavior of larger diverse groups. Promiscuity or sexual identity was not mapped, but rather the onset of AIDS in Africa raised questions about which combinations of sexual behavior, social status and poverty were contributing to patterns of high prevalence.[127]

Local Pattern

One of the central puzzles in 1990 was that at precisely the time when AIDS rates significantly increased in South Africa they seemed to decline in Uganda. Advocates of conservative approaches to the epidemic swiftly

[124] World Health Organization, "Geographical Reconnaissance for Malaria Eradication Programmes."

[125] Robert Thornton, *Unimagined Community: Sex, Networks, and AIDS in Uganda and South Africa* (Berkeley: University of California Press, 2008).

[126] D. M. Auerbach et al., "Cluster of Cases of the Acquired Immune Deficiency Syndrome: Patients Linked by Sexual Contact," *The American Journal of Medicine* 76, no. 3 (March 1984), 487–92.

[127] On the transfer of epidemiological and clinical practices from San Francisco to Uganda see also Crane, *Scrambling for Africa*.

announced the falling numbers a success for the re-established merit of a moral foundation through the Christian churches, which had supposedly increased commitment to sexual abstinence. Thornton argued instead that a shift in sexual behavior had indeed changed the statistical picture of the epidemic, but instead of general sexual restraint he called the implementation of a different attitude to be the key factor. "Zero Grazing" required communities to restrict their sexual endeavors within local circles to alter the configuration of a "sexual network," reflecting a specific kind of social structure. Thornton argued that such networks had only become visible through the onset of AIDS, as the "sexual network, although largely invisible, is unlike the invisible networks that link people in other epidemics."[128] Making these networks visible, Thornton argued, would again emphasize that the precondition for changing sexual behavior was first to establish a localized understanding of how sexual encounters are organized and how communities that had been unimagined become visible.

These approaches were accordingly used in many different settings. Elizabeth Pisani, author of the infamous study on the *Wisdom of Whores* recalls a particular scene from her work in UNAIDS, when she struggled against the official Chinese position that women in China would per se not engage in sex before marriage. She drew a sex map of a classic Chinese drama, the "sprawling sexual soap opera" "Golden Lotus," and used the generic WHO color coding for high- and low-risk partnerships to successfully contradict the official position that nonmarital sexual relations did not exist in China.[129]

Many other sexual networks were drawn in the following years to investigate, for example, the social position of sex workers and clients of sex workers; a particularly thorough study deserves more attention.[130] Stephane Helleringer and Hans-Peter Kohler mapped the sexual network of the Likoma Island on Lake Malawi. Moving away from the usual pattern that centered on high-risk groups, the authors aimed to identify patterns within a general population of young adults that illuminated the transmission routes of HIV. The resulting model shows a sexual network

[128] Thornton, *Unimagined Community*, 24.

[129] Elizabeth Pisani, *The Wisdom of Whores: Bureaucrats, Brothels and the Business of AIDS* (London: Granta Books, 2010), 195 f.

[130] C. N. Morris and A. G. Ferguson, "Estimation of the Sexual Transmission of HIV in Kenya and Uganda on the Trans-Africa Highway: The Continuing Role for Prevention in High Risk Groups," *Sexually Transmitted Infections* 82, no. 5 (October 2006), 368–71, doi:10.1136/sti.2006.020933; M. E. Gomes do Espirito Santo and G. D. Etheredge, "Male Clients of Brothel Prostitutes as a Bridge for HIV Infection between High Risk and Low Risk Groups of Women in Senegal," *Sexually Transmitted Infections* 81, no. 4 (2005), 342–4, doi:10.1136/sti.2004.011940.

composed of three patterns, each displaying a high prevalence of cycle structures. The authors conclude that a large and robust network connected a substantial portion of the island. Half of all sexually active young adults on the island were connected through one of the spatial components visualized on the map (Fig. 2.8). But HIV prevalence was highest on the margins of these larger networks, and incidence rates were higher in the sparse regions of the map, indicating an ecology of unidentified factors beyond the grasp of the mapped sexual network.[131]

These maps were technical instruments, useful to a handful of experts who were able to integrate the visualizations into arguments on possible points of intervention into the developing epidemic in Sub-Saharan Africa. To audiences beyond these cycles, the maps stand as representations of studies that had been developed to chart out the epidemic drivers in highly diverse local settings, contributing once more to a fractured, scattered and increasingly disconnected vision of AIDS around the world.

The AIDS atlas did not contain any of these systematic local mappings, as the maps' specificities did not comply with the general scope of visualizing AIDS to a medical audience. The globalizing epidemic was instead integrated into the atlas through pictures of its shifting epicenter. A focus on the changing global picture rather than particular patterns addressed the atlas's predominantly Western audience.

In Mildvans's international AIDS atlas, we find two maps with a comparably neutral vision of AIDS in the world (Fig. 2.9). This map from the 2008 edition totals 38.6 million people living with HIV, and the shading compares the ratio, the relative density of HIV prevalence from country to country. Along the national boarders, maps like this one reflect, on the one hand, the structure of national reporting to the WHO or UNAIDS and, on the other hand, give a quick impression of the shifted epicenter of AIDS today.

But how to translate these localized and highly specialized encounters into the global public arena in which AIDS was perceived from 1990 onward? And how to integrate the diverse conditions of the many local epidemics into the totalizing vision of the atlas? The diversity of the spread of AIDS as a locally different, social entity required yet another form of visualization that would both guarantee the vision of AIDS as a global entity and would allow for an immediate impression of context-dependent diversity. As the WHO assumed leadership of crafting an

---

[131] Stéphane Helleringer and Hans-Peter Kohler, "Sexual Network Structure and the Spread of HIV in Africa: Evidence from Likoma Island, Malawi," *AIDS* 21, no. 17 (November 2007), 2323–32, doi:10.1097/QAD.0b013e328285df98.

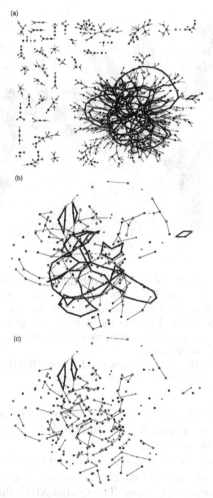

Fig. 2.8 Pattern of sexual networks in Malawi. The representations
of possible transmission routes have been made visible to identify
the conditions of HIV distribution and viable points of intervention
and regulation. The maps visualize a complex local condition that
constitute a unique ecological niche and therefore is evidently not
universally applicable.

Source: Stéphane Helleringer and Hans-Peter Kohler, "Sexual Network
Structure and the Spread of HIV in Africa: Evidence from Likoma Island,
Malawi," *AIDS* 21, no. 17 (November 2007), p. 2328. Permission granted
by Wolters Kluver Health.

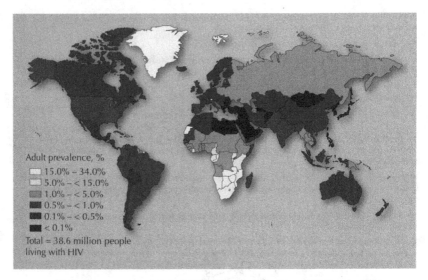

Fig. 2.9 A map of global HIV distribution from Mildvan's 2008
International Atlas of AIDS. The most common visualization of the
global burden of HIV expresses two significant aspects: It visualizes
the presence of AIDS all over the globe and draws affected countries
into comparison, revealing the now-familiar pattern of high prevalence
in Sub-Saharan Africa.
Source: Donna Mildvan, ed., *International Atlas of AIDS* (Philadelphia:
Springer, 2008), 4th ed., p. 2. Courtesy of UNAIDS.

international response characterized by diverse social responses, rather
than unified scientific principles, the multitude of spaces and places of
AIDS were given greater emphasis.

A first crucial step was to divide the world into districts: each of which
was perceived to contain shared characteristics. Such efforts defined
AIDS as a highly localized disease. The Global AIDS Policies Coalition,
founded in 1991 as a not-for-profit partnership led by Jonathan Mann,
charted out 10 different regions as the "New Global Geography of
AIDS."[132] The data was divided by indices of the estimated local start
of the epidemic, the year of the first diagnosis, the year organized data
became available, major modes of transmission, ratio of urban to rural
cases, gender-ratio of infection and responses of the national leaders.
Mann's 10 regions were made up as follows: North America, Western
Europe, Oceania, Latin America, Sub-Saharan Africa, the Caribbean,

[132] Bastos, *Global Responses to AIDS*, 52.

Eastern Europe, the South and East Mediterranean, North and East Asia, and Southeast Asia.[133] A more feasible and lasting division of the world was a three-pattern model, separating the mainly homosexual distribution of the United States and Europe (Pattern I) from mainly heterosexual transmission in Africa (Pattern II) from the Asian epidemic, which was mostly characterized by its late onset (Patttern III).[134]

Either way, the result was a devastating picture. In 1991 in almost all regions prognoses were pessimistic. Global considerations were largely structured by the impression that strategies, shown to be effective in the early appearances of AIDS, could not be translated into a global context. Where activism, community organizing and emotive mobilizations from below made a lasting impact on public health policy and public perception in some regions – mainly the United States and Europe – global challenges appearing with increasing diversity posed very different social and economic problems. The "remarkable successes in some communities contrast dramatically with a sense of threatening collective global failure," so the editors introduced the 1992 report "AIDS in the World."[135] The picture of global diversity became a representation of the developing drastic injustice caused by resource distribution and general poverty.

The most familiar visualization of the new global pattern of AIDS is this shaded global map, similar to the one printed in Mildvan's atlas series. Another example can be found already in the opening section of the before-mentioned WHO publication on the global image of the epidemic (Fig. 2.10). Visualizing the percentage of blood screened for HIV in 1992 as it was reported by nations to the WHO, the map served one crucial function: It visualized areas of relative safety as it showed how governments had reacted to the risk of transmission through blood supplies. But the maps also indicated once again that by 1994 AIDS had become a global phenomenon; a view that the WHO pamphlet photographically reiterated in its 100 pages, which divided areas of the world by their relative intensity of infection rates, case numbers or – mostly negative – outlooks.[136]

Printed in many publications these maps became ubiquitous and were placed alongside statistics, national and transnational reports on the progress of the virus.[137] Unadorned by vector markings, arrows or any

[133] Mann et al., *AIDS in the World*, 19.   [134] Patton, *Globalizing AIDS*, xii.
[135] Mann et al., *AIDS in the World*, 1.   [136] World Health Organization, *AIDS*, 10.
[137] These maps are often used to visualize the annual datasets provided by the WHO, see, e.g., the annual reports from UNAIDS "AIDS by the Numbers, 2016," www.unaids .org/sites/default/files/media_asset/AIDS-by-the-numbers-2016_en.pdf.

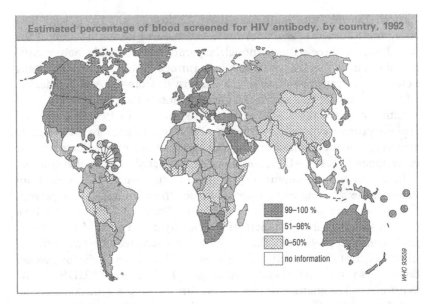

Fig. 2.10 Map of the ratio of blood supplies screened for HIV around the world from the WHO publication "AIDS: Image of the Epidemic," 1994. While the design resembles the familiar visualization of shaded global comparison, this map does not point to districts of risk but instead charts out areas of safety that may or may not resemble areas of high HIV prevalence.
Source: World Health Organization, *AIDS : Images of the Epidemic* (Geneva: World Health Organization, 1994), p. 10. Courtesy of World Health Organization.

indication of trajectories, these maps did not engage with the question of origin, nor do they make arguments about causal chains of international transmission. Instead, the shading of the *ratio* of the disease burden projects a global picture in which the epidemic is already assumed to have arrived in every place of significance, separable only through incidence or prevalence rate. Visualizing AIDS through these maps disregarded the epidemiological question of *where from* as much as it devalues the purpose of asking *what kind of disease*. These maps interrogate instead the question of *how*. Framing the conditions under which the same disease occurs in different intensities, with different impact, the shaded global map creates a vision of global AIDS, in which the different areas of the world are brought into comparison to each other. Through the lens of the everywhere-present pandemic, these maps point to separable geographical entities that invite us to engage further with the specific conditions that distinguish districts with a higher burden from those with moderate rates.

Districts of Disease

The single most important mapping instrument of colonial and, later, tropical medicine may have been maps of disease districts. The visualization was required to better understand diseases that seemed oblivious to social or racial difference yet affected only inhabitants of certain geographical places. These maps served as an essential technology in defining and verifying the specificity of yellow fever, leishmaniosis, sleeping sickness and, later, malaria or tuberculosis.[138] An instrument of surveillance, social control and hygienic principle, the map of disease districts reintroduced spatial coordinates of difference, crafting geographical entities that could easily be translated back onto social and racial relations if these failed to maintain their assumed immunity and community.

The German general practitioner Friedrich Schnurrer produced perhaps the first global map of a disease in 1827. Although deeply influenced by Humboldt's assumption of discrete natural disease identities, Schnurrer argued decisively against the contagionists and mapped cholera to demonstrate its innate relationship to regions, areas and landscapes. In his 1831 publication on the nature, distribution and treatment of cholera, he conceded that the disease might mimic the shape of a contagious disease but continued to list exhaustive examples of how cholera outbreaks remained entangled with specific qualities of districts to prove its noncontagiousness.[139] By considering the implication of water sources and humidity, he proposed that cholera was driven by an emanation of sorts, from which the disease is received by those directly affected.

While this makes for an unusual explanation for the cholera's particular relation to water, it provides a historical account of how certain diseases were perceived as illnesses of location. In this case, and against the background of his time, locales were a central aspect of how a disease worked for Schnurrer. Such early procedures for creating index locations

---

[138] Delaporte, *The History of Yellow Fever*; Saul Jarcho, "Yellow Fever, Cholera, and the Beginnings of Medical Cartography," *Journal of the History of Medicine and Allied Sciences* 25, no. 2 (1970), 131–42; Lyons, *The Colonial Disease*.

[139] Friedrich Schnurrer, "Die geographische Verteilung der Krankheiten, vorgelesen in der Versammlung der deutschen Aerzte und Naturforscher zu München den 22. Sept. 1827," *Das Ausland* 1, no. März (1828), 357–9; R. Broemer, "The First Global Map of the Distribution of Human Diseases: Friedrich Schnurrer's 'Charte über die Geographische Ausbreitung der Krankheiten' (1827)," *Medical History Supplement* 20 (2000), 176–85.

of diseases did not need vectors or other references to direction, nor were they dependent on notions of origin and distribution. Arriving at very different conclusions, Snow's map of a limited geographic cholera presence just 20 years later proved contaminated water was responsible for the local peculiarities of the disease.

A common object of pandemic mapping and modeling has been the return of bubonic plague in the late nineteenth century. Confronted with outbreaks largely beyond the European scope, plague quickly turned into a paradigm of international hygienic intervention, quarantine regulation and pandemic mapping. Maybe the first pandemic that appeared within the framework of a modern medical geography, plague captivated map makers as much as wider audiences, witnessing the return of a centuries-old pest through its mapped trajectories.[140] With the third plague pandemic, as it was officially called several decades later, originating in Hong Kong, spreading to India and from there to almost every port city in the world, the plague pandemic crafted a basic prototype for the modern global disease model. Plague's repetitive structure, appearing with a similar pattern in a variety of far-flung places, catalyzed geographical as well as epidemiological interest. Most significant outbreaks, from the early case of the Russian village Vetlianka, the onset of the epidemic in Hong Kong and continuing to the outbreaks of Porto or San Francisco attracted international teams going to sites of plague to better understand why the epidemic had appeared in these of all places, and why it had spared so many others. The plague's bacteriological agent had been identified by Yersin – with or against Kitasato, a debate we cannot linger on here – in 1894, but the specific vector of how the bacteria entered the human body remained as ambiguous as the implications of climate, poverty, dirt and international trade on the disease burden. As Barrett has pointed out, maps and geographical reasoning served in the early years of the epidemic as technologies of epidemic control, which sought to establish a scientific discourse where the laboratory had failed to provide sufficient explanations.[141]

Plague researchers such as Albert Calmette from the Paris Institute Pasteur, mobilized the scientific capacity that medical geography had established in the nineteenth century to revise scattered outbreaks of plague into a true pandemic.[142] Indicating the similarity of global

---

[140] Myron J. Echenberg, *Plague Ports: The Global Urban Impact of Bubonic Plague, 1894–1901* (New York: New York University Press, 2007); Koch, *Disease Maps. Epidemics on the Ground*, 49 ff.

[141] Barrett, *Disease and Geography: The History of an Idea.*

[142] Albert Calmette, "The Plague at Oporto," *The North American Review* 171, no. 524 (1900): 104–11.

outbreaks maps enabled a perception of plague as a global threat, traced as it was happening. Cartographic instruments could be used to tackle the transnational issues of quarantine and surveillance. The US Public Health Service produced a series of quarantine maps, visualizing the worrying plague belt of global port cities. Other global maps served to test and evaluate hypotheses on the role of climate and to demonstrate patterns of distribution over time.

Half a century later, between 1952 and 1961, Ernst Rodenwaldt, a medical geographer from Heidelberg, published the "Welt-Seuchen-Atlas." A folio atlas in three volumes, this project aimed to collect and distribute a complete archive of the medical geography of all known epidemics of the past and present. After some of the maps and their accompanying apparatuses had been published through Zeiss, a medical geographer working for the German Wehrmacht, the shelved project was picked up again in the 1950s as a collaboration between German geographers and the US Navy.[143] The remarkable atlas, unique in scope, format and technique as well as historical detail, contained an extensive section on bubonic plague and specifically the third plague pandemic.[144] The series of maps visualized the development of plague through the decades, emphasizing the distinctive shape of plague in the twentieth century.

Hans-Juergen Raettig produced this impressive map while he worked at the Robert-Koch-Institute, charged with surveillance and reportage on the global movements of the epidemic (Fig. 2.11). Raettig attributed the less lethal character of this recent pandemic from the medieval Black Death to a new awareness of the plague formula, to popular knowledge about the combination of human plague with the trajectory of bacteria through rats and fleas. Plague's animal vector came to be accepted widely by 1912, and Raettig's map draws an intriguing picture of the historical trajectory of the infectious disease.

Originating from the Asiatic realm, specifically, the central Asian elevated plateaus reaching into the Hindukush, presented an expansive enzootic area where plague was assumed to have been endemic. Unresolved conditions triggered the bacteria to reach Hong Kong in a critical mass, and the subsequent outbreak there spanned to a series of pathways reaching the shores of China, Japan, India, Australia and the South Asian Islands. Through Bombay, Raettig argues, plague came to the African

---

[143] Koch, *Cartographies of Disease: Maps, Mapping, and Medicine*, 220 ff.
[144] Ernst Rodenwaldt, ed., *Welt-Seuchen-Atlas. Weltatlas der Seuchenverbreitung und Seuchenbewegung; in drei Teilen – World-Atlas of Epidemic Diseases* (Hamburg: Falk, 1952), III/31.

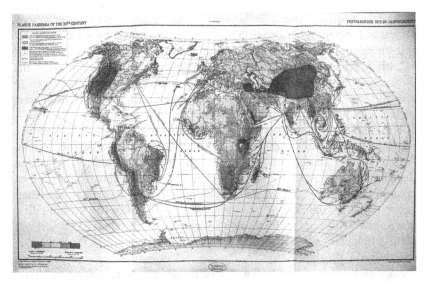

Fig. 2.11 A map of the global distribution of the third plague pandemic, published in the Rodenwaldt's *Seuchen Atlas* in 1952. The map demonstrates the global distribution of the disease, indicates endemic zones and gives a detailed impression of the vectors. An effect is the division of the world in districts of endemic presence and those of epidemic arrival.
Source: Ernst Rodenwaldt, ed., "Welt-Seuchen-Atlas. Weltatlas Der Seuchenverbreitung Und Seuchenbewegung," in Drei Teilen, *World-Atlas of Epidemic Diseases* (Hamburg: Falk, 1952), III/31. Courtesy of Falk.

continent, into the Middle East and eventually to Europe, most prominently to Porto in Portugal.[145] The map is construed by these vectors of the disease, which are drawn over a classic world map projection. The lines and arrows connecting the endemic area of origin to the outbreaks of the pandemic picture are kept in red. Shading distinguishes between active endemic appearances, newly developed enzootic outbreaks and those enzootic occurrences that seemed to continue for an unusual long time. Dots mark places in which plague appeared among considerably large groups of people confined by space and time. Dates and notes clarified the origin of certain trajectories that help to establish a particular picture of how plague conquered the world. The global vision clearly distinguished between areas assumed to have been implicated and affected by plague routinely and those places and pathways where plague arrived

[145] Ibid.

opportunistically. As Gallo mapped the history of AIDS at the end of the twentieth century, his map too suggested an area of historic origin, from which the pandemic picture developed into global extension, rendering the American epidemic an opportunistic epidemic event.

The disease district in which plague was confined as a naturalized entity bound to an endemic cycle was transgressed.[146] Both China and India are placed as the spatial and timely origins of the global vision of plague, both their implication in the large endemic district of plague as well as their mapping as points of departure divides the world into places implicated in plague all along and in new places of infection characterizing the emergency of pandemic. Within the atlas the question of how and why plague was able to stay in certain places, while others remained untouched is answered with a second diagram, adding the climatic conditions of the disease into the global picture. The atlas author's aim was to combine an Asiatic origin with an ecological disposition of the disease to certain climatic conditions. With combined application of theories, data and trajectories, the map unfolds its powerful argument, incorporating the original disease district with pathways and ecological conditions of a disease.

When AIDS became global, the contours of its original districts lost any great importance and disappeared from maps. For a while, neither the original space of the urban homosexual male, nor the later foci in the Sub-Saharan Africa worked as places that were identified as being substantially involved in fostering the disease. Between 1986 and 1995, when the disease was established as a viral infection, but medical research was unable to provide a biomedical solution or treatment, the immune deficiency was predicted to reach every possible corner of the world and was painted as a global disease without a residing "home," mirroring the absence of a culpability narrative in the interim years. While maps of AIDS – similar to the distribution model proposed by Raettig for plague – showed AIDS becoming increasingly global, they also worked to pinpoint an origin of the disease beyond the shores of the United States.

Projecting models such as the one put forward by Gallo, in which the epidemic originated decisively outside of the United States but was probably rampant long before it became visible to the eyes of Western doctors, framed the global model with a crucial twist. Whereas the globalization of the syndrome was an established assumption, its historical geography was crafted to shift the epicenters of the early 1980s

---

[146] Christos Lynteris, "Zoonotic Diagrams: Mastering and Unsettling Human-Animal Relations," *Journal of the Royal Anthropological Institute* 23, no. 3 (2017), 463–85, doi:10.1111/1467-9655.12649.

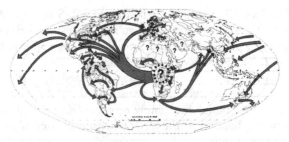

Fig. 2.12 A map of the original diffusion of AIDS from the geographers
Shannon and Pyle, published in 1989. The map deviates substantially
from Gallo's model and suggests a complex pattern of diffusion rather
than identifiable single vectors. Increasing complexity of the pathways
of original distribution would make these kinds of maps redundant.
Source: Gary W. Shannon and Gerald F. Pyle, "The Origin and Diffusion
of AIDS: A View from Medical Geography," *Annals of the Association of
American Geographers* 79, no. 1 (1989): 1–24, p. 12. Permission granted
by Taylor & Francis.

epidemic into the periphery. With Gallo's model, a vision was established
that remained resilient against future changes in the details of trajectories
and pathways. The historical and the global shape of the epidemic aligned
in these global projections, so that one disease district – the American
urban environment – disappeared, so another – the continent of Africa –
could appear as the past, present and future of AIDS.

As an alternative model to Gallo's perhaps naïve idea of singular
transmission routes, geographers Shannon and Pyle already delivered
in 1989 a model, which would replace the notion of disease distribution
pathways with a model of diffusion.[147] Their map, based on a wide range
of statistical datasets rather than guided by hypotheses and etiological
theories, serves as example to visualize the transition between pathway
mappings of the first decade of AIDS, versus maps of the AIDS areas,
separable by shading and gradient, which were important in the epidemic's second decade. With improvement in access to accurate data and
statistical instruments, pathway models were to become so detailed that
their visual representation simply ceased to make much sense.

The 1989 map, built on the WHO's quarterly statistical data publications, provides a very different image of the epidemic's movement
around the globe (Fig. 2.12). The plotted "Patterns of Spatial Diffusion"
remain notably incomplete. Question marks litter the map, pointing to

---

[147] Shannon and Pyle, "The Origin and Diffusion of AIDS: A View from Medical
Geography."

missing datasets, absent reporting among other problems. Departing from the African continent, the map visualizes a simultaneous arrival of the epidemic in Northern Europe, the United States and the Caribbean. Evidence for the epidemic's presence in Brazil, South Africa and Australia further suggest diffusion patterns well beyond the single pathways previously assumed by Gallo and others. While a later onset in Asian countries, estimated to have occurred around 1985, was assumed by the authors, the overall impression of the map resists a narrative sequential reading of AIDS's globalization. From this pattern of global diffusion, the authors claimed a so-called hierarchical-nodal pattern in which the movement of the epidemic was seen to resemble a structure in which urban centers retain centrality, while the infection jumped from large city to large city around the globe. Then, it diffused from these centers to smaller clusters of high-density settlement.[148]

Maps of the history and present of the global burden of AIDS emphasized an image of an all-encompassing presence of the epidemic, comparable to the syphilis maps, in which only fine-grained resolutions were able to separate prevalence from culture, society or life. These maps have truly turned the infectious disease into a pandemic, present in almost every part of the world and distinguishable only through its severity by comparison from one district to another. However, as the question of the origin of AIDS did not disappear from the spheres of biomedical, microbiological, anthropological and historical interrogation, AIDS inherited a new locale in Africa. Shannon and Pyle made in their paper a statement of particular significance about both the original and the new AIDS district: "The substantial amount of evidence from a variety of directions including biological, spatial and temporal, now points to Central Africa as the 'index' location for AIDS."[149] And with surprising candor, the authors marked the much sought-after location of origin and increasing AIDS burden with a large question mark.

Origins and Futures of AIDS

But what does it mean to position Africa as the "index location" of an immunodeficiency that affected the whole world? Shannon and Pyle followed the assumption raised by many epidemiologists and researchers that the epidemic must have originated at a specific time before its visibility as an epidemic in the 1980s. Where available epidemiological data increased in volume, quality and availability after the epidemic's

[148] Ibid., 13.   [149] Ibid., 7.

official birth, with increasingly accurate pictures of its actual distribution around the globe, virtually no data was available to determine the conditions that illuminated the actual inception of AIDS.

Already in Farthing's 1986 atlas, the map resembling Gallo's model was accompanied by a neutral political map of West Africa that focuses on Zaire, Uganda and Tanzania. In 1986, the editors were aware that reports of a so-called slim-disease, present throughout the 1970s, was characterized by rapid onset of emaciation in patients.[150] The atlas editors suggest that these reports indicated the presence of AIDS in this region before the beginning of the official epidemic in the United States. A further key to the inconspicuous representation of West Africa might be found in the contextualization of the map within the atlas's chapter on AIDS epidemiology. Whereas the indication of place – in this case West Africa – is achieved through a map or a cropped portion of a map, this place is similarly connected to a visualization of origin, demonstrating the historical starting point of the epidemic. Furthermore, both maps are accompanied by representations of the virus's genetic information. Diagrams, graphs and simplified trees of genetic structure, development and homology are used to draw on a natural history of HIV to position it as the uncontested deadly agent, but also a diagram in which the resemblance to simian viruses is shown to indicate the locations where HIV emerged as it crossed species in its prehistory of the pandemic.

Mildvan's atlas after 1995, more than 10 years later, integrated a map into the epidemiological chapter, in which the political borders of the African continent disappeared. Where once were national boundaries, the map separated the continent according to the favored habitats of several monkey species, each of which were at that time possible candidates for transmitting the original virus to the first human host.[151] The map (Fig. 2.13) therefore sought to visualize both a definition and the origin of HIV, while capturing the "geographic distribution of four major species of the green monkey." Accompanied by photographs of the monkey and diagrams of the phylogenetic resemblance between HIV and simian immunodeficiency virus (SIV), the visualization suggests a similarly geographic and genetic origin of HIV in the distribution areas of the monkey, while the specific conditions under which the agent mutated into a virus capable of crossing species was unknown in 1996.[152]

---

[150] David Serwadda et al., "Slim Disease: A New Disease in Uganda and Its Association with HTLV-III Infection," *The Lancet* 326, no. 8460 (1985), 849–52; Thornton, *Unimagined Community*, 12.

[151] Tamara Giles-Vernick and James L. A. Webb, *Global Health in Africa: Historical Perspectives on Disease Control* (Athens, Ohio: Ohio University Press, 2013).

[152] Mildvan, *AIDS*, 2.3.

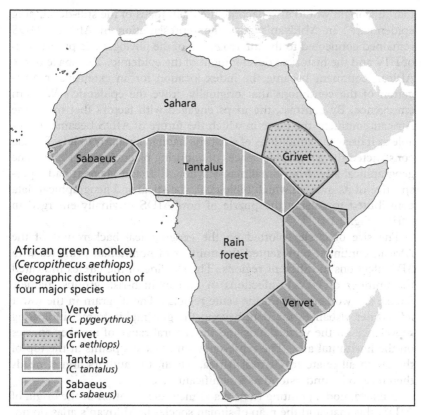

Fig. 2.13 Map (drawn after the original) showing the distribution of green monkey species in Mildvan's 1995 AIDS atlas. Charting the geographic domains of the primates serves to arrive at analytical conclusions about the highest probability for the original moment of species crossing that would have allowed identification of the conditions for the virus's transformation from SIV to HIV.

Source of original map: Donna Mildvan, ed., AIDS. Vol. 1. Atlas of Infectious Diseases (Philadelphia: Current Medicine, 1995), p. 1.4.

The powerful geographical linkage of the natural history with the developing epidemic in present prompted biologists, geneticists and virologists from the early 1990s to interrogate the African ecology for traces of how HIV crossed into human kind.[153] The extent of the epidemic sustained a belief in an African origin, and it was widely believed

[153] On the relationship of social and biological histories in the long history of AIDS in Africa see: Tamara Giles-Vernick et al., "Social History, Biology, and the Emergence of

that this origin would also become the main focus of the still-developing epidemic.[154] In Mildvan's atlas the representation of African AIDS remained connected to the interrogation of the phylogenetic progression of HIV and the historical development of the epidemic. The space of the African continent became the index location for an extensive interrogation of the conditions that originally drove the epidemic's Western emergence. By contrast, the maps engaged with factors that made the African continent the place in which the future of AIDS became inevitable as it drew the conditions of a natural habitat, similarly to how Raettig constructed the geographic spaces of enduring plague in the 1950s. The geographical atlas from Smallman-Raynor, Cliff and Haggett had a perspective of its own, in which biological, statistical and geographical data contributed to solving the puzzle of how AIDS originally emerged in Africa (Fig. 2.14).[155]

The size of circles plotted on the geographical background of the African continent represented the number of nonhuman primates with SIV infections in different regions. The shading of the circles indicated the number of HIV-1 infections in human high-risk groups, namely female sex workers, within the same regions. The diagram in the lower left corner visualizes the data beyond the geographic frame, indicating prevalence on the vertical axis and the natural range of monkey species on the horizontal axis. The representation of excess points at the top of the graph all relate to Central Africa, which, the authors argue, needs therefore to be understood as a significant place.

Unlike a model pointing to Africa as the index location or the origin of AIDS, this map and the map of simian species in Mildvan's atlas do not produce nominal representations of the presence or absence of disease. Instead, both maps work through ratios of HIV prevalence in relation to the prevalence of SIV in nonhuman carriers. Plotting both numbers onto a geographical space created a picture, in which statistical density formed spatial pattern, so that the relationship between disease and the natural conditions of its origin could be seen. A crucial aspect of geographical visualizations like these is that they do not engage with the disease and its distribution of spaces to signal impact and risk of infection in particular places, but rather visualize a space that has come into focus through an investigation into the biological, social and medical origin of AIDS.

HIV in Colonial Africa," *The Journal of African History* 54, no. 1 (2013), 11–30, doi:10.1017/S0021853713000029.

[154] Patton, *Globalizing AIDS*; Gallo, *Virus Hunting: AIDS, Cancer, and the Human Retrovirus*.

[155] Smallman-Raynor et al., *London International Atlas of AIDS*, 134.

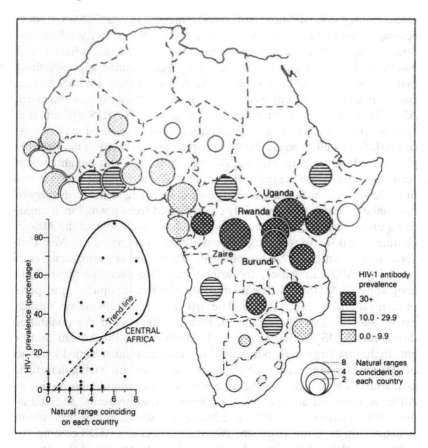

Fig. 2.14 A map on the relationship of SIV and HIV in Smallman-Raynor et al. 1992. The analytical device crafts a zoonotic argument in which the distribution of primates and human social behaviors are layered to arrive at conclusions about probable original vectors of the species crossing in Central Africa by measures of density.
Source: Matthew Smallman-Raynor, Andrew Cliff, and Peter Haggett, eds., *London International Atlas of AIDS* (Oxford and Cambridge: Blackwell Publishers, 1992), p. 134. Permission granted by Wiley.

Both maps are representative for the different approaches undertaken once the fact that AIDS "had reached" Africa was undisputed. The radically different picture of transmission (predominantly heterosexual instead of homosexual) did not allow for a clear picture of a single etiological factor, as it was in place in the early 1980s in the United States. As Bastos pointed out, it took a long time for an African AIDS epidemiology to be defined on its own terms and to establish a system of ecological surveillance "around clusters of roads, traffic, warfare, and other social variables rather than on the basis of individual behavior, as it was in the United States."[156] Beyond the sober scientific approach these maps seem to present, a problematic focus remains on the African continent as a harbor of disease. Where nature-culture barriers collapsed, Africa became the place in which a different kind of AIDS is posited, at once older and closer to an original nature when compared with American AIDS, as well as where newly mutated variants seem to flourish; the place in which poverty, cultural diversity and a lack of enlightenment seemingly disallowed the implementation of Western public health measures. Africa was and is a powerful projection, lodged in the history of colonial medicine, and never fully emancipated from postcolonial angst.

To unpack the larger implications of such visualizations of the African continent, it is worth revisiting a discussion that originated in a *New York Times* feature article in September 1990. Published as part of a series of pieces on AIDS in Africa, the article aimed to visualize the shifting geography of AIDS and to communicate the drastic epidemic in parts of Central and Western Africa. The article emphasized the yet unseen extent and invisible consequences, focusing heavily on the qualitative differences AIDS distribution seemed to maintain on the African continent. Including large-scale portraits of mothers in an unspecified location in Africa, nursing their probably infected children, having left their husbands from whom they became infected, the population at risk in Africa is portrayed as predominantly heterosexual, maternal and infantile. With estimates of the epidemic having already exceeded five million infections throughout Africa, the *New York Times* saw AIDS coming not only into a global focus, but also nesting into the fabrics of the African continent, where poverty, limited infrastructure for public health and slow response from global health institutions made AIDS a fundamentally different disease than in the United States.[157]

In a paper from 1993, Cindy Patton unpacked the implications of the *New York Times'* reporting on the new epidemic of AIDS in Africa, and she drew particular attention to a map that accompanied the 1990 article. Entitled "AIDS in Africa: An Atlas of Spreading Tragedy" the map visualized percentages of sexually active adults across the African continent who were believed to have contracted HIV. While gesturing to uncertainty about the data and its vague estimates in the text of the

---

[156] Bastos, *Global Responses to AIDS*, 57.
[157] Erik Eckholm, "AIDS in Africa: A Killer Rages On," *New York Times*, September 16, 1990.

article, the map elucidated a different picture. The ratio shading suggested a confident statement of high infection rate throughout the continent, only increasing to darker shading in Central and Eastern Africa. The absence of comparative data visualizations for other global regions and the implicit and explicit background of the US epidemic for comparison, painted a picture of a dramatic explosion of "'their AIDS', as heterosexual in comparison with 'our AIDS.'"[158] The invocation of "dangerous traffic" by a picture of trucks and the cartographic detail of "AIDS crossroads" hardly help to unpack the conditions under which the epidemic had become so virulent. The hesitation among the international community to engage preventive policies when early signs of the African epidemic were already reported in 1985 is, for Patton, integral to the dramatic epidemic development. But the map claimed a simplified polemics of distribution – and causation – through prostitution. Attached to the map is a long list of the affected African countries, ordered by estimated severity of their epidemic situation. Subtitled as an "atlas of a tragedy," the map offered a new geography of Africa. National borders, products of colonial control and conflict, become visible through their vulnerability in this new epidemiological order. In this Africa, Patton argues, disease overcomes national boundaries, and "the map of the postcolonial world has now been redrawn as a graph of epidemiologic strike rates."[159]

Frantz Fanon famously described the African continent as an interchangeable vessel with the African body, rendered as a flattened, homogenous and unified surface.[160] Mapping AIDS seemed to have enabled a similar reductive mapping of a dangerous African sexuality. Either labeled as traditional or condemned as destructive (read: prostitution), this sexuality seems to transmit the virus both across the continent and into the familiar fabrics that make up the Western imaginary of a generic African population. The appeal of early Western interventions into the projected "tragedy" of AIDS in Africa culminated in a series of attempts to proliferate the value of the traditional heteronormative and bourgeois family. Bringing together the broken social fabric of postcolonial statehood with a premodern fascination for tribal culture, the picture of AIDS in Africa was inescapably rooted in the continent's colonial past.

---

[158] Cindy Patton, "From Nation to Family: Containing African AIDS," in *The Lesbian and Gay Studies Reader*, ed. Michèle Aina Barale, David M. Halperin, and Henry Abelove (Hove, UK: Psychology Press, 1993), 127–41.
[159] Ibid., 131.
[160] Frantz Fanon, *A Dying Colonialism* (New York: Grove/Atlantic, 1994).

For Paula Treichler, the map from the *New York Times* catalyzed a broader reflection on the changing geography of the epidemic.[161] Carefully unpacking the language differences when speaking of an American or an African AIDS, Treichler noted how affected populations become "devastated" and how infected locations become "infested" once they are located on the African continent. She similarly pointed to the obscure fascination of the West with supposedly "little-known sexual practices" performed across the African continent, which in fact had been subject to a colonial obsession with the supposed exotic nature of the colonial body, leaving little room for the claimed lack of knowledge by epidemiologists. The density of cultural stereotypes about race, gender and class in the projection of the African AIDS is, for Treichler, characteristic of the chronicles of the epidemic: Women are seen as passive vessels; people of color are perceived as dependable; uneducated, illiterate people are considered immune to public health messages and the African population appears as a unified and largely homogenous body – while its cultural, linguistic, political and historical diversity is sidelined. Maps, and in particular maps of AIDS's natural history and continuous distribution in Africa, rarely address such diversity of conditions that contributed to the spread of the disease.

Megan Vaughan reminds us that the perception of diseases on the African continent cannot be disconnected from colonial heritage.[162] The vision of AIDS in Africa is equally entrenched in a tradition of colonial medicine in which the notion of the colonial people as a united community always trumped active engagement with their diversity. This notion of unity exceeded the framework of identity in which AIDS was conceived of in the urban environment of late-twentieth-century America. First, identified as part of the African people – a transliteration of the colonial people – and, second, identified as a member of a tribal culture, a larger community guided by nonmodern principles, AIDS in Africa became a naturalized disease – a disease that had returned to its origin.

The construction of a timeless "African reservoir," a place marked as AIDS's historic origin and its present epidemic is a recurrent theme in the later atlases. Repeated representations of Africa as a region of disease, of zoonotic interferences and risky social practices frame the continent as a place distinct from Europe and the United States, but also from other geographical patterns of distribution. This notion of difference,

---

[161] Paula A. Treichler, "AIDS, Africa, and Cultural Theory," *Transition* no. 51 (1991), 92, doi:10.2307/2935080.

[162] Megan Vaughan, *Curing Their Ills, Colonial Power and African Illness* (Cambridge: Polity Press, 1991).

motivated by colonial and postcolonial heritage as much as by epidemiological and genetic findings, also contributes to further separate the new, global AIDS in Africa from the old American AIDS of the early 1980s. To see AIDS as a pandemic, to invoke a borderless picture of the disease as a global threat, required a clear point of origin, a vast space of distribution and a mélange of conditions that made the history of its development from an origin feasible and graspable.

Geographic Critic

Howard Wainer, among other roles the editor of the English version of Jacque Bertin's *Semiology of Graphics*, also published a book on the graphical communication of uncertainty. The emergence of quantitative methods in the nineteenth century, Wainer wrote, gave rise to a "science of uncertainty," otherwise known as statistics. This science of statistical comparison and mathematical modeling employed graphic displays, and especially maps, to answer vexing questions and to navigate the irreducible uncertainty of human existence.[163] Uncertainty lies also at the heart of the visualizations in the maps discussed in this chapter; as a science of this communication, mapping provides pathways, propositions and visual discussions of possible ways through the open questions of original distribution, zoonotic interference, sexual communities and disease districts. In maps, one could conclude, AIDS is drawn as the bearer of uncertainty, as an epistemic anomaly, which can only be resolved through the mapping of its unique spatial patterns and through the identification of its original geographic origin.

In the epidemic's second decade, maps invoked the notion of AIDS as a global uncertainty. But crucially their purpose was to disprove and resolve outmoded concepts and models of seeing and understanding AIDS. Through mapping, the epidemic was presented first as a national crisis of the United States, then becoming a global pandemic and finally a disease of the southern parts of the African continent. Maps contributed to the problematic vision of AIDS as an exclusively African disease, repeating the colonial stereotype of Africa as a harbor for disease, which as an epidemic had contaminated the rest of the world. Geographical reasoning also applied a critical lens to Western neglect of the spiraling epidemic in Africa.

---

[163] Howard Wainer, *Picturing the Uncertain World: How to Understand, Communicate, and Control Uncertainty through Graphical Display* (Princeton, NJ: Princeton University Press, 2011), 2.

In his thesis from 1992, Paul Farmer described the efforts to find spatial coordinates in which AIDS became a disease of the Haitian village as "geographies of blame." Farmer's early ethnography details how AIDS was integrated into the existing framework of Haiti's reputation for poverty, mystical otherness and tropical climate. Maps, especially those that use vectors and arrows, remind us that the integration of global AIDS transmission routes was worked out in the existing political, economic and social networks and relationships that already crossed the oceans. Seeking causality often turned out to be a polemical rather than a critical engagement with the complexity of AIDS on the grounds. It is fitting that in 1992 Farmer rejects every account of the Haiti epidemic resembling the Pattern II of an African picture. Instead, he argues that the epidemiological picture suggested strongly that the Haitian epidemic was "American."[164]

The geographical accusation that Farmer laid out in the late 1980s in his fieldwork was that if AIDS turned out to be an African AIDS, Haiti would not only be blamed as a crucial landmark in the passage of the disease as it made its way to the United States, it would also present a chance to make the Haitian AIDS part of the invisible epidemic of "elsewhere." The idea of a Haitian AIDS was never just an identification of a transmission route but moreover was also a rejection of the global community that AIDS was on the cusp of forming: The geographical demarcation of an "African AIDS" contributed to a resolution or separation. Maps established a difference between African and American AIDS rather than a continuity. The geographical quest for a global vision of the pandemic and for increasing the visibility of its diverse conditions, AIDS's many different shapes and natures in different areas, contributed to unseeing of what would become the epidemic's locale in the late 1990s.

The work of Didier Fassin allows for a critical revision of how maps and medical geography catalyzed the radical displacement of AIDS to Sub-Saharan Africa. If we return to the beginning of the chapter, where the making of a geographical vision in maps replaced embodied representations of the patient with disease in photography, this same shifting commitment of mapping would prevent the bodies of people with AIDS in the territory of Pattern II to appear in any comparable way. Fassin has detailed how ways of seeing AIDS changed into an abstract visualization of equally abstract numbers mediated through technical and complex

---

[164] Paul Farmer, *AIDS and Accusation: Haiti and the Geography of Blame* (Berkeley: University of California Press, 2006), 177 ff.

visualizations to keep the most obvious problem out of sight: that AIDS in Africa was a global crisis.

Fassin described the effect as "cultural anesthesia": the portrayal of a decisively modern capacity to render the pain of others inadmissible to public discourse. Maps certainly played a part in this, providing the West with abstracted spatial diagrams of the tragedy "elsewhere." Extrapolating from Fassin's study, one could argue that the shaded map of distributed HIV incidence burden per nation and capita conveys an abstract picture of the millions of people who have died of AIDS around the world, but it does not invite further empathic engagement. As Fassin writes, "[W]e feel no need to know more."[165] Having established patterns of difference in which African AIDS was classified as an almost different disease – one of heterosexual transmission, linked to poverty, prostitution and an old and natural history – its contemporary development contributes to an idea of incommensurability between the social worlds in which the epidemic appeared.

A recent study, published in 2012 by Jacques Pepin, brought new significance to what is meant by the geographical origin of AIDS.[166] His combination of phylogenetic models, historical methods and anthropological expertise presents a persuasive account of the history of how AIDS turned into an epidemic, and later a pandemic. His geographical account follows the pattern of separation between the phylogenetic stages of HIV-1. The virus's genetic information is clustered according to homology and discrepancy, so that groups of ribonucleic acid (RNA) are distinguished as M (main), responsible for roughly 99 percent of worldwide cases of AIDS, the group O (outlier), the group N (non-main, non-O) and the group P. Group M has nine subtypes, which are called A-K, with E and I removed, as they turned out to be identical to other subtypes. Infections sometimes occur in combinations of these subtypes, creating so-called Circulant Recombinant Forms (CRF) infections. Each subtype is consistent in its appearance among specific risk groups and often characteristic for particular geographic spaces. The combination of their local appearance and the phylogenetical emergence allowed for a more detailed mapping of the spatial development of AIDS before 1981. Where a specific subtype is the only one found in an area like West Africa, such as CRF02_AG, it can be concluded that infection in that area happened considerably late in the natural development of HIV-1. In the United States and most of Europe, subtype B is responsible for up to 98 percent of the total cases, indicating that a relatively late variant of the

[165] Fassin, *When Bodies Remember: Experiences and Politics of AIDS in South Africa*, xii.
[166] Jacques Pepin, *The Origins of AIDS* (Cambridge: Cambridge University Press, 2011).

virus was carried across the continental divide. As these geographical indicators allow for a vague model of distribution, it would be wrong to assume that the oldest known variant of the virus would indicate the original location of species crossover. What is instead indicative of a phylogenetic index location of origin is the place with the highest divergence of subtypes and groups of HIV: Central Africa.

The highest diversity of HIV-1 subtypes was found in an area where the two Congos, Cameroon, Gabon, the Central African Republic and Equatorial Guinea meet. Not only have all known subtypes of group M been present here, but the data also indicates a higher genetic diversity within these subtypes compared to anywhere else. Pepin's conclusion, supported by many researchers working on the phylogenetic trees of HIV is clear: "HIV-1 must have originated in central Africa, where it has had more time to diversify genetically."[167] This acquired diversity is not only achieved over time, but also through the efficiency of its propagation. But furthermore, the question was how the virus eventually escaped these regions. Pepin narrowed down the list of probable places of the oldest epidemic outbreaks of AIDS, caused by HIV-1, to the two Congos and, more specifically, Kinshasa and Brazzaville.

The next pieces of the puzzle were provided by a series of assumptions about chimpanzees in Central Africa and the closest relative to the human retrovirus, which was agreed to be SIV-cpz. Combining these understandings with clinical observations from a French colonial doctor in the 1930s suggests the presence of a syndrome resembling the appearance of AIDS in Kinshasa already in the 1930s. Furthermore, Pepin used studies and data derived from "molecular clocks" to further date a common ancestor of HIV-1 in 1931, suggesting that a species crossover must have happened in the decade before. Against the backdrop of historic Kinshasa as a town of trans-African labor exchanges and a center for constructing large railway tracks, the point of departure for singular infections to become epidemic were likely be found here. As a colonial legacy, Pepin describes how the practice of mass treatments delivered by injections that were administered in conditions ignorant of sterile guidelines contributed to the proposed original spillover. He concludes that these practices, in place when a wave of mass immunization against what was feared by colonial authorities to be a syphilis outbreak among the sex workers of Kinshasa, seemed to be responsible for the first major event in HIV distribution.[168]

What Pepin brings to the discourse on AIDS's origin is a welcome suggestion that AIDS has indeed several different beginnings. When

---

[167] Ibid., 14.   [168] Ibid., 79 ff.

maps and geographical reasoning are trying to achieve a perfect alignment of the historical and geographical point of a disease's departure, or
the infectious agent responsible, the notion of the many different
moments of origin that are involved in turning a supposed single event
of a simian virus crossing species into a global pandemic with 60 million
infections is lost. Imagining a true origin – and it is worth remembering
that we do not know the true origin of most infectious diseases – seemed
to promise a full understanding of a threat that could then be dismantled.
These thoughts resonate with Nietzsche's notion of the chimera of origin
that is inextricably bound to a desire for a true essence.[169] To identify the
point of origin seems to allow a final view of the epidemic's essence, the
innermost truth of the epidemic. A quest for an epidemic's origin is
nearly always driven by the desire to resolve the epistemic anomaly that
an epidemic almost inescapably is. But Pepin, along with many map
makers and geographic modelers, points to the manifold nature of ori-
gination, in which randomness, arbitrary events and a plethora of biological, social and cultural factors contribute to a genealogy of AIDS,
equally characterized through unstable viral evolution, transnational
travel, zoonotic constellations and companion species. The origin is a
complex story of random mutations, of colonial interventions, tropical
medicine and hygienic failure.

Maps give single pictures of complex and often-contradicting stories.
The map can visualize an origin of AIDS as the collapse of categories
such as nature and culture, society and medicine, biology and anthropology. But maps can equally yield to a highly suggestive interpretation
of AIDS history, suggesting an undisclosed, inaccessible mystified point
of origin from which the epidemic found its way to the non-African
world. The discrepancies between the Gallo model (1986) and the
complex modelings of uncertainty found in the geographic atlas, and
later in Pepin's book, is foundational to a critical understanding of how
AIDS became African and how the territory of the African continent has
become a synonym for the birth and the future of AIDS in the 1990s. But
Pepin's work also shows in all clarity how the quest of defining the origin
of AIDS is increasingly consumed by the unpacking of the innermost
mechanics of HIV.

---

[169] This quality of Nietzsche's perspective onto the concept of origin in the philosophy of
history has been contrasted by Foucault with the concept of genealogy. Where the
notion of the origin inescapably insists on the notion of essence and originality
genealogy offers a history of niches and an ecology of historical development. Michel
Foucault, "Nietzsche, Genealogy, History," in *The Foucault Reader*, ed. Paul Rabinow
(New York: Pantheon Books, 1984), 76–100.

3   Seeing HIV as AIDS

"Face of the Killer." A dramatic caption in the 2007 brochure of *Europrise*, the European Vaccines and Microbicides Enterprise, stands in strange contrast to the almost peaceful impression given by the colorized electron micrograph to which it referred.[1] The brochure announces a "super-network" of scientists, funded by the European Union to defeat the AIDS/HIV epidemic. The picture is credited to Lennart Nilsson, who pioneered visualization of HIV in the mid-1980s. Nilsson's virus portraits traveled the realms of AIDS representation, as they appeared in AIDS journals, countless newspapers, posters and art galleries. The photographer recalled his first encounter with HIV when he was working with Luc Montagnier, credited as the man who discovered the virus at Institut Pasteur in Paris. "And when I pressed the button to take the pictures," Nilsson remembered, "I felt something very unusual, because this was a great killer in the world – and is still a great killer in the world."[2] What is this peculiar effect of looking at the "great killer"? And how did its visualization change the way AIDS was perceived?

To look at HIV is a radically different way of seeing AIDS compared with the photographs and maps discussed previously. Images of HIV reach the viewer through laboratory procedures of electron microscopy. Concepts relating to the virus's mechanisms can be communicated through diagrams that chart functional aspects of virility. Models of the pathogen relay understandings about receptors, binding processes and RNA cores. This virus, the single agent identified as driving the epidemic

[1] The picture was named "Life" by Lennart Nilsson, who became famous for the photographic reproduction of embryos in the 1960s, but who was also crucially involved in the visualization of HIV. This picture in particular has been reproduced for many public as well as scientific publications and is perhaps one of the more iconic pictures of HIV. Perhaps incidentally a commentary on the iconic status of such pictures, the Stockholm agency TT Nyhetsbyrån AB, which maintains the copyright for Nilsson's work, has priced his pictures far beyond the reach of academic publications.
[2] "NOVA Online/Odyssey of Life/Behind the Lens: Interview with Lennart Nilsson," www.pbs.org/wgbh/nova/odyssey/nilsson.html.

and causing those infected to require lifelong pharmaceutical management, can be visualized in a myriad of forms, shapes and models. But every picture is the result of a highly mediated process, whereby the agent's visibility is processed through a cascade of traces, references and representations.

Today, pictures of HIV are everywhere.[3] Newspaper articles on possible scientific breakthroughs, routine reports on the epidemic's status and documentaries on the history and present of AIDS have come to integrate visualizations of the virus as a permanent placeholder for the syndrome, its effects and its devastating history since the mid-1990s.[4] Crossing boundaries between media, scientific publications and artists' expressions, the visualized single entity of HIV has become the most important way of seeing AIDS, leaving photographed patients and mapped social spaces of AIDS as redundancies of the past.

The series of different visualizations of the viral agent will be addressed in this chapter as icons of HIV. In semiology, icons are understood to make immediate sense by bearing physical resemblance to their object of reference, and so the referent finds itself in a likeness to the reference. In the case of HIV, the synecdoche of the icon not only stands in for the viral agent, but also crucially for the epidemic in its entirety. Neither just the symptom as an effect of the virus, nor only the ecological sphere of the condition is implied by the icon of HIV, as with patient photographs and maps. Instead, we believe ourselves to be in the presence of AIDS when we see (an icon of) HIV.

In the visual semiotics of Charles Sander Peirce, icons imply a different mode of representation than symbols or index signs.[5] Where symptoms point to an underlying syndrome in an indexical and causal way (a skin rash as a sign of a herpes virus, for example), symbols refer to their object

---

[3] Most stock image providers and Google now return search requests for AIDS, AIDS/HIV, and, of course, for HIV with images of the virus, either illustrated models or colorized electron micrographs. See, for example, Wellcome Images, National Institute of Health Image Library, Getty Images or Stockphoto and Google Images.

[4] See, for example, a sample of the coverage of the recent turn of events, when British researchers announces that one of their patient's HIV load was undetectable. Most articles were illustrated with pictures of HIV: Fergus Walsh, "Why Talk of a Cure for HIV Is Premature," *BBC News*, October 3, 2016, www.bbc.co.uk/news/health-3754 5953; Haroon Siddique, "Scientists Testing HIV Cure Report 'Remarkable' Progress after Patient Breakthrough," *The Guardian*, October 2, 2016, www.theguardian.com/society/2016/oct/02/scientists-testing-cure-for-hiv-report-progress; "'Critical Milestones' Reached For HIV Vaccine," *International Business Times*, September 9, 2016, www.ibtimes.com/cure-aids-hiv-vaccine-eyed-broadly-neutralizing-antibodies-human-mice-2413719.

[5] Charles Sanders Peirce, *Peirce on Signs: Writings on Semiotic* (Chapel Hill: University of North Carolina Press, 1991), 252.

through a connection of social or cultural convention (such as the red ribbon for World AIDS day). Visual references to the virus can be indexical in the mechanical traces of electron micrographic imaging, and they can be symbolic in functional diagrams of the pathogen's reverse transcriptase ability. But tracing the visual history of HIV through the series of AIDS atlases reveals that pictures of HIV have lost their representational "distance" from the objects they visualize. In losing their indexical and symbolic status, this chapter shows, they have become conflated with their object, and have become canonical icons not only of the virus but also of the epidemic at large.

This chapter argues that the formation of an iconic quality has many causes. Pictures of HIV have been used first and foremost to provide evidence for the existence of the virus. Both electron micrographs and explanatory diagrams, graphs with keys and labels, have been applied to prove HIV as a single viral agency behind AIDS and to unite the scientific community's focus on a microbiological resolution of the epidemic. Embroiled in conspiracy theories and HIV denialism, pictures of HIV have been fundamental in establishing the indisputable materiality of the virus.[6] Yet the icon of HIV did more than just provide visual proof. It offered a chance to move beyond a perception of AIDS mediated by the individual patient body or the abstracted mappings of social spaces affected by viral transmission. Apparently cleansed of social, cultural and political signifiers, the icon of HIV seems to promise a neutral, value-free and emphatically scientific way of seeing the pandemic. Furthermore, sight of a microbiological object, such as the virus, remains the exclusive domain of scientific practices such as imaging technologies and diagrammatic drawings. The virus cannot ever be seen by the naked human eye, nor enhanced through optical lenses, to compare its appearance with its portrait. What is required to reproduce the traces that the virus left behind is a complex scientific apparatus of visualization. Icons of HIV always carry the insignia of complex techno-science with them; seeing HIV implies seeing science in action.

This drastic transformation in the visual configuration of the epidemic – from patient photograph, to map and then to the HIV icon – is exemplified in the atlas series by Donna Mildvan, from 1995. In its inaugural edition, the atlas set out to narrate a radically new story of AIDS, which went on to be refined and extended in three further editions. The series had ambitions to supplant all previous atlas projects and

---

[6] Nicoli Nattrass, *The AIDS Conspiracy: Science Fights Back* (New York: Columbia University Press, 2013); Seth C. Kalichman, *Denying AIDS: Conspiracy Theories, Pseudoscience, and Human Tragedy* (New York: Springer Science, 2009).

provide the twenty-first century with a scientific rather than a clinical or a geographic image of AIDS. With Mildvan's leadership as an infectious disease specialist, the large team of influential advisors, including many of the editors of previous series, steered the atlas to reflect the changing research landscape on the epidemic and adjusted its focus predominantly on the microbiology of the virus. To this end, highly specialized chapters were included that detailed the complicated microbiological outcomes of HIV infection and AIDS outbreak.[7]

A key chapter on virology opens with a collage (Fig. 3.1). In the upper-left corner there is a blurry picture, composed of gray-toned circular shapes, on the brink of merging with a larger mass below. In the upper-right corner is a higher magnification of this image, although it is unclear that anything has come into sharper focus in this close-up or what exactly the viewer is being encouraged to recognize. In stark contrast to the gray shaded picture, the lower part of the page is dominated by a colorful diagram with numerous shapes and descriptions. This simplified graphic holds a loose resemblance to the indistinct picture above it. Both the large mass that fills roughly two-thirds of the page and the smaller round structures entering and exiting or hovering above it can be made out in the graphic as in the electron micrograph. What was vague and unclear in the micrograph has become schematized and certified information in the graphic by a translation of visual information that is not readily transparent to the reader.

As the captions state, both the diagram and the electron micrograph capture the defining moment of an HIV infection in which "the virus can be seen."[8] The electron micrograph shows several viruses, the small spherical structures, budding from an infected human cell. The micrograph has been chosen to show this budding "as it happened," while the graphic delivers an explanation in the form of a functional mask, extracting key elements from the micrograph to schematize the "life cycle" of the virus. According to the simplified graphic, the cycle begins when the virus binds to the human T cell using a CD4+ receptor. On penetrating the cell membrane and entering the cytoplasm, the reverse transcription of RNA into deoxyribonucleic acid (DNA) takes place, followed by integration into the host cell nucleus. The nucleus contains machinery for its own RNA and DNA synthesis, which is hijacked by the virus to become the servant of the virus's requirements to make more RNA, which then in the host cell cytoplasm is packaged into new virions.

[7] Donna Mildvan, ed., *AIDS*. Vol. 1. Atlas of Infectious Diseases (Philadelphia: Current Medicine, 1995).
[8] Ibid., 1:2.7.

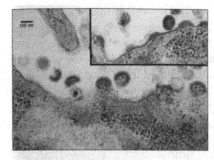

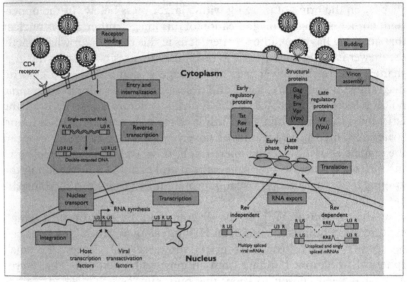

Fig. 3.1 Electron micrograph and diagram of HIV in Mildvan's 1995 atlas. While the micrograph provides a portrait of the morphology of the virus, the diagram unpacks its functionality. The combination of a picture proving the virus's existence with a diagram identifying its infectious agency is key to visualizing HIV as cause.

Source: Donna Mildvan, ed., *AIDS.* Vol. 1. Atlas of Infectious Diseases (Philadelphia: Current Medicine, 1995), 2.7. Permission granted by AAAS and Wolters Kluwer Health.

Many viral clones can now bud from the cell to infect other human cells. The cycle then repeats.

The graphic visualizes the mechanics of HIV infection. It seeks to extract and explain the primal scene, an apprehension that transformed the ways in which AIDS was confronted, understood and visualized.

Thousands of diagrams like this one were produced in the early 1990s to demonstrate newfound levels of understanding HIV's functionality. Crucial to these graphics is the message that HIV treatments can intervene at key points in this cycle. Several processes aggregated in the diagram had been successfully thwarted or at least targeted with pharmaceutical interventions, five of which were combined into HAART.[9]

Instead of engaging with affected bodies and spaces of transmission, the virus combined two cultures of scientifically encoded imagery: the electron micrograph and the microbiological diagram. The tension to be unfolded in this chapter lies within the heritage of these elements. The micrograph was placed in Mildvan's atlas as a successful capture of HIV, the diagram was taken from a textbook to summarize and generalize the electron micrograph's information to explain how HIV infection works and how it could be prohibited. But what is seen and what is known does not usually align so neatly as the atlas's juxtaposition would have us believe.

The electron micrograph from Mildvan's atlas was in fact originally produced in 1983, when it once visualized something quite different from what it was supposed to resemble through the lens of its diagrammatical explanation 12 years later. As this chapter shows, the proximity of visibility and visual functionality on this atlas page hosts a narrative of AIDS history in which the icon of HIV turns "the time of the virus" into the history of the epidemic.

What does it mean to visualize a virus? Pictures – diagrams as well as electron micrographs – do not just reveal a neutral biological entity, captured through cutting-edge laboratory technologies and diagrammatical reasoning. They visualize a disease agent, a thing, consisting of a crystalline protein structure, whose existence is determined by its new identity as the causal agent responsible for the outbreak of diseases as a consequence of a failing immune response. With its causality proven through standardized experimental procedures, HIV is assumed to have done its infectious work silently and in advance of appearances of AIDS on a single body's surface, responsible for the patterns, which went on to be isolated and plotted in disease mappings. As the causative condition behind these appearances, the virus is identified as originally responsible for occurrence of symptoms and spatial patterns. The virus is implicated in the epidemic's ever-increasing emergence and positioned to mark the

---

[9] HAART decreases the patient's total burden of HIV, maintains function of the immune system and prevents opportunistic infections that often lead to death. Its substances attack the RNA reverse transcriptase, the provision of the viral proteins or the final budding stages.

supposed true origin of the epidemic. This origin can be geographical, as we have seen in the previous chapter, but other than maps the picture of the virus brings us to a timeless and spaceless impression of origin.

Reflecting on the strange nature of viruses that exist both as biological entities and originators of social, political and cultural crises, Karen Barad has recently called the commonly implicated causality a "queer creature."[10] Given the limits of our analytical epistemology, the very concept and idea of causality seems never sufficiently approached through the perspective of a natural agent or through the perspective of socially determined factors. Neither the supposedly distilled essence of a disease, embodied through its agent nor the integration of sexuality, race or other social denominators seem to allow a sufficient understanding of causality for epidemic crisis. Neither can be deemed fully responsible for the outcome, which is AIDS.

Icons of HIV, I will show, evade the dichotomy between single agent theories and social denominators, a strict causality and a broad disease ecology. They even escape the strict confines of a representational setting in which the picture refers to a fixed underlying original object. The perspective of visualization enables escape from the well-trodden discourse of origin yet enhances understanding of how the virus and the concept of a causal agent became entangled through their visual configuration in electron micrographs and diagrams. Visibility and functionality become entwined in the icon of the virus. The combination of functional and structural, diagrammatic and electron microscopic images merged seeing and knowing AIDS within a single iconic figuration. Accordingly, photographs of patients and mappings of the AIDS space were undone in their acquired meaning and came to be seen as mere traces of viral activity. Fittingly, one could argue, these icons take center stage in a time when AIDS is increasingly referred to as HIV/AIDS or HIV disease.

In line with the previous chapters, it is tempting to argue that the virus managed to embody AIDS as a microbiological agency. Accordingly, this would mark the crucial point in AIDS history where the perspective shifted from an epidemic of AIDS to the chronic condition of an HIV infection, from the catastrophic first decade to a time of increasing control and successful strategies of containment, from the problematic body of the person with AIDS and the problematic space of AIDS ecology to the artificial, scientific and inherently neutral body of the virus. Departing from the unusual appearances captured through

---

[10] Rick Dolphijn and Iris van der Tuin, eds., *New Materialism: Interviews and Cartographies* (Ann Arbor, MI: Open Humanities Press, 2012), 57.

photographs in their ambiguous appearance to the geographical and biopolitical abstractions of the epidemic's accumulated and calculated effects, the icon of the virus reinstates the full force of exactitude, accuracy and empirical vision. With the visualization of the virus, the very epistemology of scientific knowledge that seemed destabilized by the epidemic in the first place reinstates itself as the pivotal condition through which every facet of the epidemic – in past and present – is to be reckoned with.

As the chapter draws out, the ubiquitous presence of the icon of HIV since the mid-1990s had the effect that past appearances and previous images and imaginations became impressions of the epidemic's archive. In so doing, the complex history of AIDS is also replaced by a narrow and flattened version that seems to evade human influence and social determinism. The virus is not only placed at the beginning of the individual history of each single case of an infection, which would eventually develop into AIDS, but also is effectively placed at the historical origin of the epidemic. The icon of the virus invokes a specific narrative structure of the epidemic's history, a structure that made other histories and their visual archives unseen.

It is important to note that pictures of the virus were present in atlases from Farthing's 1986 first edition onward. As an illustration of Farthing's virology chapter, a blurred electron micrograph was accompanied by a few simplified diagrams, visualizing the probable structure of the virus to explain the way it was assumed to enter and destroy the T cells of its host. Moving from a larger view of the T cell, to an enhanced close-up of the budding of viral particles to a functional diagram and a schematic picture of the viral RNA, the atlas suggests an ever-increasing proximity to the internal mechanics of the epidemic.[11]

In Friedman-Kien's atlas, published first in 1989, again a single virus picture points to the causal agent of the epidemic. The electron micrograph's placement seems incidental, at the margin of a detailed text on the presumed virology of AIDS. The overall composition suggests a certain disregard for the benefits that the visual representation of HIV could deliver to the clinical picture in this atlas, which is dominated by the rationale of clinical photography as discussed in Chapter 1.[12]

But Mildvan's atlas changed this picture drastically from 1995 onward. The virology page that opened this chapter is accompanied by more than a hundred pages of diagrams explaining the binding of HIV to

[11] Charles F. Farthing et al., eds., *A Colour Atlas of AIDS (Acquired Immunodeficiency Syndrome)* (London: Wolfe Medical Publications, 1986), 14.
[12] Alvin E. Friedman-Kien, ed., *Color Atlas of AIDS* (Philadelphia: Saunders, 1989), 129.

CD4-receptors, the "envelope glycoprotein complex" and "loop regions in env and antigenic variations."[13] The following section on immune responses contains a dozen descriptions of HIV, each detailed with a diagram and illustrated occasionally by electron micrographs.[14] After chapters on classification and bodily appearances, the 1995 atlas closes with another chapter on the viral nature of AIDS, using the same diagram discussed previously, but this time layered with possible targets for treatment and pharmaceutical intervention in the life cycle of the virus.

While the second edition does not change the majority of this orchestration of the visual representation of the virus, these pictures become ubiquitous throughout subsequent editions. Almost every chapter is, from the third edition onward, accompanied by one or more diagrams that explain how the virus and its structure contributes to immunology, early symptoms of the infection, how antibodies might relate to virility, how antiretroviral therapies work and even how the exact "site of action of the reserve transcriptase inhibitors" can be understood and visualized before "attractive targets for antiretroviral therapy" are introduced.[15] In the final edition of 2008, the virus has become the dominant icon in and beyond the atlas. Scattered among the arrangement of bodily representations and numerous maps, the virus seems to be everywhere present and everywhere implied. Not only has it become the predominant pathway for seeing AIDS, it also welcomed the overarching presence and importance of scientific methods applied to tackle the epidemic crisis: The virus has become an image in and of the science of AIDS.[16]

This development mirrors the grand historical narrative of how the laboratory and the introduction of bacteriology – and later virology – into medicine supposedly revolutionized how we think about diseases in the twentieth century. Turning several diseases into infectious diseases bound to microbiological entities shifted public health strategies, cultural imaginations and social behavior on large scales. While "magic bullets" remained largely a fantasy of the early days of the bacteriological revolution, the dream of halting an epidemic through microbiologically facilitated deactivation of its causal agents lingered throughout the twentieth century as a rich source of research and funding for disinfectants,

---

[13] Mildvan, *AIDS*, 1:2.7.   [14] Ibid., 1:16.

[15] Gerald L. Mandell and Donna Mildvan, eds., *Atlas of AIDS*, 3rd ed. (Philadelphia: Springer, 2001), 303.

[16] Bernd Hüppauf and Peter Weingart, "Images in and of Science," *Science Images and Popular Images of the Sciences*. Vol. 8, ed. Bernd Hüppauf and Peter Weingart (New York: Routledge, 2008), 3–31.

vaccines and cures.[17] At times successful, as in the case of smallpox, at times humiliating failures, as in the case of malaria eradication, today the single agent has lost most of its "magic" as ecological, vector-based and epigenetic questions have prompted new pathways of reasoning through the complexity of infectious diseases.[18]

In the history of AIDS, pictures of the virus have worked from early on as powerful icons to signal unity and to emphasize evidence supporting the viral entity of AIDS to the wider public. Already in 1985, a remarkable cover of *Time* magazine used one of the earliest visualizations of the virus, simply entitled "AIDS. The Growing Threat – What's being done." The cover page contained a gray visualization of a T Cell with small round particles attached to it, described as a 150,000 times magnified virus, caught in the act of "destroying T cell."[19] This picture of the virus seems already in 1985 to be trusted with the representation of a vague but extensive epidemic threat, the endeavors of bringing the disease under control and demonstrating the unseen mechanisms of how exactly the virus caused immune systems to collapse.

But what does it mean to trust a picture of a virus to represent the full array of social, medical and political aspects that were at that time attributed to the epidemic? Were the motives of the editors at *Time* magazine, with its venerable history of significant and poignant visual representations of pressing social issues, different from those motives in the sciences and in medical practice who sought to visualize the virus? To carry forward a concern of the previous chapters, the question can be updated to ask what kind of disease do virus pictures present and what is the mode of thinking through which such pictures engage with the crisis of AIDS?

In fact, the virus does not embody the epidemic in a comparably intuitive way to the social space in maps or the patient's body in clinical photography. The structure of this book resists a strict triptych of three

---

[17] Allan M. Brandt, *No Magic Bullet: A Social History of Venereal Disease in the United States since 1880* (New York: Oxford University Press, 1987); Andrew Cunningham, "Transforming Plague: The Laboratory and the Identity of Infectious Disease," in *The Laboratory Revolution in Medicine*, ed. Andrew Cunningham and Perry Williams (Cambridge: Cambridge University Press, 1992), 209–44.

[18] Christoph Gradmann, "A Spirit of Scientific Rigour: Koch's Postulates in Twentieth-Century Medicine," *Microbes and Infection* 16, no. 11 (November 2014): 885–92, doi:10.1016/j.micinf.2014.08.012; Mark Honigsbaum, "'Tipping the Balance': Karl Friedrich Meyer, Latent Infections, and the Birth of Modern Ideas of Disease Ecology," *Journal of the History of Biology* 49, no. 2 (2016): 261–309; Michael Kosoy and Roman Kosoy, "Complexity and Biosemiotics in Evolutionary Ecology of Zoonotic Infectious Agents," *Evolutionary Applications*, June 29, 2017, doi:10.1111/eva.12503.

[19] Time Magazine, August 12, 1985, content.time.com/time/covers/0,16641,19850 812,00.html.

equal embodiments and periodization of the epidemic, in part because the virus does not relate to the same genera as the body and the space; it does neither reveal an individual nor a social affection from a disease or an epidemic. The virus's problematization of the epidemic is crucially different from those of affected bodies and ecological conditions, as it erases the individual experience as well as the social realms to enfold a logic of its own onto our perception of the disease. It shifts attention from epidemic to chronicity, from cultural excess to scientific rigor, from external conditions onto inherent structures, and from a disposition onto an AIDS ontology. The ensuing normalization of AIDS is organized and captured in the ever-present icon of HIV, which populated AIDS history since the virus's inception. The icon draws its authority from medical traditions of visualizing disease agents, earns its versatile nature from the particular history of HIV discovery and inherits its cultural pervasiveness from the larger frame of an AIDS history beyond the medical realm.

Tracing the Pathogen

In the years preceding the discovery of HIV from 1981 to 1984, comparisons to the work of Robert Koch were a common occurrence. Richard Krause, Director at the National Institute for Allergies and Infectious Diseases at National Institutes of Health, drew heavily on Koch's work on tuberculosis to bring the attention of the International Congress of Infectious Diseases in Vienna in 1983 to the ambivalences of identifying causal agents. A much-desired breakthrough, it would enable full comprehension of the nature of AIDS and, even more crucially, Krause argued, laboratory-based testing of a patient would enable diagnosis before the disease even appeared. In 1983, the diagnosis along the existing outlined diagnostic manuals relied solely on clinical appearances and thus were often followed by a timely death of the patient "[d]iagnosing AIDS at this stage," he remarked, "is similar to diagnosing tuberculosis when there is open cavitation and the sputum is flooded with the hemorrhage of arterial blood."[20]

But Krause drew on an even more complex version of Koch's postulates, exceeding the often-simplified assumption that finding the virus would necessarily yield to a quick fix. Knowing that the agent would not immediately lead to the end of the developing epidemic, Krause argued that comparisons to the historic case of tuberculosis could be drawn fruitfully because at least the overall shape of the epidemic would change.

---

[20] Richard M. Krause, "Koch's Postulates and the Search for the AIDS Agent," *Public Health Reports* 99, no. 3 (1984): 294.

When Koch looked back on his identification of the tubercle bacillus, the agent that caused tuberculosis, he was well-aware that almost 30 years later, no treatment had been found to attack the bacterium he identified. Despite this, tuberculosis mortality in Prussia had declined, and Koch was convinced this should be attributed to changes in hygiene, diet and the development of treatment routines in the sanatoria. Emphasizing the utility of epidemiological research and a deep understanding of the disease's natural history, Koch retrospectively broadened his own view and conceded that success in lowering mortality rates was not strictly dependent on knowing a disease's bacterial cause. Discovering the agent of AIDS requires an application of Koch's postulates, Krause concluded in his speech, but curtailing the epidemic required a deep appreciation of epidemiology and natural history.[21]

In hindsight, Krause's words entail a story that relates to the historic examples of AIDS and tuberculosis and speaks to the subject at the heart of this chapter. Bacteriology has arguably reorientated the outlook on diseases and epidemics but also drastically changed medical practice, epidemiological research and the conception of public health. What Krause reiterates by alluding to Koch is the puzzling phenomenon that knowing the cause, identifying the agent behind the appearance of symptoms and the impact of infectious diseases on demographic developments, seems to promise an immediate pathway to the disease's resolution, yet rarely has that ever played out in practice, as numerous epidemic histories remind us.[22] Krause's motivation in diluting the enthusiasm of the discovery of the AIDS virus might have been to keep a broader perspective alive, through which to emphasize the enduring need for a variety of public health interventions even beyond the expected successful identification of the virus and to moderate expectations for an immediate resolution of the epidemic.

But invoking Koch's sense for the broader epidemiology of tuberculosis brought another aspect to light that, knowingly or otherwise, drew attention to the utility of identifying an epidemic's necessary cause beyond imminent destruction of the agent. In the years following

---

[21] Ibid., 299.
[22] Owen Whooley, *Knowledge in the Time of Cholera: The Struggle over American Medicine in the Nineteenth Century* (Chicago: University of Chicago Press, 2013); Myron J. Echenberg, *Plague Ports: The Global Urban Impact of Bubonic Plague, 1894–1901* (New York: New York University Press, 2007); Sanjoy Bhattacharya, Mark Harrison, and Michael Worboys, *Fractured States: Smallpox, Public Health and Vaccination Policy in British India 1800–1947* (New Delhi: Orient Longman, 2005); René Dubos and Jean Dubos, *The White Plague: Tuberculosis, Man, and Society*, 3rd ed. (New Brunswick, NJ: Rutgers University Press, 1996).

Krause's call for methodological variety, the discovery, identification and establishment of HIV led to a drastic new way of seeing and understanding AIDS. This would eventually lead to substantial changes in AIDS's local and global treatment, to an unparalleled expansion of research activities and to a successive unseeing of clinical appearances, demographical impacts and social challenges. The visualization of HIV played a profound role in this transformation. The icon of the virus streamlined research processes and presented the spectacular scientific resolution of AIDS to the world. Koch had already acknowledged in 1881 that seeing the bacteria and capturing it through micro-photography had powerful effects, far exceeding immediate results achieved within the laboratory.

The Pathogenic "Photogramm"

Koch's findings in bacteriology were based on visual evidence, and photographs, he argued, were integral to apprehend the "Tuberkelvirus." To be a viable agent it not only needed to be measured *in situ* with a repeatable method for the bacterium to be isolated, it needed to become visible (Fig. 3.2).[23] This process started with concerted filtering of organic material, the specific development of staining the solutions, so that the bacteria would become a visible objects in the contrasts delivered through the lens of a microscope to the emulsions on photographic plates. The visualization was a conditional element in positioning the concept of bacteria at the causal origin of a broader understanding of diseases as well as providing a foundation for the experimental system established to reveal a new origin for *every* specific disease.[24]

In his fascination for photography, Koch did not disregard traditional ways of drawing microscopic findings by hand. Influenced by his friend, the botanist Ferdinand Cohn, Koch published most of his early findings on the bacillus that caused splenic fever (anthrax) through structured analytical drawings. Detailed portrayals of the different shapes and forms of the bacillus were brought together to demonstrate the characteristic shapes, transformations and their functions in the service of illustrating

---

[23] Robert Koch, "Zur Untersuchung von pathogenen Organismen," *Mittheilungen aus dem Kaiserlichen Gesundheitsamte* 1 (1881): 123.

[24] Thomas Schlich, "'Wichtiger als der Gegenstand selbst' – Die Bedeutung des fotografischen Bildes in der Begründung der bakteriologischen Krankheitsauffassung durch Robert Koch," in *Neue Wege in der Seuchengeschichte*, ed. Martin Dinges and Thomas Schlich, Medizin, Gesellschaft und Geschichte (Stuttgart: Franz Steiner Verlag, 1995), 143–52.

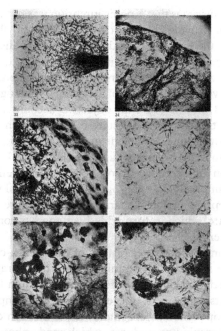

Fig. 3.2 Micro-photographs of the "Tuberkelvirus" in Koch's publication on pathogenic organisms from 1881. Not only did Koch insist on keeping photographs as untouched as possible, he also delivered detailed description of the process for producing the photographic visualizations of the pathogen, so the picture would be seen as a convincing trace of the pathogenic properties of the bacteria. *Source:* Robert Koch, "Zur Untersuchung von pathogenen Organismen," *Mittheilungen aus dem Kaiserlichen Gesundheitsamte* 1 (1881): 112–63 (p. 123). Courtesy of the Wellcome Collection.

and convincing an audience of the etiology of the "Milzbrandkrankheit."[25] But Koch's appreciation of the genre of scholarly guided drawings had certain limitations: "Drawings of microscopic objects are almost never true-to-life (naturgetreu)" he wrote, "their beauty always exceeds the appearance of the original."[26] Much like the clinical doctors confronted with the increasing availability of mechanical objectivity introduced in Chapter 1, Koch grew suspicious of artistic expressions as convincing evidence.

[25] Robert Koch, "Die Ätiologie der Milzbrand-Krankheit, begründet auf die Entwicklungsgeschichte des Bacillus anthracis," *Cohns Beiträge zur Biologie der Pflanzen* 2, no. 2 (1876): 277–310.
[26] Koch, "Zur Untersuchung von pathogenen Organismen," 33 (my translation).

Thomas Schlich argues that Koch's intention was not only to develop a scientific rigor in proving the agency of a bacterium through its functional position in the history of the development of a disease, but also to represent its shape and appearance in a way that would resist any objection.[27] The "convincing proof afforded by photographic illustration"[28] superseded the vague aesthetics of drawings. Photographs, as Koch wrote, succeeded in delivering an objective account of the objects in place, and given the controversial state of the research field invested in understanding pathogenic organisms at that time, Koch considered the "Photogramm" to deliver a true image, free from any intention or unintended deception of a prepared solution to an indefinite amount of observers.[29] Additionally, the photograph's mechanical production integrated the perception of the bacterium as it imprinted itself onto the photographic plate, which in turn added yet another convincing trace of the microscopic entity.

As Tucker pointed out in her history of nineteenth-century scientific photography, the impact of these microscopic photographs and the fact that they traveled quickly across Europe and around the world was immense. Objects, unseen by the eye, often even impossible to track through microscope lenses, were made visible through complicated and fine-tuned photographic procedures, which made photography the very reason for their discovery.[30] But skepticism and outright suspicion not only fell toward drawings but affected photography too. The photographs of bacteria produced and circulated at the end of the nineteenth century often lacked sharpness and contrast, which drawings had delivered beautifully. In catalogs, compendia and atlases of the many different bacteria, illustrations could provide clearly recognizable shapes that distinguish the bacteria from human tissue whether through color or delineation. Tucker draws attention to the rising demand for explanatory diagrams to accompany the blurry pictures deriving from microphotography, so that medical students and teachers alike could begin to make sense of the novel organisms to which the photographs bear witness.[31]

[27] Thomas Schlich, "Repräsentationen von Krankheitserregern. Wie Robert Koch Bakterien als Krankheitsursache dargestellt hat," in *Räume des Wissens – Repräsentation, Codierung, Spur*, ed. Hans-Jörg Rheinberger, Michael Hagner, and Bettina Wahrig-Schmidt (Berlin: De Gruyter, 1997), 171.

[28] Crookshank quoted in: Jennifer Tucker, *Nature Exposed: Photography as Eyewitness in Victorian Science* (Baltimore: Johns Hopkins University Press, 2005), 122.

[29] Koch, "Zur Untersuchung von pathogenen Organismen," 123.

[30] Jennifer Tucker, "Photography as Witness, Detective, and Impostor: Visual Representation in Victorian Science," in *Victorian Science in Context*, ed. Bernard Lightman (Chicago: University of Chicago Press, 1997), 392.

[31] Ibid., 394.

Similarly, Koch used extensive descriptions to elucidate his first set of published photographs in 1881. He explained the meaning of shadows and the different shades of gray. He defined blurry areas as deliberate removals of focus controlled by the microscope to draw attention to the sharper elements of the picture so that the bacteria could more readily be seen. He explained in detail his particular staining technology to assure possible comparisons with the same technology of counterstaining the tubercle bacillus with a brown dye, while the photographs were taken with blue light. Furthermore, he referred to the remaining scratches, blind spots and stains on the photographs as proof of the pure and objective character of the photographs. Any kind of "retouche"[32] would have compromised their capacity of truthfulness. With the rise of photography, drawings were demoted to a subsidiary, explanatory, clarifying function to make seen what the photographs were showing.

Nevertheless, an imagination that the bacterium was visualizing itself using a photographic representation remained a guiding principle for Koch's work. The photograph's need for further explanation was not considered problematic but contributed to the idea of a nature imprinting itself onto the passive surface of the photographic plates, maintaining its transferred requirement for description and analysis.[33] Here, Koch again emphasized the utility of photography as a medium of objective truthfulness. Its vulnerability to blurred lines, weak contrasts and particular frequencies of light forced the researcher to assert tight control in preparing the original and to challenge his own observations carefully through the results he achieved on a photographic plate.[34] The photograph was never just an instrument to distribute the bacteriological concept into the world, like photographs of moulages presented in Chapter 1, but was integral to the experimental setup and an essential indicator of its scientific rigor.

Critics of the new photographic medium opposed Koch's technology for several reasons. Some insisted on the poorly conceived status of mechanical reproductions, pointing to possible future enhancements, while others outright rejected the usefulness of representations that claimed to be true to nature. Drawings, much in the spirit of those that depicted pathological specimens in the nineteenth century, remained for

---

[32] Koch, "Zur Untersuchung von pathogenen Organismen," 152.
[33] Lorraine Daston and Peter Galison, "The Image of Objectivity," *Representations*, no. 40 (1992): 81–128.
[34] Koch, "Zur Untersuchung von pathogenen Organismen," 123.

many the preferred and trusted source with the capability of teaching to see.[35] Photography of bacteriological specimen might have been useful to popularize the very idea of bacteriology or establish the authority of the emerging science, however, it lacked other capabilities. By the end of the nineteenth century, a physician spoke for many when he emphatically argued: "All illustration for the purpose of elucidation should be diagrammatic."[36] The drawing, and its modern successor, the diagram, remained the trusted medium in teaching how to understand, differentiate and place bacteria within the process of developing diseases.

As seen in the atlas page introduced in the preceding text, HIV visualizations routinely rely on the combination of mechanic representation and diagrammatic interpretation, where the one serves as an imprint of the virus activity and the other as an explanatory device. But their combination also elucidates the scientific processes that allow the virus to become visible and to contribute to our understanding of its functionality. But furthermore, this combination was necessary to achieve not only a visualization of a biological artifact, but also to orchestrate the visual presence of a pathogenic organism, the agent behind a disease.

Tucker points to a similar issue in the history of scientific photography. Many agreed on the usefulness of photography to propagate new scientific methods to the general public, but doubts grew around the capacity of the new medium to visualize what was most important about the new scientific methods when applied to medicine. "Photographs of bacteria did not show those things about which scientists and lay people disagreed most by the 1880s and 1890s," Tucker writes, "that is, whether or not, and how, bacteria caused disease."[37] The crucial question of causality, supposedly embodied in the microscopic agent, was not unpacked by the new medium for and in itself.

Koch argued that representing bacteria through photography was not about identifying different biological microscopic objects, but rather arresting a causal agent for diseases such as tuberculosis. Schlich has argued that the photographs produced by Koch need to be understood therefore as a discrete element within an ordered chain of representation.[38] Looked at the chain from its end, the photograph points to a bacteria, which has been made visible in a complex procedure, which was found in a concoction and which has been taken from a body that

[35] Tucker, *Nature Exposed*, 174–5.
[36] William Keiller, "The Craze for Photography in Medical Illustration," *New York Medical Journal* 59 (1894): 789.
[37] Tucker, *Nature Exposed*, 187f.
[38] Schlich, "Repräsentationen von Krankheitserregern."

has presented symptoms of a disease, lending reason for bacteriological analysis in the first place. By layering and condensing functional representations, such as morphological descriptions, or diagrams detailing the procedures of infection with microphotographs of the bacteria, the concept of a microbiological causal agent is processed as both the origin and the result of the embodied experience of a disease. Only if the photograph was embedded within this circular chain of references between a disease and its cause, was it turned into a visualization of an agent and not just a neutral biological specimen. To make the photograph work as a visible trace of the activity it has captured, it is turned into a mere visible trace that needs to be accompanied by precise descriptions and explanatory diagrams, which in turn become part of the reference processed in the photograph.

The question as to how micro-photographic pictures of the causal agent have come to be read, understood and accepted as representations of the disease leads us back to the case of visualizing HIV. How do photographs, such as those produced by Koch as part of creating the new concept of a cause for diseases, as a singular point of departure in a chain of references become an icon empowered to visualize the complex world of a disease? How does the micro-photograph contribute to the transformation of the bacteria from a controversial concept into an epistemic thing whose authority claims to explain and define the disease it causes?

Microbes have captivated the imaginations of many historians of science and medicine. Viruses and bacteria cannot be seen without sophisticated instruments of visualization, and the proof of their existence as veritable objects in the world has always been mediated through complex scientific practices. However, their impact on individual lives, on the social fabric, and on the genealogic trees of evolution is palpable, substantial and undeniable. Among the highly artificial procedures through which unseen enemies became visible was the colorization of cells, the filtering of light spectra, freezing the specimen to prevent their movement and, in the later electron micrographic practices, the staining of organic matter in silver to produce a trace. Latour has referred to these practices as black boxing: They allow us to see but are obscured in the visual product.[39] Once a procedure has yielded the desired results with repeatable steps reliant on agreed-upon concepts, the practices that process the realness of the microscopic entity did not require permanent repetition but would become the accepted condition for this entity to be established

---

[39] Bruno Latour, *Pandora's Hope: Essays on the Reality of Science Studies* (Cambridge, MA: Harvard University Press, 1999).

within the cultures of scientific practice and beyond. The visible trace of a virus signaled the success of a visualization method that at the same time proved the realness of its viral concept. But the laboratory procedures, the technical and conceptual details of the visualization, become invisible as a result of that success. "Paradoxically," Latour argues, "the more science and technology succeed, the more opaque and obscure they become."[40] Pictures are identified with the object they have made visible and conceal the means by which an outsider could argue against their veracity. To align Latour's description with the argument of this book, we can agree that the visualization of HIV almost always rendered the technical, conceptual and practical circumstances of its visualization unseen.

But this process also integrates a notion of time into our perception of agents of disease. Pictures of bacteria and viruses often come into being before the particular agent is fully understood, defined, classified and "black boxed." The 1986 electron micrograph in Farthing's atlas, for example, presents us with the visualization of human T-lymphotropic virus III/lymphadenopathy associated virus (HTLV-III/LAV) – a combination of concepts that would later be unified into HIV. As such, the visual product tends to inhabit a strange position, embodying both the origin and the result of an experimental process. The microbes' excess, breaking through the fabrics of what is known and what is accepted, calls for further research as well as it signals the very success of such endeavors. The electron micrographs used in the 1995 atlas from Mildvan were produced long before the entity they show was agreed and defined. At the time of its production in 1983, it merely showed some unidentified viral particles in the lymph node tissue of a suspected AIDS patient. So how exactly can a visual representation, a mechanically produced trace of an object, exist before the object is defined and understood? It is this operation, the visible invocation of an object before it came fully into existence that contributes to the iconic capacity of pictures of HIV.

At the heart of this iconization, a positivist account might conclude that the object is already "out there," waiting to be discovered, understood and integrated into the ranks of scientific knowledge. Such an arrangement would see the visualization as a capture of nature, which is indifferent as to whether we understand it. But electron micrographs are not accidental snapshots, in which a virus is fortuitously captured. On the contrary, the visualization of a specific viral object begins with a series of

[40] Ibid., 304.

assumptions about the properties and capacities of that object, which inform a lengthy process of calibration, adjustment and correction until the visualization of the object appears as expected. Every electron micrograph carries not only a visual reference of the object it presents, but also remains inextricably attached to a representation of scientific activity and experimental procedures, of which the image is equally a result. But, paradoxically, it is the visualized object that determines how we recognize the circumstances of its visualization to secure its persistence as a natural entity, not primarily crafted through social procedures or cultural conventions but indeed discovered. This visual looping effect, where the virus defines how it was made visible and where the visual representation shapes a perception of how the virus became seen, resonates with what Rheinberger has called the "historiality" of epistemic things.[41] The capacity of a natural entity is not only bound to historic circumstances, but also invokes a history of its own, determining a specific time expressed through the time of the experimental system, set up to find the epistemic object to which it is tuned.[42]

Making the Virus Seen

In a comparable case, Rheinberger has demonstrated this "historiality" in the extensive history of discovering the virus that caused a malignant tumor in chickens at the start of the twentieth century. Encapsulated in the history of searching for the agent responsible for this commonly occurring disease known not to be a bacteria, the question of the emergence or discovery of something new is deeply entangled with the transformation of a very old idea: the virus. The word *virus* had been used historically to denote anything malicious, such as bad air or foul smells, and *virus* became in the late nineteenth century an umbrella term to describe bacteria, fungi and protozoa.[43] The circumstances under which *the virus* was separated from its previous generic meaning to become a unique biological class are puzzling. Viruses were suddenly, as Andre Lwoff in his famous 1957 lecture on the concept of viruses has argued, "deprived of their ancestral right to be called viruses."[44] The virus's

---

[41] Hans-Jörg Rheinberger, *Toward a History of Epistemic Things: Synthesizing Proteins in the Test Tube* (Stanford, CA: Stanford University Press, 1997).

[42] Hans-Jörg Rheinberger, "Difference Machines: Time in Experimental Systems," *Configurations* 23, no. 2 (2015): 165–76, doi:10.1353/con.2015.0013.

[43] Owsei Temkin, *The Double Face of Janus* (Baltimore and London: Johns Hopkins University Press, 1977).

[44] André Lwoff, "The Concept of Virus," *Journal of General Microbiology* 17 (1957): 241.

passage from its etymological Latin origin as poisonous substances to become a type of an infectious agent is not so much of a story of increasingly refined terminology, but bound to the inherently fluctuating process of research on the chicken sarcoma – a story that resembles some of the key characteristics of how HIV came into being.

The cause of the sarcoma was initially defined as a substance that escaped filtering but remained invisible to available microscopic technology. In the early twentieth century, "the virus" first became several things within the setting established to define its nature. In 1910, Peyton Rous tried to isolate the substance responsible for the chicken sarcoma, arguing for a nonbacterial cause and therefore insisting that this disease should be removed from the field of cell pathology. His argument later became embroiled in a controversy about the nature of viruses altogether, ignited by Stanley's discovery of the Tobacco Mosaic Virus.[45] The open question was, whether the particular behavior assumed to characterize the nature of viruses stemmed from a soluble biochemical substance, or from an ultra-microscopic matter foreign to the host's body yet distinct from everything known about parasitic agents to that date.

In the 1920s, this controversy led James Murphy to revive Rous's experiments and to argue that an endogenous substance needed to be responsible for the transmission of the disease from chicken to chicken. Contesting the organic stability of this substance, which underwent a series of stringent purification procedures, Murphy in collaboration with Albert Claude would later argue the possibility of its identity being a "transmissible mutagen, chemical in nature and endogenous in origin."[46] Later on, this mutagen came to be assumed as being another enzyme, defined as a protein and a lipid in 1935. Over the next decade, Claude developed a complex theory of "microsomes," a submicroscopic cancerous agent that derived from ultra-centrifugal fractionating of cytoplasm. This research moved the field of oncology closer to ideas of cytomorphology by suspecting that the causal factor for the chicken sarcoma was due to random cell mutation.

---

[45] Angela N. Creager, *The Life of a Virus: Tobacco Mosaic Virus as an Experimental Model, 1930–1965* (Chicago: University of Chicago Press, 2002); Andrea Sick, "Viren 'bilden.' Visualisierungen des Tabakmosaikvirus (TMV) und anderer infektiöser Agenten," in *Sichtbarkeit und Medium. Austausch, Verknüpfung und Differenz naturwissenschaftlicher und ästhetischer Bildstrategien*, ed. Anja Zimmermann (Hamburg: Hamburg University Press, 2005), 257–87.

[46] Hans-Jörg Rheinberger, "Experimental Systems: Historiality, Narration, and Deconstruction," in *The Science Studies Reader*, ed. Mario Biagioli (New York: Routledge, 1999), 73.

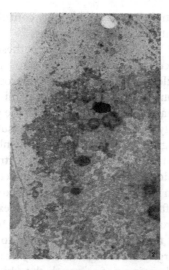

Fig. 3.3 Electron micrograph of the chicken tumor from 1947 that was suspected to be caused by a variety of endogenous and exogenous substances. The experimental system would finally determine that the uncertain cause was a virus, of which this picture became subsequently a portrait.
Source: Albert Claude, Keith R. Porter, and Edward G. Pickels, "Electron Microscope Study of Chicken Tumor Cells," *Cancer Research* 7 (1947): 421–30 (p. 427). Permission granted by AACR.

In the early 1940s, Claude introduced the electron microscope into his ongoing yet unsuccessful research on the agent responsible for chicken sarcoma (Fig. 3.3). As Rasmussen has since convincingly shown, it took enormous translational endeavor to integrate the new technology of visualization that was mostly apt for the physical world to work within the realm of microbiology. The crystalline structure of the virus, "occupying the borderlands between physical and biological phenomena" and invisible to most microscopes, provided an ideal testing ground.[47] Furthermore, throughout the 1940s and 1950s virus research and electron microscopy became mutually dependent, as virus research further integrated the technology, while the refinement of the apparatus was increasingly adjusted to the requirements of its biological application. Rasmussen concludes that "the electron micrograph of a virus was its

---

[47] Nicolas Rasmussen, *Picture Control: The Electron Microscope and the Transformation of Biology in America, 1940–1960* (Stanford, CA: Stanford University Press, 1999), 198.

official, definitive portrait," as the technology contributed predominantly to the identity, integrity and clarity of viruses.[48]

Applying the new technology to his hypothesis of cancer-causing elements within the cell, Claude was unable to prove the existence of any particles that would support his idea of a microsome, an endogenous substance to be responsible for the disease transmission. The absence of endogenous agents made his research return to the possibility of exogenous agents. He finally arrived at a suspicious substance that he had witnessed multiplying in malignant cells. Rheinberger recalls: "The cancer-inducing agent gained identity only as a structure that could be detached from an endogenous component of the cell not known before, the microsome, which in turn had gained identity only in the search for a cancer agent."[49] Shifting between internal and external agents of the cancer, a series of procedures were put in place to identify substance, that never turned out to be what it was assumed to have been.

The point Rheinberger forces us to take away from this parable, points to the visualization changing not so much the object, but transforming the system in which it is integrated as a new way of seeing: "For forty years the experimental system was in a sense oscillating around an 'epistemic thing' that constantly escaped fixation; and by transplanting new methods into the setup – ultracentrifugation, electron microscopy – the system itself constantly shifted its borders." The virus, as it was named in 1947, became the condition for seeing the agent, Rous had tried to identify a few decades earlier, precisely as something that it had not then been. Rheinberger insists we must accept that the agent visualized in the 1940s through some of the very first electron micrographs was not, at that point, what it would later become. The experimental system in which it was procured has produced a whole series of significant material, but with each new layer of traces and representations introduced into the system, the old traces are enlightened as something they had never been.

From the standpoint of medical history, these entities – Koch's bacteria and Rous's virus – share the particular quality that they emerged not only as microscopic or submicroscopic particles, but also as agents at the origin of a chain of causalities leading to the appearance of disease. Throughout the process of their introduction into the textbooks of microbiology and medicine, they became agents by being proven to be present at the origin and thus at the timely and causal derivation of the disease. The appearance of tuberculosis in a patient and the growth of a

---

[48] Ibid., 219; See, e.g., Kurt Herzberg, *Virus-Atlas* (Transmare-Photo, 1951).
[49] Rheinberger, "Experimental Systems," 76.

specific tumor in chickens share with each other and with a series of processes in the research endeavor – biochemical reactions, colored stains – that they are traces of an agent, whose inherent qualities lead to symptoms of diseases as much as it led to visual traces in specialized procedures. The picture of the tubercle bacillus or the chicken sarcoma virus have become traces of a newly emerging concept, introduced into the existing frames of tuberculosis and fowl cancer, while it signifies both the origin of what is visualized, as well as what has led to a disease outbreak. Rheinberger has called these procedures "recurrent": The virus becomes a virus precisely by yielding a number of material traces that process the virus as the recurrent origin of the trace – "It is only the trace that will remain which creates, through its action, the origin of its nonorigin."[50] Visualizing a virus through an electron micrograph does indeed teach us that the historiality inscribed into the picture-as-trace inherits a diagrammatic function, bearing witness to the virus that has caused its own image.

It is this historiality, the dissolution of causal and linear time scales, that makes representations of viruses become icons of the diseases they cause. They can lend to a disease a clear etiological origin, and they produce in a Nietzschean sense a visual "essence" of the disease they originate, as much as they originate their own visual traces. Researchers have put their faith repeatedly in this potency of the image, of the visual representation of the virus that causes AIDS, in accordance with the viral hypothesis of the epidemic's early years. Their reasoning, arguments and proofs implicitly and sometimes explicitly relate to the visual strategies applied by Koch and his descendants in microbiology.

The visualization of HIV was never a project to add yet another element to the larger picture of the epidemic, but rather to fundamentally transform how AIDS was to be perceived by patients, understood by clinicians and interpreted by researchers. Indeed, it provided – much like in the case of tuberculosis – a powerful way to disattach the immune deficiency from social or cultural causes. As with Rous's chicken virus, AIDS was bound to a larger setting of causes, here ranging from internal, lifestyle-related aspects to external factors to be found in various retroviral entities. The picture of AIDS came to be transformed from a lifestyle hypothesis and condition to a viral infection, from an endogenous to exogenous entity and from an inconceivable epidemic of signification to become a topography of traces pointing to a single origin of HIV.

---

[50] Ibid., 69.

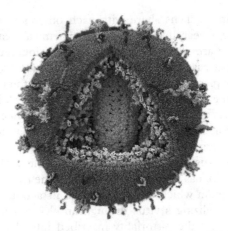

Fig. 3.4 Model of HIV and winner of Science's 2010 visualization
competition. The model resembles the characteristic shape of the virus,
familiar through electron micrographs. Every detail of this visualization
has been modeled based on research hypotheses about the molecular
structure of the virus.
Source: visual-science.com/projects/hiv/illustrations/. Permission granted by
Visual Science.

The AIDS Virus

The annual International Science and Engineering Visualization Challenge – a cooperation of the US National Science Foundation (NSF) and
the journal *Science* – gave its prestigious award in 2010 for the category of
illustration to a model of HIV (Fig. 3.4). The picture, which subsequently appeared on the title page of *Nature*,[51] enjoyed a metaphorically
viral distribution and became the go-to illustration for journals, newspapers, blogs and books concerned with AIDS. Stunning in its design,
aesthetics and implications, it is easy to agree with the committee's
decision to pronounce the picture as the apotheosis of making HIV
visible, graspable and knowable. The picture shows the virus in the shape
of a ball, sliced opened in a segmented manner to allow a sight of its inner
mechanics. The unusual, but all the more convincing, coloration in
shades of orange and gray allow different protein components to be
recognizable. The meticulous design of the numerous elements and
details is informed by extensive research data taken from an impressive

---

[51] *Nature Medicine,* September 8, 2010, Special Issue for the Scientific Strategic Plan of the
Global HIV Vaccine Enterprise.

list of papers, each of them anchored to its corresponding detail in the online interactive model of the virus.[52] This approach to modeling HIV successfully merged evidence-based research on the function of its molecular elements with a visible representation, combining the construction of dense scientific insights with the depiction of an object, whose gestalt seems to derive equally from what we know and what we see.

The design of this model of HIV stands in stark contrast to blurry electron micrographs and simplistic diagrams first published in 1983 and 1984. While the characteristic form and behavior of the virus was a subject of vast speculation in the early 1980s, it has become a widely agreed upon, intensely stylized, intricate figuration by 2010. But this award-winning picture can hardly be approached as just a picture. Applying a prudent typography of visual representation, it would need to be understood as a diagram, as it derives its authority predominantly from discursive rather than from aesthetic orders. It assembles elements of knowledge and data into a scheme. It remains an abstraction in the realm of generic expressions, delivering an archetype of how things are, rather than how things *might* appear.

According to the German *Bildwissenschaftler* Dieter Mersch, visual artifacts like these can be seen as visual references that veil their own diagrammatic nature. Their smooth aesthetic seems to point to a material referent, which in his perspective makes the genre noteworthy. He argues that the transposition of discrete graphical structures into ontological entities is based on a visual switch from a diagrammatic to a mimetic appearance, where a visible and graspable thing is constructed to turn a concept into an epistemic thing.[53] Crowning the history of understanding the etiology of a terrifying epidemic, the virus has in the shape of the award-winning model become an entity whose representation does not need to look like the virus. Its diagrammatic visualization has already achieved an iconic status in which the epidemic in its personal, global, social and political dimensions has been integrated and made unseen. To understand how a model of HIV could have reached this status, I would like to draw on a genealogy that combines the historical formation of bacteria and viruses as outlined previously, with the ways in which seeing HIV has become the ultimate successor to several ways of seeing AIDS.

---

[52] For an interactive digital version see visual-science.com/projects/hiv/illustrations/.
[53] Dieter Mersch, "Visuelle Argumente. Zur Rolle der Bilder in den Naturwissenschaften.," in *Bilder als Diskurse, Bilddiskurse*, ed. Sabine Maasen, Torsten Mayerhauser, and Cornelia Renggli (Weilerswist, Germany: Velbrück, 2006), 111.

In April 1983 and then in May and August 1984, three independent teams published their research on a regularly observed viral activity in patients with AIDS. The teams, led by Françoise Barré-Sinoussi in France and by Robert Gallo and Jay A. Levy in the United States managed to establish three different variants of the virus, they believed was responsible for the immune deficiency. The three articles were by no means the only hypotheses published on the viral etiology.[54] But as they arrived at different conclusions, and as they mark the beginning of a long-standing and often difficult academic and political dispute, they all share a common but at the time unusual feature: Each of their arguments is accompanied by diagrams and electron micrographs of the virus.

The French article, published on May 20, 1983 in *Science*, was the first ever to argue for the possibility of a human retrovirus, and part of the family of HTLV viruses. The team, led by Barré-Sinoussi, had isolated a "t-lymphotropic retrovirus" from the lymph node of a patient. "We report here the isolation of a novel retrovirus from a lymph node of a homosexual patient with multiple lymphadenopathies. The virus appears to be a member of the human T cell leukemia virus (HTLV) family."[55] The accompanying description reveals the story of the patient, a 33-year-old homosexual man who sought medical assistance due to a severe lymphadenopathy. Having been treated for gonorrhea and syphilis, he had a record of STD infections: "During interviews he indicated that he had more than 50 sexual partners per year and had traveled to many countries including North Africa, Greece, and India. His last trip to New York was in 1979."[56] Fitting the epidemiological profile of the time, which was to come under critical scrutiny in subsequent years, the sexual lifestyle of the patient worked here as evidence for the characteristic patterns of an immune deficiency to arrive at a diagnosis of AIDS. The virus was isolated from the patient's tissue, cultivated with the lymph tissue and observed to show signs of continuing reverse transcription, the established microbiological index marker for multiplying retroviruses. The data that was collected and analyzed was then turned into a diagram, framed by an extensive description of their experimental

[54] See, for example, the list of papers Preda has analyzed in his study of medical rhetoric in early AIDS research. Alex Preda, *AIDS, Rhetoric, and Medical Knowledge* (Cambridge: Cambridge University Press, 2005), 156 ff.

[55] F. Barré-Sinoussi et al., "Isolation of a T-Lymphotropic Retrovirus from a Patient at Risk for Acquired Immune Deficiency Syndrome (AIDS)," *Science* 220, no. 4599 (1983): 868.

[56] Ibid.

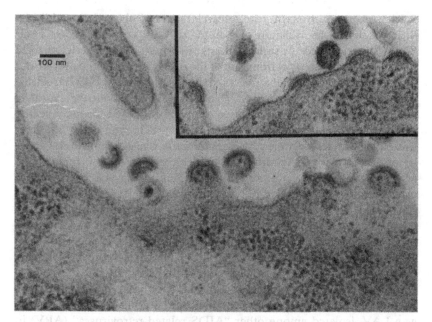

Fig. 3.5 Electron micrograph of HTLV in Barré-Sinoussi's paper from
1983. The micrograph was included to demonstrate the unique shape
of the virus particles budding from a T Cell. In this original outing,
the picture could not show anything but a suspicious virus in a single
patient, who seemed to show the characteristic clinical patterns
of AIDS.
Source: F. Barré-Sinoussi, J. C. Chermann, F. Rey, M. T. Nugeyre et al.,
"Isolation of a T-Lymphotropic Retrovirus from a Patient at Risk for Acquired
Immune Deficiency Syndrome (AIDS)," *Science* 220, no. 4599 (1983), 869.
Permission granted by AAAS.

system and accompanied by an electron micrograph of the infected
umbilical cord lymphocytes, which shows a virus at various stages of
budding from the cell surface (Fig. 3.5). The paper ends with a rather
vague statement: "The role of this virus in the etiology of AIDS remains
to be determined."[57] Based on a single case, the French team did not
make any clear statement on the causal involvement of the virus but
showed the presence of a virus in one patient suspected to show the
characteristic signs of AIDS.

---

[57] Ibid., 870.

In the same *Science* issue, the research team of Robert Gallo published their results on an isolation of a human T cell virus in AIDS. Their findings were based on three patients, in whom HTLV antigens were found, and then the virus from one of the three patients was cultured and examined. The morphology seemed to resemble a type-C retrovirus, distinguishable from other HTLV viruses.[58] Vague about the causative involvement of this particular virus, the team proposed further research with larger representative samples. As in the article from Barré-Sinoussi, this paper was accompanied by diagrammatic visualizations of the activity of the retrovirus (Fig. 3.6) and an electron micrograph. In a second article proposing the same viral candidate, published a year later, another electron micrograph was added to demonstrate the "fairly uniform morphological appearance of HTLV-III."[59] They showed the budding of the virus from a T cell in three different resolutions. Gallo and his team believed they had found a characteristic morphology in the cylindrical shape at the core of the virus, and the paper finally concludes a high probability of a "causative involvement of the virus in AIDS."[60]

Jay A. Levy published his research a year later on August 24, 1984 and in *Science*. A variant of the virus he had been following was framed loosely as a LAV, isolated among other "AIDS related retroviruses" (ARV) in 22 of 45 randomly selected homosexual men from San Francisco.[61] Similar to the two earlier publications, the argument was supported by a diagram of reverse transcriptase and an electron micrograph of the virus particles budding from a T cell. Acknowledging previous research and results from around the world, the authors were convinced about the causal position of their virus in the etiology of AIDS but remained skeptical about the exact identity of the virus and its relations to other known and already-published candidates.

Three different teams had during 16 months published three different and unique research results, stemming from comparable experimental systems and yielding almost similar structures of visually supported

---

[58] R. C. Gallo et al., "Isolation of Human T-Cell Leukemia Virus in Acquired Immune Deficiency Syndrome (AIDS)," *Science* 220, no. 4599 (May 20, 1983): 866, doi:10.1126/science.6601823.

[59] Robert Gallo et al., "Frequent Detection and Isolation of Cytopathic Retroviruses (HTLV-III) from Patients with AIDS and at Risk for AIDS," *Science* 224, no. 4648 (1984): 502.

[60] Ibid., 503.

[61] Jay A. Levy et al., "Isolation of Lymphocytopathic Retroviruses from San Francisco Patients with AIDS," *Science* 225, no. 4664 (1984): 840–2.

Fig. 1. Reverse tran-
scriptase   activity
from lymphocytes es-
tablished in cell cul-
ture from a patient
with pre-AIDS. Via-
ble cell number and
Mg^{2+}-dependent RT
activity were deter-
mined by established
procedures (13). Sym-
bols: O, viable cell
number in 1.5 ml of
growth medium; ●,
RT in 5 μl of fivefold
concentrated condi-
tioned medium sam-
pled at the indicated
time. A sudden verti-
cal drop in the dashed

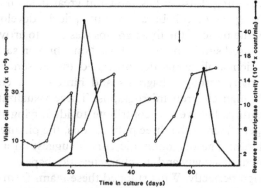

curve indicates the time of subculturing of cells to the indicated cell number. Arrow indicates
the time of addition of rabbit antiserum to α-interferon to a portion of the cultured cells (also see
legend to Table 1).

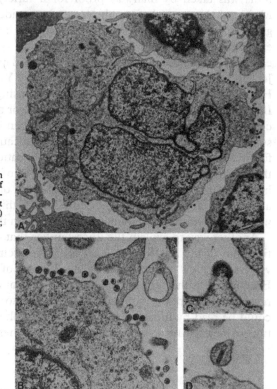

Fig. 2. Transmission
electron micrographs of
fixed, sectioned lym-
phocytes from a patient
with   pre-AIDS.   (A)
×10,000; (B) ×30,000;
(C and D) ×100,000.

Fig. 3.6 An electron micrograph together with a typical diagram to
demonstrate reverse transcriptase activity from Gallo's paper in 1984.
Arranged with the electron micrograph, these diagrams suggested that
the entity visualized in the electron microscope might be a retrovirus.
Source: Robert Gallo, Syed Z. Salahuddin, Mikulas Popovic, Gene M. Shearer
et al., "Frequent Detection and Isolation of Cytopathic Retroviruses (HTLV-III)
from Patients with AIDS and at Risk for AIDS," Science 224, no. 4648 (1984),
501. Permission granted by AAAS.

reasoning. Epstein has shown in great detail how these teams started in the spirit of collaboration, but quickly developed competing models. While none of the three groups was able to arrive at a definitive etiology, all used similar methods. Based on a human sample of male homosexual patients, all teams demonstrated the presence of reverse transcriptase activity through diagrams and hinted at a characteristic morphology through electron micrographs. These visualizations arrested additional features believed to contribute to identifying the precise nature of the agent. Across the three publications, the pictures seem to show the same things: The diagrammatic curves suggest an almost identical measurement of activity and the characteristic shape of the viral particles seems to align perfectly. What stopped these teams from combining their hypotheses and comparing their research results to one common end?

Epstein suggests that the appearance of AIDS through multiple symptoms was taken by many as proof for a variety of underlying causes. Multicausal approaches to the emerging epidemic were quite usual, given that the doctrine of specific etiology had been abandoned by many epidemiologists, who preferred ecological and synergistic models of diseases. In September 1982 community-based physicians, such as Dr. Joseph Sonnabend who worked for the New York City Department of Health, voiced a common concern about focusing on a single viral agent. If this virus was assumed to be carried by one or more minority groups, it could yield tragic political outcomes. Sonnabend insisted that, so far, no sufficient proof had carried further a single cause model. His research found support, which led to a medical publication in May 1983: AIDS, the authors argued, is caused by a variety of causes, reaching from hormonal alterations, malnutrition to the use of opiates and a series of acute viral infections.[62] A single cause model, this article suggested along with others, was not self-evident to everyone in the research community.

Another way to explain the uncertainties that overshadowed the identification of the AIDS virus, derived from circumstances of how retroviruses became an acknowledged element of biological knowledge. Established in the early 1970s, the discovery of an enzyme that enabled reverse transcriptase, copying viral RNA into host cell DNA, which could be read by the host cell, established a blueprint for the reproduction of new viruses. A large team of researchers, among them Robert

[62] J. Sonnabend, S. S. Witkin, and D. T. Purtilo, "Acquired Immunodeficiency Syndrome, Opportunistic Infections, and Malignancies in Male Homosexuals: A Hypothesis of Etiologic Factors in Pathogenesis," *JAMA* 249, no. 17 (1983): 2370–4, doi:10.1001/jama.1983.03330410056028.

Gallo, set out to understand possible connections between these new types of viruses and a series of cancers. Association between AIDS and homosexual lifestyles did not ignite Gallo's curiosity for the emerging epidemic. In his own recollections, his interest was sparked only when a CDC epidemiologist emphasized the reoccurring effect on T cells in cases of AIDS in accordance with theories about a single viral agent. Having worked on HTLV viruses, whose inference with T cells was already proven, Gallo turned his attention to a member of the HTLV virus family being implicated in AIDS. This research led to his publication in *Science*.[63]

In France, a group of immunologists were convinced they could demonstrate a cause other than homosexuality for the occurring epidemic.[64] Together with a leading viral oncologist at the Institut Pasteur, Luc Montagnier, they focused on acute lymphadenopathy, swollen lymph glands, to draw attention to the initial stages of AIDS. They managed to capture viral particles budding on a T cell in the electron micrograph shown in the preceding text. Epstein and others have reported on this turn of events, when Montagnier contacted Gallo with initial findings in 1982.[65] Hoping for collaborative publications in *Science*, Gallo reviewed Barré-Sinoussi's paper and added an abstract, claiming a shared identity between both his and their viruses. Barré-Sinoussi and Montagnier removed Gallo's abstract and later went on to prove their suspicion that the virus they had found did not in fact belong to the HTLV family, as their photographs did not closely resemble the morphology of Gallo's pictures. They went on to call their virus LAV.[66]

The ensuing conflict is history. Both laboratories followed different routes. Montagnier's group seemed to have sent a sample of LAV to Gallo's laboratory for further analysis. Gallo ran into trouble when he was unable to find HTLV in other AIDS patients, and in his 1983 publication in *Science*, he renamed his virus HTLV-III, which in fact, as another researcher proved in 1985, was identical to LAV: "Whether the consequence of accidental contamination of viral cultures – a common problem in virology labs – or of outright theft and misrepresentation, the

---

[63] Robert Gallo, *Virus Hunting: AIDS, Cancer, and the Human Retrovirus* (New York: Basic Books, 1991).

[64] Steven Epstein, *Impure Science: AIDS, Activism, and the Politics of Knowledge* (Berkeley: University of California Press, 1996), 69.

[65] Mirko D. Grmek, *History of AIDS: Emergence and Origin of a Modern Pandemic*, trans. Russell C. Maulitz and Jacalyn Duffin (Princeton, NJ: Princeton University Press, 1993), 47 ff.

[66] Preda, *AIDS, Rhetoric, and Medical Knowledge*, 165 ff.

Pasteur Institute's LAV had found its way into Gallo's cultures. Almost beyond a doubt, Gallo had in fact 'discovered' Montagnier's virus."[67]

The San Francisco–based researcher Levy, whose candidate was the AIDS-associated retrovirus, might have come closest to calling his variant a causal agent. But none of these papers and their underlying research managed to fulfill the benchmarks of proof set out by Robert Koch 100 years earlier. All the information published by 1984 suggested a regular appearance of one or more viruses in people with AIDS. If these were in fact opportunistic infections or causative agents was not proven. The open question was, therefore, to what end did visualizing the viruses help to prove and establish its causative function?

As shown in the case of Koch and tuberculosis, visualization is not a representation. To visualize the cause is an integral element in the chain of events within an experimental process to reveal a disease's cause. If we recall Schlich's interpretation of Koch's procedures, a specific layering of functional and visual representation was required to allow Koch's audience to see not just a microbial object, but also a disease agent. Accordingly, the micrographs printed in the three papers cited were not to be seen as portraits of the virus behind AIDS. At the time of their publication, they were mere traces of viruses more or less regularly observed in patients with the puzzling immune deficiency. The electron micrographs did not attempt to designate a final causative agent. They remained traces of objects emerging through the repetitions of a research process, which was not yet fixed on its outcome: the AIDS virus.

Against this backdrop it seems hardly surprising to find the electron micrograph published in the first AIDS atlas in 1986 with a caption of HTLV-III/LAV. While Charles Farthing referred to the controversy that predated the publication of the atlas, the editor's based their political and scientific decision to use a combination of both viral hypotheses in the eventuality that both isolates were found to be identical just before the atlas went to print. Therefore, they decided to stick with the combination of two acronyms as the unified acronym HIV had not been widely accepted.[68]

It cannot be emphasized enough how puzzling the ensuing picture of the virus is, presented by the atlas in 1986. Embedded within the authority of a medical publication, especially an atlas, this combined nomenclature is unusual. While every virological picture, every model and every piece of information within the atlas points to a single entity, naming it as two draws our attention to the more ambiguous discursive conditions

---

[67] Epstein, *Impure Science*, 74.   [68] Farthing et al., *A Colour Atlas of AIDS* (1986), 10.

of sciences such as microbiology. What shines through here is the fact that naming plays a crucial role in the provision of a unique, coherent and unified signifier, which is in turn necessary to empower a virus to become the performative agent driving an epidemic. Furthermore, the ambiguity expressed in the combination of two virus-concepts sheds light on the difficult historical conditions that allowed HIV to appear in the first place.

The Value of Unification

Treichler, in her later writing on the AIDS virus, reflects on the prevalent usage of a combined acronym in the years leading up to the agreed-upon name of HIV. Departing from Taussig's understanding of a "clinical construction of culture"[69] in which the Western medical system is experienced by its practitioners and patients as inescapably natural, she demonstrates that the AIDS virus was condensed into an ever-increasing reality, emphasizing its overarching usefulness for a variety of scientific, political and social causes. To become the unquestionable agent, citation patterns, research results and publications needed first to find unity. Within this process it was ambiguities such as the double naming that pointed to the "apparatus of production, to the practices through which facts are fabricated."[70] And it is precisely the division between the uncertain entities of HTLV-III and LAV where the virus identity was marked as contentious and where the resulting HIV becomes readable as a "consequence of a dispute rather than its cause."[71]

For a scientific object to be the result of a controversial process is nothing unusual. Nor does it mean the virus's materiality as an epistemic object, as a real agent, was in question. On the contrary, it can be argued that HIV's strength as a causative agent and immensely powerful cultural signifier derived from the virus's capacity to integrate the difficult history of AIDS, while establishing continuity as the structuring agent that drove the epidemic all along. The dispute ended to a large extent when the Subcommittee for Retroviruses from the International Committee on the Taxonomy of Viruses adopted an internationally acceptable name for this group of viruses in 1986. The aim was to unify what circulated under several scientific names, predominantly the compound used in the atlas:

---

[69] Michael Taussig, "Reification and the Consciousness of the Patient," *Social Science and Medicine* 14B, no. 1 (1980): 3–13.

[70] Paula A. Treichler, *How to Have Theory in an Epidemic: Cultural Chronicles of AIDS* (Durham, NC: Duke University Press, 1999), 161.

[71] Bruno Latour and Steve Woolgar, *Laboratory Life: The Social Construction of Scientific Facts* (Princeton, NJ: Princeton University Press, 1979), 167.

HTLV-III/LAV. They also sought to leave behind the colloquial name, favored by the press, of the "AIDS virus." Conforming to a system of nomenclature, the name began with the host species ("human"), contained a word that denoted a major although not its exclusive pathogenic property ("immunodeficiency") and ended with the pathogenic species ("virus"). Following widespread concern of clinicians, the use of AIDS in the naming of the virus was avoided. The paper documenting this bureaucratic decision was published in *Science* as a letter, signed by Levy as well as Barré-Sinoussi and Luc Montagnier, while Gallo and his colleagues declined their support.[72]

Consequently, the second edition of Farthing's atlas in 1988 used the newly agreed upon name for the virus behind the acquired immune deficiency syndrome. Identical pictures, the same layout of zooming into the genetic architecture of the virus, were now framed through a single entity of HIV. The editors wrote that "AIDS is defined as *a disease* indicative of a defect in cell mediated immunity occurring in a person with no known cause for immunodeficiency *other than the presence of HIV.*"[73] The textual account of the nature of the epidemic has aligned with the visual proof. HIV had escaped its conceptual status and could now be successfully identified with the visual traces it had already produced before it came into full existence.

The dermatologically oriented atlas by Friedman-Kien gives a slightly different picture. References to the virus remain rare and decentered in the overall atlas structure. Visual references to HIV can be found, but their placement, contextualization and interpretation make clear that no further knowledge could be gained by close inspection of the virus's morphology, structure and functionality. The focus in Friedman-Kien's edition from 1989 hinged on the epidemic's perception and full comprehension through symptoms on the skin; its contribution to the field and to understanding the disease remained attached to the accumulation, interpretation and cataloging of variations of KS and associated skin conditions (as laid out in Chapter 1). The atlas acknowledges the virus as the evident causal factor but sidelines it to a chapter away from the editor's center of attention. Accordingly, the virus is visually presented through an electron micrographic portrait, which merely illustrated its textual presentation, while any diagrammatic explanations are absent. To take up an argument made by Weingart and Mitchell, the electron micrograph here signifies predominantly the scientific practice carried

---

[72] J. Coffin et al., "Human Immunodeficiency Viruses," *Science* 232 (May 9, 1986): 697.
[73] Farthing et al., *A Colour Atlas of AIDS* (1986).

out to identify and arrest the agent, which remained untreatable at the date of the atlas's publication.[74]

But this picture changed drastically in the second edition of Friedman-Kien's atlas, published in 1996. Dedicated now to HIV-related diseases, the atlas incorporated the virus in its central argument. The chapter on virology, previously located at the end of the first edition, was now moved to the beginning of the series and placed ahead of the chapters with clinically relevant photographs. Seemingly, the clinical photographs have moved into a second order of seeing AIDS, moving behind the viral agent's primacy. The arrangement asked the reader to see the clinical photographs now as an aftermath of the virus, which has been moved to a point of origin within the narrative presented by the atlas. Similarly, the question of clinical diagnostics has a secondary importance, while the virus and its diagnostic capabilities have moved to the fore. Given the continuous absence of diagrammatic explanations or interpretations of the virus, shown in the electron micrographic portrait, the overall structure of the atlas suggests another diagrammatic interpretation. Where the virus chapter lays out the structure, functionality and history of the virus, the following chapters work as visual traces of the virus, rendering KS, herpes or PCP as effects of their common causal origin, HIV.[75]

But what happened after the virus was integrated into the medical canon after 1985, unified in 1986 as HIV, that led to these significant shifts of attention in the epidemic's visual economy? According to the 1996 atlas, it is clearly the unprecedented increase in the "acquisition of knowledge about the molecular foundations and clinical expressions"[76] that set this edition of the atlas apart. Since the virus was established, the research arena for AIDS has greatly expanded. Journals were founded, and a variety of research laboratories as well as big pharmaceutical companies began work on a biomedical solution for the epidemic. Knowing the causal agent, its biomolecular structure and its mechanism led to the mapping of an immediate plan for the virus's destruction. Acknowledged in the example of the geographic atlas from London, the growth of scientific literature on the epidemic increased to roughly 30,000 papers by 1991, and by 1992 a paper on AIDS was published every half hour.[77] For the London atlas, as well as for Friedman-Kien's atlas, this meant a

---

[74] W. J. T. Mitchell, "Image Science," in *Science Images and Popular Images of the Sciences*, ed. Bernd Hueppauf and Peter Weingart (New York: Routledge, 2008), 55–68.
[75] Alvin E. Friedman-Kien and Clay J. Cockerell, eds., *Color Atlas of AIDS* (Philadelphia: W. B. Saunders, 1996).
[76] Ibid., xi.
[77] Matthew Smallman-Raynor, Andrew Cliff, and Peter Haggett, eds., *London International Atlas of AIDS* (Oxford and Cambridge: Blackwell Publishers, 1992), viii.

drastically transformed research landscape. The slow-moving and totalizing format of the atlas became an impossible dream, outpaced by vast
and fast developments in the field, propelled by the unified research
object of HIV. By the time of publication, every atlas was already out
of date.

In 1995, the history of AIDS was marked by the arrival of HAART. To
many, particularly in the history of medicine and science, this symbolized
a turning point in the epidemic, as the infection seemed to become
manageable. The politics directed at AIDS had to change rapidly from
research-based funding to the overarching task of global distribution,
thus laying ground for a new direction in global health.[78] HAART was
based on the successful development of protease inhibitors, the first
designer drug based on a structural and functional analysis of HIV.
Martin Delaney has stressed that the familiar story of a unique discovery,
largely accomplished by a groundbreaking research team, is more complex than often told and should instead be seen as collaborative efforts
between private pharmaceutical researchers, basic science and continuous clinical testing in dozens of institutions. The successful treatment
became available by 1996, which consisted of two NRTIs (nucleoside
reverse-transcriptase inhibitors) and various protease inhibitors.[79] The
impact of this "triple-therapy" was immense, expanding the life span of
those infected with HIV by an average of 13 years at the time of the
treatment's introduction, but through further development longer
latency was achieved by the end of the century. AIDS had been successfully converted, so the story goes, by pharmaceutical intervention into a
chronic disease.

This development set the backdrop for Mildvan's atlas series. The first
edition established a different approach to covering the epidemic. It
focused heavily on analysis, management and treatment of HIV, integrating vast clinical, geographical and even political complexity. Over the
course of the following decade, Mildvan established a picture of AIDS
that did both justice to the rapid development of its surrounding research

---

[78] Allan M. Brandt, "How AIDS Invented Global Health," *New England Journal of
Medicine* 368, no. 23 (June 6, 2013): 2149–52, doi:10.1056/NEJMp1305297.
[79] For an in-depth description of the circumstance under which activists, patient
organizations and the industry collaborated to get the drugs through approval, see
David France, *How to Survive a Plague: The Story of How Activists and Scientists Tamed
AIDS* (London: Pan Macmillan, 2016), 485 ff. Martin Delaney, "History of HAART –
the True Story of How Effective Multi-Drug Therapy Was Developed for Treatment of
HIV Disease," *Retrovirology* 3, no. Suppl 1 (December 21, 2006): S6, doi:10.1186/1742-
4690-3-S1-S6; Steven Epstein, "Activism, Drug Regulation, and the Politics of
Therapeutic Evaluation in the AIDS Era: A Case Study of DdC and the 'Surrogate
Markers' Debate," *Social Studies of Science* 27, no. 5 (1997): 691–726.

landscape while carrying on the unique character of earlier AIDS atlas series. Gerald Mandell, the editor of the series of infectious disease atlases in which this series first appeared, pointed out that the new atlas worked as a "vivid indication" of the "unique and atypical" manifestations seen in HIV patients.[80]

Throughout the series, HIV was visually presented in a recurring arrangement. Electron micrographs were contextualized with countless diagrams, which, according to the steadily growing research field, increased in complexity from edition to edition. The iconographic elements of the diagrams often sought resemblance to the shapes and forms given in the electron micrographic portraits. The virus was plotted in its activity through life-cycle diagrams, visualizing the process of the virus infecting a cell, exploiting the host's replication machinery, transcribing RNA into DNA by reverse transcriptase activity and transforming the nucleus and host ribosomes into a factory for virions, budding out of the cell to infect other cells. The proximity of these diagrams to an electron micrograph invites a reading in which the mechanical picture becomes the momentous close-up of the virus in its deadly activity, which is powerfully visualized in diagrams. Different from Farthing's atlas, where the electron micrograph and its close-up were at the center of a visual argument that sought to demonstrate the virus's existence, Mildvan's series is set up to demonstrate visually *what* we know about the virus.

The shift in the epidemic's visual economy, already evident in Friedman-Kien's second edition, is here developed through a reorganization of the relationship between mechanical reproductions and their diagrammatical counterparts. Both visualizations, as the history of disease agents shows, are necessary elements in the chain of traces that need to be produced to make the agent emerge as the causal origin. The mechanical reproduction serves as evidence for the entity in its morphology, while the diagram brings a functional layer to turn the discrete biological object into the origin of disease. While this holds true, the history of AIDS gives a remarkable example of the extraordinary appeal of electron micrographs even before their diagrammatic counterparts could be conceptualized. Their accumulated traces were later used to construct a linear explanatory narrative necessary to transform every visual representation into a trace, a recurrent effect of a natural agent that had been "out there" all along. The 1983 electron micrograph, unlike photographs and maps of that time, is not of its time. It never gets old.

---

[80] Mandell in: Mildvan, *AIDS*, 1:v.

The Recurrence of the AIDS Virus

In a 2008 issue of *HIV Plus*, another of Lennart Nilsson's early portraits of the virus was printed on a full page. The image, called "HIV Virus on the Surface of a White Blood Cell," had been included in a traveling exhibition that opened in June 2008 at the University of California, Los Angeles's Fowler Museum. The picture is of a large orange amorphous mass with tiny blue dots scattered across its surface that gives a highly stylized and three-dimensional impression of a cell overrun and subsequently destroyed by a myriad of viruses. "The unseen can be scary," Nilsson is quoted saying in the journal, and he continues to explain the purpose of his artful craft: "Images like this one help everyone let go of unfounded fears they have about HIV by allowing them for the first time to visualize what is otherwise invisible and unknown."[81] The portrait of the virus was to Nilsson never just an act of merely visualizing the unseen, but was also one of familiarization with the unseen enemy and the promise of knowing what was previously unknown.

But as Karlheinz Lüdtke wrote in his short history of the early research on viruses, electron micrographs often do not seem especially helpful in establishing the virus as a scientific concept. Lüdtke argued that the blurry pictures and the many complex conditions required to arrive at a sensible image did not withstand criticism and scrutiny. Many researchers in the 1930s and 1940s were skeptical about the new technology's utility in furthering their research, as they thought the images clouded rather than clarified the nature of viruses.[82] Once again, these visualizations did not contribute to particular understanding of how a virus worked, how its attachment to human cells was organized, how it replicated and how it was to be defeated. The beautiful electron micrographs seem to have no further purpose but to prove the existence of a submicroscopic entity and to redirect understanding, perception and the ways of seeing a disease, like AIDS. This applies to all electron micrographs in the AIDS atlases, which point to an out-of-focus object that might be seen as a discrete entity. The pictures did not necessarily contribute to a deeper understanding of what was crucial to audiences, researchers and clinicians: an understanding of how the virus works. So, what do the portraits of the virus do and why do we find them in every atlas of AIDS and, since the mid-1990s, in increasing quantities of popular publications about the epidemic?

---

[81] Nilsson quoted in: *HIV Plus* (Los Angeles: Here Media, 2008), 44.
[82] Karlheinz Lüdtke, *Zur Geschichte der Frühen Virusforschung* (Berlin: Max-Planck-Inst. für Wissenschaftsgeschichte, 1999), 52.

A clue is given in the source of the electron micrograph in Mildvan's atlas (Fig. 3.1). As pointed out in the introduction to this chapter, the picture was first published in the 1983 paper from Barré-Sinoussi and Montangier (Fig. 3.5). Apart from the remarkable fact, that the source of the individual pictures printed in this and other atlases is rarely ever given – a point to be taken up later – the source here is a paper that did not have HIV as its explicit topic. The paper in question was embroiled in the early stages of a difficult research controversy in which the identity of the virus was far from unified. Clearly, the editors of Mildvan's atlas saw the controversy resolved, and followed the global research community that had decided to grant the true origin of HIV to the candidate published by Barré-Sinoussi in 1983, originally named LAV. It makes sense to follow the narrative implied by the atlas and assume that the virus was originally named in error. As tempting as this narrative might be, it relies precisely on the kind of smooth historical emergence of epistemic objects that Rheinberger has objected to in his work. Finding the picture that shows HTLV in 1983 in an AIDS atlas from 1995, where it is used to demonstrate both HIV and the history of its discovery, creates a particularly complex visual formation of the virus's representation that needs to be further unfolded.

First, it is critical to acknowledge that the different names for the virus were also related to a different conceptual framework in which Barré-Sinoussi and her colleagues initially invested their research. Suspecting a qualitative relation between the virus and the manifestation of lymphadenopathy in *one* patient led the team to a particular viral candidate, which crucially had not been proven to have any causative involvement in the development of AIDS. The regular association of this undetermined agent to persons with AIDS suggested a causal involvement, but other publications, in particular the ones from Gallo and colleagues, overshadowed Barré-Sinoussi's paper and deepened skepticism about the validity of the French researcher's results. It is fair to say that in 1983 the virus candidate found by Barré-Sinoussi and Montagnier seemed to be the most unlikely of those proposed in the field.

Second, the atlas from 1995 referred to the electron micrograph as a timeless picture. Its caption is written in present tense, describing the viral particles and its qualities as if the picture were a snapshot, displaying a process that happened in the same way countless of times, regardless of circumstance or context. Within the authoritative capacity of an atlas, the electron micrograph was transformed into a representation of the virus, whose visible appearance, movements and virility were not dependent on the single case of the specific patient at risk of AIDS analyzed by Barré-Sinoussi and her team. The picture is invoked as a rather diagrammatic presentation of the virus as a concept as well as a material object.

Third, the combination of mechanic representation with the illustration in the following text stabilizes this double meaning and establishes a diagrammatic fissure in which both the particular object – the unknown virus of 1983 – and the system of HIV – the virus responsible for every outbreak of AIDS – become one, combined in a single visual argument. Whereas the diagram constitutes the virus beyond its particular materiality, breaking it down to its constitutive elements with each responsible for a specific function that the virus maintains, the electron micrograph grounds the virus in empirical endeavors, as evidence for a virus that has been found, captured and understood.

If we were to approach this picture in isolation, it has little to reveal to an expert eye and even less to teach a lay audience. But the way in which this electron micrograph altered its visual argumentation – or augmentation – between 1983 and 1995 says a great deal about how AIDS came to be seen and unseen. What was useful in 1983 to visualize a mysterious viral agent taken from a particular case that resembled an emerging immune deficiency with an appearance of lymphadenopathy, became a picture representative of the virus causing AIDS. In this very sense, Rheinberger's analysis holds true that the new, at the moment of its appearance, cannot possibly be what it will have been.[83]

The new, Rheinberger reminds us in the case of the chicken tumor agent, is at the moment of its appearance nothing but an irritation. To acknowledge it, make sense of it, frame and name it requires recurrence. Only the knowledge about the product – here HIV – grants access to the conditions of its emergence – here the 1983 paper concerned with LAV. The recurrence of the electron micrograph in 1995 as a picture and a historical trace bore witness to both the original object of HIV and the controversial circumstances of its identification, which never was HIV. This historiality of HIV is empowered through the combination of the electron micrograph with the diagram, presenting the picture as a timeless capture of an ever-repeating natural process. Drawing a line from the 1983 findings to the 1995 established concepts, distorts the picture of history further. It invokes the image of an undistorted past, constituted through a clear teleological line, so that the science of today represented through diagrams – always inescapably anchored to the past – is symbolized through the "snap shot" of the historic virus from 1983. The atlas in this way has become a truly historical work, as it established the acknowledged identity of the virus through the cleansed version of the

[83] Rheinberger, "Experimental Systems."

past of its discovery. To distinguish this history – what "really happened" as presented in the atlas – from the historiality of the recurrence of the virus in its electron micrographic actualizations is crucial to understand the nature of these pictures as traces.

Rheinberger's reading of the concept of traces as developed by Derrida is deeply informative for arguments about the nature of icons of HIV. The trace is not to be understood as a causal outcome of its origin, but as the only access, the exclusive approach to what could be understood as an origin. Pictures such as the electron micrograph are never to be seen as a clearly defined trace – an electron mechanical passive reflection – that maintains a logical relation to its origin or the virus as a presupposed entity.[84] The picture used both in the paper of 1983 and in the atlas from 1995 guarantees the very existence of the origin to which it bears witness. Only because the micrograph exists can we agree upon the natural entity it claims is already there. The picture does even more: If we understand it as one of the means by which the text was written for the paper in 1983 and continuously so as a means by which the atlas chapter was conceptualized and written, we have to integrate the pictures' capacity for excess: "[G]raphic entities ... contain more and other possibilities than those to which they are actually held to be bound."[85] Rheinberger rightly insists. It is here that the electron micrograph turns its origin into a causal agent, emerging in its visibility as it made an epidemic emerge from individuals to reach a global scale.

The Viral Temporality of AIDS

So how does the atlas make AIDS seen, and what is made unseen in this particular configuration of the page on viral reproduction? Given the recurrence of the AIDS virus as a necessary element of its introduction and establishment as HIV, it is in the temporal structure of its traces that the icon of HIV unfolds its signifying potency. This particular present of HIV as visualized in Mildvan's atlas from 1995 is the future of a past that has never happened. It presents itself as the logical repetition of a virus first captured in 1983 but ignores the ambiguous circumstances, the particularities and even the researchers' intentions of the original, to

---

[84] On a discussion of the physical intricacies of electron micrographic imaging and the entanglements between apparatus and phenomenon see Karen Barad, *Meeting the Universe Halfway: Quantum Physics and the Entanglement of Matter and Meaning* (Durham, NC: Duke University Press, 2007).
[85] Rheinberger, "Experimental Systems," 71.

instead invoke a history in which an almost magical telos of rationality
unfolded against all circumstantiality. Orchestrated in this way, the electron micrograph enfolds a history of its own origin that erases its origin by
making it unseen. "The trace is not only the disappearance of the origin,"
writes Derrida, "[it] thus becomes the origin of the origin."[86]

The electron micrograph processes the virus's existence beyond the
unstable experimental system in which it was conceived. The recurrence
of the electron micrograph in 1995 gives the reader insight into a space in
which the virus, independent of epidemic events, theories of causation
and social and cultural determinants of health, always already persisted.
It is here where the visual faculty of the diagram and the electron
micrograph achieve something very different. Beyond just proving the
existence of the virus, the electron micrograph creates a notion of the
virus's activity, placing it among many causal outcomes identified in
the origin of the virus. The diagram relies on this temporality established
through the micrograph as trace, so that it can successfully achieve the
visualization of the properties of a virus and not just of a related concept
or mere theory.

The temporality this visual configuration achieves could be called an
evolutionary or natural time of the epidemic. This is a time in which the
phylogenesis of HIV and the circumstantial point of its discovery become
key elements of an epidemic seen through the emergence of its agent.
Calling AIDS an emerging epidemic, phrasing its appearance in a world
that assumed itself in an age beyond infectious diseases, firmly attaches it
thoroughly to the agency of the agent as its own origin. Contrary to the
visualization of persons with AIDS or the mapping of spaces that show
AIDS, the icon of the virus shifts the conditions of how AIDS came into
our world, integrating the epidemic into the other, foreign world of the
virus and its capacity to make an epidemic emerge. The notion of
emergence, in other words, naturalizes the narrative of how AIDS came
into being. It shifts its origin as well as its driving forces into an effect of
what a virus has done. Yet, this very virus in its emergence can only be
perceived through its graphematical traces, its numerous recurrences,
which can be electron micrographs, but its traces might as well be maps
of its distribution and symptoms captured in a clinical photograph.

Turning these images of an emerging epidemic into an icon of the
"AIDS virus" depends on the diagrammatical framing of the atlas. In
editions following the first publication by Mildvan, this framing becomes
the key instrument to make sense of the virus. Crucially, the editors add

---

[86] Jacques Derrida, *Of Grammatology* (Baltimore: Johns Hopkins University Press,
1998), 61.

more than just an analysis of the virus's structure and phylogenetic genealogy. Diagrams point to possible points of attack in the life cycle of the virus, transforming in-depth analysis into a plan of action to enact against the agent of the epidemic. Chapters on therapeutic strategies were added, diagrams of the functionality of protease inhibitors and other medications were included and the overall vision of a manageable virus was refined from edition to edition.[87]

Pictures of the virus become attached to strategies of containment, to mechanisms of treatment, to visions of the inner life of the epidemic, to the driving forces of its emergence and the virus was claimed as the causal origin of symptoms, devastating deaths, social disruptions and political crisis. These pictures have become iconic, precisely because they replace and diminish other historical, social and political accounts of the epidemic from the mid-1990s. Unlike the photographs of patients, the maps of spaces, which enfold references to conditions, circumstances and contexts implicated and affected by the epidemic, the icon of the virus seems to show nothing but itself. In its entangled state between graphematical and diagrammatical forms, it claims to show everything that drove the epidemic in the past, that is characteristic of it in the present and that will lead to its resolution in the future. In this way, the picture of HIV makes AIDS in its endless facets and countless dimensions unseen, leaving it as a cleansed, unified and inherently normalized object of knowledge.

Canguilhem concluded his thesis on the normal and pathological with a thought about crafting norms: "To set a norm (normer), to normalize, is to impose a requirement on an existence, a given whose variety, disparity, with regard to the requirement, present themselves as hostile, even more than an unknown, indeterminate."[88] Iconization achieves precisely this result. An icon of HIV did not just replace an existing way of seeing, a previously working visual representation, but claimed a position within the visual economy of AIDS in which all other visualizations became necessarily secondary traces of this original trace of the actual agent, the virus. The hostile indeterminate in Canguilhem's argument is here the broad history of AIDS as presented through the photographic portraits of a lifestyle hypothesis, through maps of the epidemic's social dimension and historical narratives and, in short, through every

---

[87] The chapter is tentatively called "Treatment and Prophylaxis of Opportunistic Infections in the Era of Highly Active Antiretroviral Therapy." Mandell and Mildvan, *Atlas of AIDS*, 213 ff.

[88] Georges Canguilhem, *On the Normal and the Pathological* (Dordrecht, the Netherlands: Reidel, 1978), 239.

element that has been visually foregrounded in the spirit of testing, evaluating and understanding its causal involvement in the epidemic. The icon of the virus removed these disparities, cutting the historical variety of the epidemic and crafting a streamlined linear history to make traces of social practices and cultural denominators unseen. AIDS through the lens of HIV has been turned from epidemic to disease, from affliction to infection and from disposition to HIV-as-AIDS, or as we tend to say today: HIV/AIDS.

The Past of HIV

You have this gaping mouth that almost looks like it's ready to eat you the way AIDS is eating away at society.[89]

Tom Wagner, member of the panel judging the winning picture of the 2010 challenge (Fig. 3.4), demonstrates here that the criteria for awarding the prize exceeded questions of scientific accuracy, modeling skill or visualization methods. Traces of the virus's impact and the disastrous effects of the epidemic seem to shine through the rigorous technical modeling of this HIV icon. At first sight, affect contradicts the idea of a cleansed gaze onto the history of AIDS as a microbiological tale of emergence in which the icon of HIV stands for science's triumph over the epidemic. However timeless and abstract this particular model of HIV might appear, it seems incapable of escaping the traces of the painful and traumatic epidemic. Indeed, it might even have won the favor of the jury as a result of its intimacy with the haunting pasts of AIDS.

To approach the past of HIV, it is not enough to focus on its phylo-genetic or geographic history (see Chapter 2), but rather requires raising the question about what kind of AIDS commemoration is preserved in the icon of HIV. Is this a history of scientific breakthrough that overcame challenges in the field? Is this a streamlined history that turned every aspect of the epidemic's past into traces of the teleological object that HIV turned out to be and, in so doing, declaring every other way of seeing and knowing AIDS mere errors of history? Or does HIV present us with a story of AIDS in which the beginning, middle and end of the epidemic become feasible elements of a straight narrative, preferable to the chaotic "epidemic of signification" suggested by Treichler in 1986?

---

[89] Tom Wagner, panel of judge member of the "International Science and Engineering Visualization Challenge 2010" about the winning HIV-Modell, see www.nsf.gov/news/news_images.jsp?cntn_id=118720&org=NSF.

The particular version of AIDS history proposed by the icon of HIV is attractive for many reasons. Seeing AIDS as the result of a clear causal agent served various agendas. First, it gave to researchers and scientists a unifying object, through which to focus research resources and the scientific community's efforts, leading to a tangible resolution for the AIDS crisis. Second, it represented a scientific understanding of an epidemic that had up until then been perceived through individual suffering, risk groups and stereotyped sexualities. Third, for the first time the icon of HIV allowed a visual grasp of AIDS in a coherent qualitative difference to social spaces and individual patients, revealing a unique figuration of the epidemic that was previously unseen. Reaching far beyond a community of researchers, HIV was, as Epstein puts it, "not simply a scientific powerhouse. It was also – crucially – a social phenomenon."[90] Precisely because it proved useful for campaigners as much as researchers, patients as well as politicians, HIV as icon won the encapsulating status it continues to enjoy today.

But first and foremost, the icon of HIV always doubled as an icon of scientific knowledge. As far as a medical and scientific history of AIDS remains separate from the social and cultural history of AIDS, this dichotomy has been a guiding principle for those experiencing the epidemic in "the trenches."[91] In her study, "AIDS and the Body Politic," Catherine Waldby accordingly focuses on the biopolitical violence implicated in the scientific research on AIDS. Her account frames the early 1990s as a time of scientific takeover in which war on the epidemic was turned into a war against the virus. Visual representations were understood to be a crucial condition for this, as it "is science's capacity to visualize the virus at the molecular and cellular level which secures its claim to wage war at the appropriate level of scale."[92] Turning AIDS into a scientific problem to tackle in the laboratory was often felt as a neglect of the devastating situation on the ground. Waldby's conclusion, after discussing the scientification of AIDS on various scales, is that she has come to see "AIDS as a symptom, not of the activity of a virus, but of a particular moment in the history of sexual politics."[93] Contradicting the icon's supposed capacity to include the epidemic's many histories,

---

[90] Epstein, *Impure Science*, 92.
[91] Vito Russo, speech, see: www.actupny.org/documents/whfight.html.
[92] Catherine Waldby, *AIDS and the Body Politic: Biomedicine and Sexual Difference* (London: Routledge, 1996), 2.
[93] Ibid., 130.

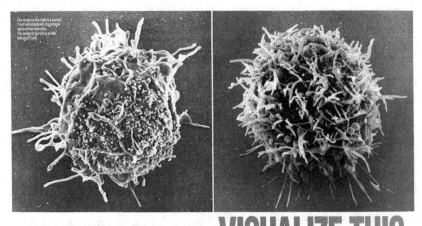

Fig. 3.7 Poster by Nancy Burson and Kunio Nagashima called
Visualize This from 1991. The artist's collaboration with a
microbiologist led to a diptych of a healthy and an infected T cell,
addressing the pervasive power of scientific visualizations and calling
for the visual identification of the actual enemy, the original disease.
Courtesy of the artist, Nancy Burson.

Waldby explicitly distances her account from the simplified narrative
suggested by the virus.

Nancy Burson, an acclaimed visual artist, took a different route on the
scientification of AIDS and produced a collaborative project entitled
"Visualize This" (Fig. 3.7) with Creative Time in 1991. The microbiologist Kunio Nagashima collaborated with Burson to bring together two
electron micrographs on a poster, one presenting an infected and one a
normal T cell. The artist's call for the visualization of complex microscopic representations, hence the caption *Visualize This,* is intriguing.
Partly an indication of resistance against other modes of representation
such as photography that were considered harmful and incorrect, she
also seeks to engage artistically with the black-boxed world of science
visualizations. Furthermore, her ambiguous positioning of the imperative
to visualize underneath the picture of the healthy T cell, along with the
order of the two pictures from left to right suggest a plea to engage with
the ways in which the virus was to be challenged, overcome and besieged.
This juxtaposition argues emphatically for a replacement of false representations of AIDS patients with the image of the epidemic in its medical abstractions, through the utilization of the transformative power of

scientific visualization.[94] *General Idea*'s emblematic "imagevirus," an adaptation of Robert Indiana's *LOVE*, by exchanging those four letters with AIDS, can be read as one of the many metaphoric appropriations of the virus circulating in the early 1990s.[95]

Reflections of HIV cannot possibly be exclusively contained within a scientific or medical history of the epidemic. AIDS has changed the ways in which epidemics and their driving factors are appreciated and communicated within society. Several years before HIV became the agreed-upon icon of the AIDS epidemic, Charles Rosenberg had already noted the epistemological shifts AIDS had imposed on thought in the social sciences and humanities. Perspectives of social construction were not sufficient for thinking through and acting upon the deadly epidemic. "The biomedical aspects of AIDS can hardly be ignored," he writes. "[I]t is difficult to ignore a disease with a fatality rate approaching 100 percent." This emphasizes that interpretations of AIDS as a mere social product were unacceptable, insensitive and dangerous in the eyes of activists. "AIDS has, in fact, helped create a new consensus in regard to disease," Rosenberg continues, "one that finds a place for both biological and social factors and emphasizes their interaction."[96]

Continuing where Rosenberg left off, Treichler has given a brilliant account of the versatile nature of the icon of HIV in her essay on "AIDS, HIV, and the Cultural Construction of Reality." Confronted with a towering model of HIV at the 1989 AIDS conference in Montreal, she presents her reader with a detailed analysis of how the virus and its icons have been players in the story of the epidemic. She explains to what end this history provides further insight into understanding AIDS, and how this history holds particular lessons for any rejection of simplified social constructionism, as well as the shortcomings of a cultural analysis that does not appreciate the many cultures of science.

A scientific culture, Treichler argues, is what contributed to the reality of the virus and what "most effectively disguises its existence as a cultural construction."[97] The shifting literature on the sociology and history of scientific facts, spanning from Fleck, Kuhn, Knorr-Cetina, to Latour and Woolgar, to Haraway and beyond, has offered many ways to give justice both to the static and the dynamic nature of scientific knowledge, to accommodate both the fabrication of facts and of facts being the opposite

---

[94] Sophie Junge, *Art about AIDS, Nan Goldin's Exhibition Witnesses: Against Our Vanishing* (Berlin: De Gruyter, 2016), 98, doi:10.1515/9783110453072.
[95] Gregg Bordowitz, *Imagevirus: General Idea* (London: Afterall Books, 2010).
[96] Charles E. Rosenberg, "Disease and Social Order in America: Perceptions and Expectations," *The Milbank Quarterly* 64, no. 1 (1986): 34–55.
[97] Treichler, *How to Have Theory in an Epidemic: Cultural Chronicles of AIDS*, 172.

of fabrication. Both the collapse of *"the AIDS virus* and *the cause of AIDS,"* HIV was installed as an interchangeable entity in the epidemic, as well as its cause. As a viral agent, HIV exhibited its singular significance for reordering AIDS discourse as the result of "merged" and "muddled" realities.[98] The arguments about the virus have been silenced to leave us with a taken-for-granted reality and a lived experience for researchers and people with AIDS. HIV has turned into a powerful and important weapon to attack false assumptions and current politics.

Furthermore, the virus seemed to embody the nature of the epidemic in an inert, almost radically artificial way. Epstein identified its appeal by noting that while "talk about lifestyle had seemed to lay the groundwork for victim blaming in the larger society, the viral hypothesis had more neutral moral implications."[99] It guaranteed public health campaigns, gay safer-sex proponents, policy makers and patients a valuable and morally incontestable notion of a cause, precisely because it represented a natural object, washed of cultural assumptions and social constraints. "Both fabrication and fact," Treichler concludes, "HIV has become, in short, a reality that is too costly to give up."[100] This reality is secured, I argue, through the two visual operations – electron microscopy and graphic diagram – that make up the pervasive icon of HIV.

These two visual operations, the diagrammatic simplification and the electron micrograph of the virus, reach the level of iconicity precisely by resisting a mediated mode of representation. Instead of presenting an object, a symptom or a cluster of streets and spaces, this pair of pictures point to an entity that cannot be seen with the naked eye and that can only become real through its familiar traces. The infection of HIV, yielding to the onset of AIDS, skin lesions of KS, characteristic patterns of distribution in space as well as micrographs and diagrams all become traces of the viral entity that causes AIDS *and* its own traces. The icon of the virus thus inherits a likeness to the virus that does not rely on regimes of representation implied by patient photography or geographical mapping. The icon shatters any idea of representing AIDS in a clear and comprehensible system of signification, but rather brings about a sense of the syndrome.

Rheinberger has argued in a recent paper that such reference systems between structural and functional traces should not be valued along the lines of their representational qualities. The purpose of oscillating reference systems, in which diagrams and electron micrographs rely on each

[98] Ibid., 169.   [99] Epstein, *Impure Science*, 93.

[100] Treichler, *How to Have Theory in an Epidemic: Cultural Chronicles of AIDS*, 173.

other rather than on an external entity is simply to make sense.[101] Their
epistemic usefulness derives not from their ability to represent a natural
entity but from their capacity to reveal a coherent object that aligns with
the system in which it is found. Diagrammatical configurations of data,
on the one hand, and structural models, on the other, need to be aligned
to process a stable entity that is considered useful with regard to its
function, rather than its shape, structure and visibility.

Over the years, the AIDS atlas has shaped an icon of HIV that folds its
visuality into a reference for its function. Every picture in the atlas has
become a recurrent trace of HIV, which proves its own function as bearer
of traces. The status of a picture as a revelation of the agent was a key role
granted to both diagrams and electron micrographs that sought to reveal
the virus as a neutral, inevitable causative entity. Exhibiting variations in
quality, origin and framing throughout the atlas editions and series, a
single, centrally important aspect of the icon remained unchanged, which
set this genre of visualization apart from all others. In each and every
atlas, the virus has been captured in just one electron micrograph. There
are not series of these images, as there are grids of photographs showing
one AIDS-related symptom from a variety of perspectives. Nor is the
micrograph displayed like a developing series of maps that track growth
distributions and mobility of the epidemic. From this status of singularity, the electron micrograph is not included in the atlas to reveal *information* about the shape or structure of the virus. It is not a telling portrait.
It does not contribute to a deeper understanding of the molecular configuration of the virus. The blurred gray shapes of these electron micrographs do not aid understanding of the clinical appearance of AIDS; they
do not contribute to greater insight about how AIDS affected social
groups; they do not enhance knowledge regarding how the virus buds
from T cells. The sole purpose of the electron micrograph within the
fabric of the atlas is to anchor the virus as leading protagonist in the
historical, biological and visual order of the epidemic. In other words,
the iconicity of the virus as established cause is achieved precisely at the
point at which every other visual reference to the epidemic becomes a
trace of the recurrence of the virus.

Diagrams, unlike electron micrographs, contributed to a practical
understanding of the virus. They appear in large variety to demonstrate
the workings of HIV as a human retrovirus, revealing its functionality,
components, life cycle and intimate relation to host cells. Where the

[101] Hans-Jörg Rheinberger, "Preparations, Models, and Simulations," *History and Philosophy of the Life Sciences* 36, no. 3 (January 2015): 321–34, doi:10.1007/s40656-014-
0049-3.

electron micrograph established HIV as the object of interest, the diagrams translated the virus's presence into a system of relations and emphasized its processual nature. Working like blueprints of the virus, diagrams toggle between HIV as an object in nature and a result of practices of fabrication, outlining the characteristics of an epistemic object carved out in the laboratories of HIV research.

If we return to the page in Mildvan's atlas from the start of the chapter (Fig. 3.1), a key element is the iconic resemblance between diagram and electron micrograph. Here, the second-order feedback between the two visual operations is crucial to visualize function rather than just an object. The timeless caption of a virus from 1983, the life cycle diagram from a 1995 textbook and the reproduction of both in edition after edition of the atlas contribute to an impression of a reference to HIV that constantly references itself. The singularity of the electron micrograph, on the one hand, and the endless multiplicity of diagrams, on the other, refer to a system of reference in which the model resides in the oscillation between configured data and mechanical trace. "Here we are less concerned with how a referent relates to its reference, where in the end one asks for its *meaning*," argues Rheinberger on such models, "but rather with the relationship between different referents, where something ... makes, or does not make, *sense*."[102] We tend to forget that this is the virus picture's most obvious position in the fabric of the AIDS atlas: to present a concept, a model and a referent that makes sense as a causal agent of the epidemic.

In dialog with Canguilhem, Rheinberger reminds us that such models present nothing but a function. But within the realm of the atlas, pictures of HIV become readable beyond their functional position. In the atlas, a value of representation is ascribed and the virus visualization is installed as a canonical.[103] When models cease to be a productive element of an experimental system they become iconic, representing not a particular object but the whole reference system that has allowed them to make sense in the first place. When a diagram becomes iconic it "takes on the characteristics of an object in the world," claims Anthony Vidler.[104] The icon of HIV is both a diagram and an electron micrograph, both fabrication and fact, both a structural and a functional model, which encompasses the history, the present and the future of the epidemic. It takes its significance and its iconic capacity from the many operations that stabilized the virus at the origin of the pandemic, and it has become the single

---

[102] Ibid., 328.   [103] Ibid., 330.
[104] Anthony Vidler, "Diagrams of Diagrams: Architectural Abstraction and Modern Representation," *Representations*, no. 72 (2000): 17, doi:10.2307/2902906.

most exclusive vantage point that makes sense not only in reference to other references, but also to make sense of the epidemic.

Nowhere has this been brought to closer visual cohesion than in the prize-winning model from 2010 (Fig. 3.4). The diagram has been transformed into a visual object, an iconic body of the virus in which the calculations, fabrications and algorithmic models arrived at a graspable figuration of the virus. What is known about its functionality became what is seen. A graspable body has been made visible that aligns the image taken from electron micrographs with knowledge produced by an enormous research enterprise. HIV has been fully understood, the icon tells us, and the gap between seeing and knowing has been closed. This is the end of the history of AIDS.

Epilogue: The End of the AIDS Crisis?

The term "para-epidemic" has been used to describe society's response to AIDS as a new infectious disease, emerging without history or precedent and spreading to create a worldwide pandemic. ... Because the events and ramifications of the para-epidemic have had singular influence on the advances made for this disease, they represent an integral component for the history of AIDS. For this reason, the fourth edition now includes a new chapter, "Social Repercussions of an Epidemic."[1]

Donna Mildvan, the editor of the last AIDS atlas, emphasized in her 2008 preface that the success in resolving the AIDS crisis was not due to biomedical progress alone. Her atlas's final chapter integrates an unusual perspective into this predominantly medical publication with its highly specialized sections on the sciences of virology, genetics and the mechanics of HAART. In the concluding segment the reader all of a sudden encounters artistic photographs entitled "Fear and Uncertainty," reproductions of public health campaign posters from 1983 and 1984 that appeal against the stigmatization of children and against attempts to exclude people with AIDS from workplaces.[2] The next subsection in this final chapter is on "Loss and Bereavement," which assembles pictures of a candlelight vigil from 1983 in New York's Central Park, honoring the memories of lost friends and partners next to an aerial view of the "AIDS Quilt," which between 1987 and 2000 stitched together the names and memories of almost 20 percent of people who have died from AIDS in the United States. Below that, on the same page, we find a photograph of a funeral of a mother of four children somewhere in Sub-Saharan Africa, the caption tells us, bringing attention to the epidemic of orphanage in the shadow of AIDS.[3] Another page details "Social Disobedience," remembering the protests at the CDC in Atlanta in 1990, an undated

---

[1] Donna Mildvan, ed., *International Atlas of AIDS*, 4th ed. (Philadelphia: Springer, 2008), v.

[2] Ibid., 349 f.   [3] Mildvan, *International Atlas of AIDS*.

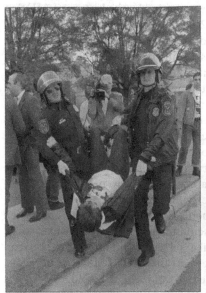

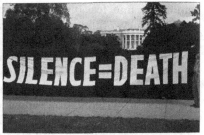

Figure 19-7. AIDS protest. Gay activists stormed the doors of the Centers for Disease Control and Prevention in Atlanta in 1990. The protestors demanded that the definition of AIDS be expanded to include women and heterosexuals so that more people afflicted with the disease would be identified and thus become eligible for medical care.

Figure 19-8. AIDS slogan. This powerful slogan was created by ACT-UP, the AIDS Coalition to Unleash Power. Founded in 1987, ACT-UP was one of the many effective organizations to evolve from the AIDS crisis in order to pressure the government into dedicating more resources toward fighting the AIDS epidemic.

Fig. E.1 A page on "Social Repercussions" in Mildvan's AIDS atlas from 2008. These pictures of protest have lost much of the urgency in the original photographs. Their inclusion in a medical atlas on AIDS makes a strange impression, as their value for teaching doctors and students how to see AIDS exceeds the usual framework and scope of the genre.

Source: Donna Mildvan, ed., *International Atlas of AIDS* (Philadelphia: Springer, 2008), 4th ed., p. 352. Permission granted by Getty Images.

photograph of ACT UP's slogan "Silence = Death" in front of the White House and a recent picture taken at a student protest against AIDS in 2005 (Fig. E.1).

The atlas moves to closure by raising the image of the "Global Impact of HIV," pictures of public health training, distribution of leaflets and medication, before a final section discusses "Living With AIDS," which guides the gaze from an annual AIDS walk to a photograph of a handful of pills, to the final picture – the last picture in the atlas: a red AIDS ribbon pinned to a doctor's white coat, encircled by a stethoscope.[4]

[4] Ibid., 357.

The perspective in this book has been guided by the history of AIDS as visualized in the atlas from 1986 to 2008. Of concern were visual instruments of knowledge production and how they integrated, distilled and structured the perception and understanding of AIDS through and in the atlas. I questioned how the atlas contributed during that period not only to making AIDS visible, but further to how unseen aspects of AIDS were produced and established through the atlas. My archaeology of AIDS knowledge asked how practices of visualization, and how a relationship between the seen and the unseen, were organized and transformed in the AIDS atlas. As my argument developed from edition to edition, visualization became feasible as an instrument of transformation in which AIDS was never fully exposed, but rather subjected to particular embodiments and spatializations before the syndrome became iconized in pictures of HIV. Archives of visual practices in medical history and a rich corpus of literature on visual representations of AIDS in a wider social and cultural context helped to make sense of intentions, effects and aesthetics of visualization practices in the AIDS atlas. The atlas, I showed, shared a mode of problematization of the epidemic with a wider context, which allowed for a tentative clustering of the epidemic's history in a photographed history of the person with AIDS, a geographical history of the local and global spaces of AIDS and of the detached, ubiquitous pictures of HIV as the causal agent of AIDS. What is left now to consider is what this changing relationship of the atlas's visualization can tell us about the conditions of the epidemic's normalizations and if the atlas contributed to a visual resolution of AIDS as crisis.

To begin the story from its preliminary last act, the question is how to make sense of Mildvan's visualization of the social and cultural history, the story of stigmatization, mourning, disobedience, activism and global health policy within the rationale of the atlas. Was an atlas not precisely the place in which these "repercussions" were meant to be removed from the epidemic's history, where a reader instead expects the biomedical consolidation of AIDS? Even in this concluding section, the atlas stayed true to its didactic and syntactic form: Each of the photographs of activists, social unrest and even the posters are presented as figures accompanied by a brief anchoring caption. Continuing the design established through the editions of this medical publication suggests that these final snapshots of the "para-epidemic" somehow too have become significant to seeing AIDS in similar ways to the genetic structure of HIV, the skin rash on persons with acute infections or the maps that detail the diverse patterns of AIDS's occurrence around the world. In fact, have these photographs of AIDS activism become characteristic pictures of AIDS?

Mildvan's choice of the term *para-epidemic* proposes a parallel world of social and cultural reactions to AIDS, suggestive of a secondary epidemic that followed the impacts of the disease. The title "Social Repercussions" has an interesting resonance as a recoil that follows an impact, it is both an unintended consequence of an event and an inevitable outcome. The term also has an etymological echo in older medical texts, where tumors or morbid humors were repercussed, pushed or driven back into an original shape.[5] As used by Mildvan, the term resembles a common rhetorical figure in contemporary medicine whereby the status of social impacts, cultural interpretations, and individual experiences of pain and disease tend to be seen as a secondary symptom of a diseases. This fallout grants the medical humanities their research field, as it finds cumbersome acknowledgment in the medical profession.

But Mildvan went further: In the preface she attributed agency to activism, community organization and social deliberations of the epidemic's impact on individuals, social fabrics and political systems. The epidemic's ramifications, Mildvan argues, have had "singular influence on the advances made for the disease."[6] Not only did the outstanding history of AIDS activism and campaigning in 2008 find its way into the section of the atlas detailing the epidemic's history, it is also characterized as a significant contributor to the resolution of the AIDS crisis. In a kind of circular argument, the inclusion of activists' historical impact on how medical research was conducted, how public health policies were formed and how global health was reinvented means that they too have become an element in the medical definition of AIDS. Their inclusion in the oeuvre of the AIDS atlas is symbolic for the significance of history for our contemporary understanding of the epidemic.

Historical sections, albeit small ones, had a place in all atlas editions. In 1986 and 1988, these passages were part of general epidemiology and explanations of immunology;[7] "historical perspective" is provided in the introduction of the atlas from 1989 and becomes a chapter, written by Charles Farthing for Friedman-Kien's second edition in 1996.[8] In Mildvan's series, the historical development of the epidemic remains a part of

---

[5] "Repercussion, N.," *OED Online* (Oxford University Press) (accessed June 11, 2018), www.oed.com/view/Entry/162762.

[6] Mildvan, *International Atlas of AIDS*.

[7] Charles F. Farthing et al., eds., *A Colour Atlas of AIDS (Acquired Immunodeficiency Syndrome)* (London: Wolfe Medical Publications, 1986), 6–8; Charles F. Farthing, ed., *A Color Atlas of AIDS* (Chicago: Year Book Medical Publishers, 1988), 6–8.

[8] Alvin E. Friedman-Kien, ed., *Color Atlas of AIDS* (Philadelphia: Saunders, 1989), 1–4; Alvin E. Friedman-Kien and Clay J. Cockerell, eds., *Color Atlas of AIDS* (Philadelphia: W. B. Saunders, 1996), 1–8.

the introduction as well as the epidemiology and virology of AIDS, before becoming a fully fledged chapter on AIDS repercussions in 2008. From short narratives of how the epidemic was discovered, to discussion about how it became entangled with social and sexual identities; from overviews of how the virus's origin moved to the African continent to how AIDS became global, the short history of this disease was thought to matter in teaching doctors and medical students how to see, to understand what AIDS was and to appreciate what it had become. "Social Repercussions" were now among the many characteristic signs and patterns unique to AIDS history.

The AIDS atlas had always had a relatively small print run and most volumes have probably become reference copies in medical libraries, used by a narrow medical audience. It is notoriously difficult to claim that the analysis of such an atlas can provide a general argument about the resolution of a crisis as complex and manifold as AIDS. The chapter on "Social Repercussions" in this final atlas edition seems furthermore to contradict my initial claim that the AIDS atlas's visualization should be understood as one of stringency and distillation, in which, over two decades, AIDS was presented in narrowing and increasingly specialized ways of seeing. It seems rather that here, at the end of this history of visualizing AIDS in a medical (or rather biomedical) structure, the scope is opening. If the atlas's aim is to leave its reader with a clarified, unified vision, to inform and to teach how to see AIDS, a historico-political section does not seem to align with this aim. The final section seems to "mop up" the nonmedical aspects of AIDS history, which might (but I think in the end does not) yield to a neat argument about medicalizing forces in our time.

Instead, the presentation of these symbols of activism, unrest and disobedience have – like other images in the atlas – become ruins of their original function. In 2008, neither the posters, nor the emotive photographs of candlelight vigils, nor activists manhandled by policemen communicate the sense of urgency and crisis that these pictures once propagated. That these figures appear in a similar material configuration as the diagrams of retroviral transcriptase, the maps of global distribution and the clinical photographs of KS on the preceding pages emphasizes a commonality in which these pictures have become part of the historical archive of AIDS. It is as if placing these pictures within the confines of this medical atlas takes away the last doubts about the state of crisis of AIDS today. In this last atlas, Mildvan seemed to make a final act of closure, in which not only nonmedical intervention is acknowledged, but also a picture of the history of AIDS emerges that is not purely driven by biomedical progress.

Can the history of AIDS ever be told without repeating dichotomies – medicine versus culture and politics – that were set up as the epidemic emerged and developed? This is a history with opposition to the medical establishment, mistrust in national and international public health institutions and experiences of stigmatization, ignorance and neglect, on one side. On the other side, we find enlightenment parables of how a few doctors confronted the uncertainty of the early years, how scientists dedicated their lives to understanding and deciphering the microbiological and macropolitical challenges of AIDS to lay the grounds for a remarkable biomedical endeavor. Two separated and often partisan historical narratives of how AIDS was overcome. A *social history* of AIDS usually focuses on activism, on patients and sometimes doctors' experiences; a *cultural history*, aligned with the perspectives in social histories, looks to the aesthetics and curative concepts of AIDS art and its presence in film and TV; while a *medical history* is particularly concerned with (and often skeptical of) a narrative of scientific and clinical progression. As indicated previously, these narratives are not arbitrary remnants of a bygone past but are traces of struggles over causality and responsibility deeply entrenched in the fabric of how AIDS came into being, how knowledge about the disease was forged and how politics of the epidemic were formed. Subsequently, these narratives were part of how these issues were overturned, upended and resolved.

If we were to accept that the AIDS crisis has been resolved, then we might ask who performed this resolution and who earned the legacy of having normalized the epidemic? Was it doctors, scientists and research institutions, or activists in the trenches working against homophobia, extortionate medication prices and discriminatory patent regulations? Will the history of overcoming the AIDS crisis be a tale of the biomedical defeat of a looming pandemic catastrophe or a plethora of microhistories in which a global transformation of social behavior, cultural attitudes and ethical guidelines contained the epidemic?

Mildvan's final chapter seems to offer a diplomatic solution to this bipolarity of the structure of telling the history of AIDS. Her conciliatory, but by no means toothless, gesture points to the inconsistencies of attributing a cause for the resolution of AIDS to either a group of scientists or to transnational activism and social movements. The laboratory is not a space isolated from social influence, nor do social movements act in a space free from medical definitions, scientific objects and research practices. There are questions – ethical, political and philosophical – about what it means to make a disease that straddle both spheres historical. It is not even evident who can best assess the end of a disease: whether it is when no more clusters of symptoms appear, no "dis-ease" is experienced or once its causal agent is eradicated from the world, such as smallpox. These ends may be localized, won in different stages, as was the case for polio. This book argues that AIDS stands apart here, and that this disease has started to become history with the resolution of its appearance as a crisis. In this process, AIDS becomes unseen, and we are left with its medicalized historical narratives in which signs of crisis, despair and conflict are put to rest in the archives.

But claiming that the crisis of AIDS has been resolved is today a baldly cynical statement. The latest addition to the series of atlases on AIDS is an atlas on co-infection, signaling the dramatic and complex consequences of tuberculosis or Hepatitis B infection in people with positive HIV sero-status.[9] As of 2016, resource scarcity and healthcare shortcomings continue to structure the lived reality for a staggering 36.9 million people infected with HIV globally, of which 22 million still wait to be treated and approximately 17 million are reported to be unaware of their positive status.[10] Speaking of the end of AIDS, or of a "world without AIDS," has acquired traction as a questionable political agenda. As the Global Fund, the WHO, the Bill & Melinda Gates Foundation and many national governments push for distribution of biomedical solutions – both treatment and prevention, for which the keyword is PrEP, Pre-Exposure-Prophylaxis – the epidemic is forecast to end in the same manner in which it was supposedly brought to its knees: through large-scale pharmaceutical intervention. Nguyen has argued that the latest medications, made available through private-public partnerships in the service of "biocapitalism," have established the dependence of millions of currently infected and yet-to-be-infected individuals on global funds and the pharmaceutical industry. He has convincingly shown that buying into the narrative of a technical fix – both as a history of the epidemic's past and as a projection of its future – seems all too often to be built on a vision that has forgotten the legacy of activism, global alliances of patient organizations and the essence of political struggle that sought to, in its own way, defeat the AIDS epidemic.[11]

[9] Lukas Engelmann and Janina Kehr, "Double Trouble? Towards an Epistemology of Co-Infection," *Medicine Anthropology Theory* 2 (2015), 1–31; Liu Jinxin and Tang Xiaoping, *Atlas of AIDS Co-Infection* (Berlin and Boston: De Gruyter, 2015), doi:10.1515/9783110353945.

[10] See "AIDS by the Numbers" (accessed June 11, 2018), www.unaids.org/sites/default/files/media_asset/AIDS-by-the-numbers-2016_en.pdf.

[11] Vinh-Kim Nguyen, Pierre-Marie David, and Gabriel Girard, "AIDS and Biocapitalisation: The Ambiguities of a 'World without Aids,'" *Books and Ideas*, November 12, 2015 (accessed June 11, 2018), www.booksandideas.net/AIDS-Biocapitalisation.html.

A visual history, I have argued, escapes these partisan perspectives and provides two points of nuance. First, it is a history that works on sources that never belong exclusively to one or another perspective. Second, a visual history makes it difficult to follow narratives of simplified historical causation. The methods I have applied here value the complex networks of forces that have contributed to the resolution of AIDS, which cannot exclusively be attributed to either science or activism, medicine or prevention politics.

Perhaps the pressing question today is not what the history of AIDS will be, but what kind of picture of this history will prevail? So what kind of image of the epidemic's past do we find in the AIDS atlas? While the last section in Mildvan's most recent edition invites associations in its explicit picturing of the epidemic's social and political fallout, I have shown in this book that photography, mapping and virus pictures each process their own vision in a unique section of AIDS history. While the atlas editions each integrated an explicit reference to the historical conditions under which AIDS appeared, they also produced a series of now-historical versions of a visualized AIDS. This changing picture of AIDS, its iterative resolutions, is answerable to a notion of AIDS as crisis.

As the chronological structure of my argument suggests, the history of this visualization begins with photographs, moves to maps and then arrives at the virus icon. These three visual genres neatly fold into three modes of interrogating epidemics: Photography shows the person affected by the disease and asks *who* is at risk. By default, this also identified who posed a threat to others, which revealed an increasingly complex demographics of risk. This heralded a visualization that could question *where* the epidemic was, originated and was heading to. Maps placed the epidemic on the ground and looked for the ecological conditions under which a picture of AIDS in place X deviated from the picture of AIDS in place Y. But when these maps seemed to point everywhere, and so nowhere particular, virus pictures were the final visualization that could approach *what* AIDS is, which could visualize the essence of AIDS without the distractions of embodiments and local variation.

In the spirit of Foucault, we could think these ways of seeing as forms of embodying disease in specific spheres. The first is the world of the clinic, in which a disease is assessed and conceptualized in its acute entanglement with a person's body. The clinical gaze and its capacity to recognize patterns across different patients, each in its variation around an ideal appearance is captured in photographs. Maps ask for the whereabouts of the disease and thus provide a meaningful picture for epidemiological intervention and public health. The disease is no longer a single case but embodied in the biopolitics of series of incidences, patterned locally but joining up to become a global epidemic. And third, the microbiological icon of the virus appears as a scientific embodiment of the disease, removed from bodies and spaces but visualized as a paradigmatic entity of the laboratory that appears to the eyes of microbiologists as an abstract, but tangible agent of the disease.

Embedded into the wider frame of medicine's historical visual archive, the atlas's visualizations as visual instruments enact a vector in which a status or mode of thinking about AIDS is transformed into a different one. It would be a mistake to think of this transformative capacity exclusively as a translation of the unseen into the visible. Photographs were, of course, taken to visualize the unseen syndrome, to demonstrate the realness of its uncertain shape and unusual occurrence, but they also worked to turn the variety of experienced symptoms into a class of diseases indicative of the underlying immunodeficiency: Through photographs, the experience of illness became disease. Maps were crucial to a spatial vision of the disease that exceeded the social framework in which AIDS was initially thought to belong, but maps undid the errors of seeing AIDS as a condition endured by a select demographic and transformed it into an epidemic that scaled to a pandemic. Pictures of the virus most clearly show the transformation of AIDS as a disease that affected individuals, to an epidemic affecting populations throughout the world, to become the chronic condition of HIV, invisible to the naked eye.

These vectors of transformation were in their historical moment resolutions to the ongoing and shifting crisis of AIDS. These visualizations can be thought of as propositions through which seeing and thinking about AIDS was organized to establish an order from the crisis of an epistemic anomaly. To visualize here means to visually represent crisis as the moment when order has been disturbed, where the world has lost its familiarity and new difficulties have appeared. All three modes of problematizing thus captured and communicated a unique notion of AIDS as crisis. Photographs put the body of people suffering from AIDS on display and left detailed records of fragmented subjectivities governed by infection. Maps demonstrated the loss of spatial and biopolitical certainty; diagrams showed populations at risk and proved that national borders and continental divides faltered against the force of the pandemic. Virus pictures, however, let us see the immune system in crisis and showed, to quote Lennart Nilsson, the "face of the killer," the origin and cause for crisis.

These three visualizations go on to show how each of these moments of crisis were reconciled and resolved. Photographs contributed to new rules of seeing disease by framing the unusualness of AIDS. Combining discrete and well-established disease entities in their relation to the new syndrome in young, otherwise healthy homosexual men, photographs resolved the invisibility of AIDS by crafting, as Preda called it, an "usual unusual" disease. Maps extended the frame and scaled the disease all the way from individual cases to local patterns, then to national emergency and international crisis. They became the key instrument to visualize the quest for finding a natural origin of the global pandemic and produced representations of the epidemic origin beyond its "birth" in 1981 America. Turning Africa into a complex ecological niche and the index location into the "heartland" of AIDS, maps facilitated the original origin of AIDS.

But pictures of the virus visualize the epidemic without requiring the iconography of bodies in crisis or the spatial coordinates of disease-ridden districts or networks. Through the combination of electron micrographs with explanatory diagrams surfaced an agent of disease that represents nothing but itself. Virus pictures processed the new entity of HIV both as signs of its unique morphology and as schematized plans of its functionality to guarantee its specificity. The origin that is envisioned in the portrait of the unseen agent responsible for the disease is rather, as I have argued in the preceding text, concerned with its own "historiality" – a process in which we learn to see the traces of a natural entity as recurrent productions of the origin of its own nonorigin. The tautological turns, which Hacking has described as looping effects,[12] provide us with a representation of the epidemic that encircles the virus. Instead of providing a vector in which a previously health body is infected by disease, or a mapping of space that is overcome and restructured by the impact of an epidemic, the virus picture refers to nothing but itself. Not the "unusual usual," or the "original origin," these pictures seem rather to resemble the famous verdict of Andre Lwoff, when discussing viral nature in 1957.

In his formative paper on the concept of viruses, Lwoff not only argued about how this new genera of pathogenic microbe was to be integrated into the nomenclature of microbiology, he also described his vision of how viruses should be visualized. "Some scientists visualize the virus as an ill-defined shape emerging bashfully out of a dense and golden cloud," he said lyrically. "This is a beautiful and romantic vision." His grounds to reject a flattering portraiture of the pathogen were founded in his belief that a "portrait of a virus should not produce an aesthetic emotion by means of an organic disturbance" as the visualization's

---

[12] Ian Hacking, *The Social Construction of What?* (Cambridge, MA: Harvard University Press, 1999), 34.

purpose would be to make the virus "amenable to intellectual analysis."[13] In Lwoff's approach, the visualization of the virus should resemble what he described as the virus's conceptual nature. "[T]he virus has been unveiled," he continued. "Now, it stands before you, naked. Do not turn your eyes away, it is only a concept. And the concept of a virus, just as any other concept, the concept of a lecture, the concept of woman, is not as difficult to handle as the real object."[14] While we would not want to excuse the crude sexism of this 1950s argument, the metaphorical point Lwoff makes is essential to AIDS's visualization through pictures of HIV.

What we can glean from Lwoff is that the virus should never be mistaken with an organic disturbance, that its visualization should remain concerned with the virus and not its possible effects. Unlike photographs of patients, or maps of territories and populations, virus pictures remain dedicated to the conceptual entity that is the virus; they point to nothing but themselves. Lwoff thus concluded that "viruses should be considered as viruses because viruses are viruses."[15] Reflecting on the kind of abstraction with which virus pictures engaged with the crisis of AIDS, Lwoff's conceptual analysis resonates with the history of AIDS. Not a sign of organic or social disturbance, the virus takes the conceptual abstraction from photographs of mostly homosexual men (not woman), the concepts of spatial mappings (not lectures) and leaves us with a visualization of the concept, epitomized and rendered back into a materiality of the icon of the virus. In this disappearance of crisis from the picture of AIDS, the normalization of AIDS has been achieved.

Janet Roitman has argued that claims to crisis are a judgment of history; to diagnose and to claim the crisis means to define the mode of critique that is applied for the crisis's resolution. By determining the extent of crisis we judge the significance of a history.[16] But we would end up nowhere if we were to separate a state of crisis from a state of noncrisis through some kind of empirical assessment. Rather, Roitman argues, crisis entails the practice of critique as a distinction beyond dichotomies, oppositions and factions.

But if we take crisis to be a blind spot, or a distinction, which makes certain things visible and others invisible, it is merely an a priori. Crisis is claimed, but it remains a latency; it is never itself explained because it allows for the further reduction of "crisis" to other elements, such as capitalism, economy, politics, culture, subjectivity. In that sense, crisis is not a condition to be observed (loss of

---

[13] André Lwoff, "The Concept of Virus," *Journal of General Microbiology* 17 (1957), 251.
[14] Ibid., 252.   [15] Lwoff, "The Concept of Virus."
[16] Janet Roitman, *Anti-Crisis* (Durham, NC: Duke University Press, 2013).

meaning, alienation, faulty knowledge); it is an observation that produces meaning. More precisely, it is a distinction that secures "a world" for observation.[17]

The Hippocratic heritage of the Greek word *krisis* as a "decision" indicates a medical understanding of crisis as a point of irreversible transformation and decisive action, rather than interruption or a lack of order.
Foucault argues that crisis was for Hippocratic medicine the moment at
which a disease revealed its inner truth, its intrinsic nature. "The crisis is
the reality of the disease becoming truth, as it were," he wrote.[18] Before
modern medicine was born, the "crisis days" of a disease were thought
part of its natural rhythm, characteristic of a particular disease in its
contours and appearances. In crisis, the perception of the shape and
emergence of a disease, its trajectory and, finally, its resolution were
forecasted.

In the archive of the AIDS atlas, certain aspects of the crisis become
visible, while others become unseen. Photographs, maps and virus pictures each expressed and claimed crisis at a time. With Roitman, the
crisis of AIDS could never be seen as an observed condition that ultimately comes to light. As abstractions, the visualizations point to and
beyond the crisis, which remained a latency. As reductions, the pictures
have offered placeholders for the crisis: bodies that suffer and spaces
marked by the epidemic's impact. The icon of HIV reduced the notion of
crisis to an absolute past, and as a placeholder for the end of crisis it
becomes the icon of AIDS when clinical latency becomes the epidemic's
status quo. Seeing HIV stabilizes the notion of difference that separates
the person with HIV from what is assumed to be a healthy person,
despite the fact that in the very definition of the term, the HIV-positive
person is not suffering from any dis-ease. As recognizable indices of the
pathology of AIDS disappear and the latency of HIV infection assumes
new normality, it is the icon of HIV that maintains the nature of the
positive sero-status as a different normality.[19]

*

Mildvan defines AIDS in her preface as "a new infectious disease,
emerging without history or precedent."[20] Although the atlas genre

---

[17] Ibid., 39.
[18] Michel Foucault, *Psychiatric Power: Lectures at the Collège de France, 1973–1974* (New
York: St Martin's Press, 2008), 243.
[19] Conversations with and incredibly valuable feedback from Brigitte Weingart have
contributed substantially to this perspective on the pictures of HIV in relation to the
virus's clinical latency.
[20] Mildvan, *International Atlas of AIDS*, v.

marks a return of a familiar medium of medical classification, its visualization of AIDS needed to be as unique and unprecedented as the syndrome, and as such it too becomes "a medium without history or precedent." Inconspicuous at first sight – a picture book for interested medical professionals and students – it is a medium that, like its mythological namesake titan, bore the ambition to carry the world of AIDS on its shoulders. Yet the editors held fast to the august traditions of the genre, with stringent, concise and definitive measurements of the epidemic's significance. AIDS marked a return to the catastrophic times (which many thought were over) of untreatable infectious diseases, the fallout of which caused a crisis of Western epistemology, an epidemic of signification. The atlas of AIDS is striking in its efforts to balance the inclusion of everything deemed significant about a disease while establishing normative ways in which traces of AIDS were to be seen and understood.

This rationale cannot be summed up as a medical perspective or even a medicalization of AIDS. Neither does black boxing, cleansing or Latour's sieving the "chaff of ideology" from the kernel of meaning bring us closer to how the atlas visualized the epidemic. Instead of a scientific object whose definition of AIDS would be complete, or whose appearance would be widely resistant to the changes of time, the atlas created a vision of AIDS that admitted the indeterminacy of patients' bodies, was stretched in the complex spaces of ecological variety and then stabilized in the timeless scientific icon of HIV.

Between 1986 and 2008, we see eight iterations of the same atlas. The picture of AIDS that emerges from the pages of each edition changes, but as a collection they achieve an apparent completeness by visualizing the different conceptions of the disease across its three decades. As indicated previously, the changes are structured by shifting modes of seeing. But what holds these editions (from different editors), medical advisory boards and publishing houses together is that from the first to the last atlas, these three modes of seeing and understanding AIDS are positioned in constellation with each other. Accordingly, the atlas's historical transformation does not allow for a reading of progressive cleansing, in which first photographs and then maps were used only to be outdated, or deemed erroneous representations of AIDS, trumped by the virus icon. Rather their immediate function to express crisis and to make sense of the epidemic has faded, and these visualizations moved from being instruments of interrogation in experimental systems to become representations of how AIDS was seen.

In positivist readings, science and medicine are often praised as endeavors of inquiry that sustain an ability to accept error and mistaken assumptions. Internal acknowledgment of sciences own shortcomings within its allied disciplines is intended to shore up the narrative of progress. Accordingly, only the most recent state of knowledge can be counted as accurate and valid, while the past becomes an archive of inaccuracy, misguided conceptions and false belief. This presentism of scientific enquiry is encapsulated in the timeless frame of the electron micrograph, which veils its own historical insignificance in previous times when photographs and maps structured different ways of thinking through the opportunistic diseases and the epidemic risks of AIDS.

A medical history that would endorse this vision of science relegates itself to a museum of science and medicine's errors. Part of the AIDS atlas's unique resemblance to AIDS history is what prevents this perspective from being successful. With the inclusion of a final chapter on the epidemic's social repercussions, Mildvan effectively concedes to the failure of a simplistic positivist narrative. Instead of drawing a teleological line from vague notions of what AIDS was in its first years, to be interrogated and refined into the mechanics and effects of a retrovirus, Mildvan makes an important intervention. The enterprise of systematizing and classifying the AIDS epidemic is not presented as a long-anticipated revelation of truth, but rather as contested terrain on which nonmedical and nonscientific actors had decisive influence in how knowledge was formed.

The AIDS atlas thus stands as testament to another, and perhaps more important, legacy of AIDS. In presenting a changing image of the crisis structured by different ways of seeing, through photographs, maps and virus pictures, even the latest edition presents itself as an abundant catalog of the many theoretical possibilities of visualizing an epidemic. Rather than just a snap shot of how cutting-edge microbiological analysis brings us a perception of AIDS's now-familiar techno-scientific present, the atlas still contains photographs and maps for problematizing the epidemic that have become less familiar with time. As a repository of the possibilities through which AIDS could be thought and seen, the atlas refrains from claiming the end of AIDS. Nine years have passed since the last AIDS atlas was compiled, which begs the question whether this is in fact the last atlas – the final – or merely the last atlas – the most recent. Mildvan's series may continue, or a new one might emerge, but the 2008 edition chooses a wise note on which to close: seeing the archive of AIDS as characterized by incompleteness.

Bibliography

Ackerknecht, Erwin H. *Geschichte und Geographie der wichtigsten Krankheiten.* Stuttgart: Enke, 1963.

Ackermann, Michael J., Judith Folkenberg, and Benjamin Rifkin. *Human Anatomy: Depicting the Body from the Renaissance to Today.* London: Thames & Hudson, 2006.

Aggleton, Peter, Peter Davies, and Hart Graham, eds. *AIDS: Safety, Sexuality and Risk.* London: Taylor & Francis, 1995.

Åhrén, Eva. "Figuring Things Out." *Nuncius* 32, no. 1 (2017): 166–211. doi:10.1163/18253911-03201007.

Altman, Lawrence K. "Rare Cancer Seen in 41 Homosexuals." *New York Times,* July 3, 1981.

Ansary, M. A., ed. *A Colour Atlas of AIDS in the Tropics.* London: Wolfe, 1989.

Aterman, K., and J. A. Grimaud. "The Brothers Lumière: Pioneers in Medical Photography." *The American Journal of Dermatopathology* 5, no. 5 (1983): 479–81.

Atkins, Robert. "Difficult Subject: Photographing AIDS." *Village Voice,* June 28, 1988.

Auerbach, D. M., W. W. Darrow, H. W. Jaffe, and J. W. Curran. "Cluster of Cases of the Acquired Immune Deficiency Syndrome: Patients Linked by Sexual Contact." *The American Journal of Medicine* 76, no. 3 (1984): 487–92.

Bachelard, Gaston. *The Formation of the Scientific Mind.* Manchester, UK: Clinamen, 2002.

Back, Les, and Vibeke Quaade. "Dream Utopias, Nightmare Realities: Imaging Race and Culture within the World of Benetton Advertising." *Third Text* 7, no. 22 (1993): 65–80.

Baechi, Thomas. "Visualisierung von Viren? 'Seeing Is Believing.'" In *VirusExpress: Rendez-Vous Im Überall,* edited by Matthias Michel and Isabelle Köpfli, pp. 30–1. Zürich: Edition Museum für Gestaltung, 1997.

Barad, Karen. *Meeting the Universe Halfway: Quantum Physics and the Entanglement of Matter and Meaning.* Durham, NC: Duke University Press, 2007.

Barfoot, Mike, and A. D. Morrison-Low. "W. C. M'Intosh and A. J. Macfarlan: Early Clinical Photography in Scotland." *History of Photography* 23, no. 3 (1999): 199–210. doi:10.1080/03087298.1999.10443322.

Barnett, Richard. *The Sick Rose, or, Disease and the Art of Medical Illustration.* New York: Distributed Art Publishers, 2014.

Barré-Sinoussi, F., J. C. Chermann, F. Rey, M. T. Nugeyre et al. "Isolation of a T-Lymphotropic Retrovirus from a Patient at Risk for Acquired Immune Deficiency Syndrome (AIDS)." *Science* 220, no. 4599 (1983): 868–71.

Barrett, F. A. "August Hirsch: As Critic of, and Contributor to Geographical Medicine and Medical Geography." *Medical History. Supplement*, no. 20 (2000): 98–117.

Barrett, Frank A. *Disease and Geography: The History of an Idea*. York, UK: York University Press, 2000.

Barthes, Roland. *Camera Lucida: Reflections on Photography*. New York: Farrar, Straus and Giroux, 1981.

Bastos, Cristiana. *Global Responses to AIDS: Science in Emergency*. Bloomington: Indiana University Press, 1999.

Bayer, Ronald, and Gerald M. Oppenheimer. *AIDS Doctors: Voices from the Epidemic*. Oxford: Oxford University Press, 2000.

Berhouma, Moncef, Julie Dubourg, and Mahmoud Messerer. "Cruveilhier's Legacy to Skull Base Surgery: Premise of an Evidence-Based Neuropathology in the 19th Century." *Clinical Neurology and Neurosurgery* 115, no. 6 (June 2013): 702–7. doi:10.1016/j.clineuro.2012.08.005.

Berkowitz, Carin. "The Illustrious Anatomist: Authorship, Patronage, and Illustrative Style in Anatomy Folios, 1700–1840." *Bulletin of the History of Medicine* 89, no. 2 (2015): 171–208. doi:10.1353/bhm.2015.0028.

"Introduction: Beyond Illustrations." *Bulletin of the History of Medicine* 89, no. 2 (2015): 165–70. doi:10.1353/bhm.2015.0057.

Berridge, Virginia. *AIDS in the UK: The Making of a Policy, 1981–1994*. Oxford: Oxford University Press, 1996.

Bersani, Leo. "Is the Rectum a Grave?" In *AIDS, Cultural Analysis, Cultural Activism*, edited by Douglas Crimp, pp. 197–222. Cambridge, MA: MIT Press, 1988.

Bertin, Jacques. *Semiology of Graphics: Diagrams, Networks, Maps*. Translated by William J. Berg. Redlands, CA: ESRI Press, 2011.

Bhattacharya, Sanjoy, Mark Harrison, and Michael Worboys. *Fractured States: Smallpox, Public Health and Vaccination Policy in British India 1800–1947*. New Delhi: Orient Longman, 2005.

Biehl, João Guilherme. *Will to Live: AIDS Therapies and the Politics of Survival*. Princeton, NJ: Princeton University Press, 2007.

Bleichmar, Daniela. *Visible Empire: Botanical Expeditions and Visual Culture in the Hispanic Enlightenment*. Chicago and London: University of Chicago Press, 2012.

Bleker, Johanna. "Die Idee einer historischen Entwicklung der Krankheiten des Menschengeschlechts und ihre Bedeutung für die empirische Medizin des frühen 19. Jahrhunderts." *Berichte zur Wissenschaftsgeschichte* 8 (1985): 195–204.

Bloch, Iwan. *Der Ursprung der Syphilis. Eine Medizinische und kulturgeschichtliche Untersuchung*. Jena, Germany: Fischer, 1901.

Board, Christopher. "Cartographic Communication." *Cartographica: The International Journal for Geographic Information and Geovisualization* 18, no. 2 (1972): 42–78.

Bordowitz, Gregg. *Imagevirus: General Idea.* London: Afterall Books, 2010.

Bowker, Geoffrey C., Stefan Timmermans, Adele E. Clarke, and Ellen Balka. *Boundary Objects and Beyond: Working with Leigh Star.* Cambridge, MA: MIT Press, 2016.

Bramwell, Byrom. *Atlas of Clinical Medicine, Volume I.* Edinburgh: Constable, 1892.

Brandt, Allan M. "How AIDS Invented Global Health." *New England Journal of Medicine* 368, no. 23 (June 6, 2013): 2149–52. doi:10.1056/NEJM p1305297.

The Cigarette Century: The Rise, Fall, and Deadly Persistence of the Product That Defined America. New York: Basic Books, 2007.

"AIDS in Historical Perspective: Four Lessons from the History of Sexually Transmitted Diseases." *American Journal of Public Health* 78 (1988): 367–71.

"The Syphilis Epidemic and Its Relation to AIDS." *Science* 239 (1988): 375–80.

No Magic Bullet: A Social History of Venereal Disease in the United States since 1880. New York: Oxford University Press, 1987.

Branwyn Poleykett, Niccolas H. A. Evans, and Lukas Engelmann. "Fragments of Plague." *Limn,* March 4, 2016. http://limn.it/fragments-of-plague/.

Braun, Marta, and Elizabeth Whitcombe. "The Photography of Pathological Locomotion." *History of Photography* 23 (1999): 218–23.

Brier, Jennifer. *Infectious Ideas: U.S. Political Responses to the AIDS Crisis.* Chapel Hill: University of North Carolina Press, 2009.

Broemer, R. "The First Global Map of the Distribution of Human Diseases: Friedrich Schnurrer's 'Charte über die Geographische Ausbreitung der Krankheiten' (1827)." *Medical History Supplement* 20 (2000): 176–85.

Brookmeyer, Ron, and Mitchell H. Gail. *AIDS Epidemiology: A Quantitative Approach.* Oxford: Oxford University Press, 1994.

Brown, Theodore M., Marcos Cueto, and Elizabeth Fee. "The World Health Organization and the Transition from 'International' to 'Global' Public Health." *American Journal of Public Health* 96, no. 1 (2006): 62–72.

Burk, Tara. "Radical Distribution: AIDS Cultural Activism in New York City, 1986–1992." *Space and Culture* 18, no. 4 (November 1, 2015): 436–49. doi:10.1177/1206331215616095.

Butler, Judith. *Frames of War: When Is Life Grievable?* London: Verso, 2009.

Calmette, Albert. "The Plague at Oporto." *The North American Review* 171, no. 524 (1900): 104–11.

Campbell, Catherine, Flora Cornish, and Morten Skovdal. "Local Pain, Global Prescriptions? Using Scale to Analyse the Globalisation of the HIV/AIDS Response." *Health and Place* 18, no. 3 (May 2012): 447–52. doi:10.1016/j.healthplace.2011.10.006.

Campbell, David. *The Visual Economy of HIV/AIDS,* 2008. www.visual-hivaids.org.

Canguilhem, Georges. *On the Normal and the Pathological.* Dordrecht, the Netherlands: Reidel, 1978.

"Monstrosity and the Monstrous." Translated by Therese Jaeger. *Diogenes* 10, no. 40 (December 1962): 27–42. doi:10.1177/039219216201004002.

Cartwright, Lisa. *Screening the Body: Tracing Medicine's Visual Culture*. Minneapolis: University of Minnesota Press, 1995.

Casey, Edward. *The Fate of Place: A Philosophical History*. Berkeley: University of California Press, 1997.

Castiglia, Christopher, and Christopher Reed. *If Memory Serves: Gay Men, AIDS, and the Promise of the Queer Past*. Minneapolis: University of Minnesota Press, 2012.

Centers for Disease Control. "HIV Surveillance – United States, 1981–2008.' *Morbidity and Mortality Weekly Report* 60, no. 21 (2011): 689–93.

"Pneumocystis Pneumonia – Los Angeles." *Morbidity and Mortality Weekly Report* 30 (June 5, 1981): 250–2.

Chang, Yuan, Ethel Cesarman, Melissa S. Pessin, Frank Lee, Janice Culpepper, Daniel M. Knowles, and Patrick S. Moore. "Identification of Herpesvirus-Like DNA Sequences in AIDS-Associated Kaposi's Sarcoma." *Science* 266 (1994): 1865–9. doi:10.1126/science.7997879.

Cliff, Andrew D., and Peter Haggett. *The Geography of Disease Distribution*, edited by R. J. Johnston and Michael Williams. Oxford: Oxford University Press, 2003.

Cliff, Andrew D. *World Atlas of Epidemic Diseases*. London: Arnold, 2004.

Atlas of Disease Distributions: Analytic Approaches to Epidemiological Data. Oxford: Basil Blackwell, 1988.

Coffin, J., A. Haase, J. A. Levy, L. Montagnier, S. Oroszlan, N. Teich et al. "Human Immunodeficiency Viruses." *Science* 232 (May 9, 1986): 697.

Cohen, Cathy J. *The Boundaries of Blackness: AIDS and the Breakdown of Black Politics*. Chicago: University of Chicago Press, 1999.

Cohen, Jon. *Shots in the Dark: The Wayward Search for an AIDS Vaccine*. London: Norton, 2001.

"The Rise and Fall of Projet SIDA." *Science* 278, no. 5343 (1997): 1565–8. doi:10.1126/science.278.5343.1565.

Cohn, Susan E., Jonothan D. Klein, Jack E. Mohr, Charles M. van der Horst, and David J. Weber. "The Geography of AIDS: Patterns of Urban and Rural Migration." *Southern Medical Journal* 87, no. 6 (1994): 599–606.

Condrau, Flurin. "The Patient's View Meets the Clinical Gaze." *Social History of Medicine* 20, no. 3 (2007): 525–40. doi:10.1093/shm/hkm076.

Cooter, Roger, and Claudia Stein. "Visual Imagery and Epidemics in the Twentieth Century." In *Imagining Illness. Public Health and Visual Culture*, edited by David Harley Serlin, pp. 169–92. Minneapolis: University of Minnesota Press, 2010.

"Coming into Focus: Posters, Power, and Visual Culture in the History of Medicine." *Medizinhistorisches Journal* 42, no. 2 (2007): 180–209.

Coppock, J. Terry, and David W. Rhind. "The History of GIS." *Geographical Information Systems: Principles and Applications* 1, no. 1 (1991): 21–43.

Corea, Gena. *The Invisible Epidemic: The Story of Women and AIDS*. New York: HarperCollins, 1992.

Crane, Johanna T. "Viral Cartographies: Mapping the Molecular Politics of Global HIV." *BioSocieties* 6, no. 2 (2011): 142–66.

Scrambling for Africa: AIDS, Expertise, and the Rise of American Global Health Science. Ithaca, NY: Cornell University Press, 2013.

Creager, Angela N. *The Life of a Virus: Tobacco Mosaic Virus as an Experimental Model, 1930–1965.* Chicago: University of Chicago Press, 2002.

Crewe, M., and P. Brouard. "Film as an Educational Medium – a Review of Four HIV/AIDS Films: Continuing Education." *AIDS Bulletin* 3, no. 3 (1994): 12–13.

Crimp, Douglas. "Portraits of People with AIDS." In *Melancholia and Moralism: Essays on AIDS and Queer Politics*, edited by Douglas Crimp, pp. 83–107. Cambridge, MA: MIT Press, 2002.

———. "AIDS: Cultural Analysis/Cultural Activism." In *AIDS: Cultural Analysis, Cultural Activism*, edited by Douglas Crimp, pp. 3–16. Cambridge, MA: MIT Press, 1987.

———, ed. *AIDS: Cultural Analysis, Cultural Activism.* Cambridge, MA: MIT Press, 1988.

Crimp, Douglas, and Adam Rolston. *AIDS Demo Graphics.* Seattle, WA: Bay Press, 1990.

Cruveilhier, Jean. *Anatomie pathologique du corps humain ou descriptions avec figures lithographieés et coloriées des diverses altérations morbides.* Paris: Baillière, 1829.

Cunningham, Andrew. "Transforming Plague: The Laboratory and the Identity of Infectious Disease." In *The Laboratory Revolution in Medicine*, edited by Andrew Cunningham and Perry Williams, pp. 209–44. Cambridge: Cambridge University Press, 1992.

"Current Trends: Prevention of Acquired Immune Deficiency Syndrome (AIDS): Report of Inter-Agency Recommendations." *MMWR: Morbidity and Mortality Weekly Report* 32, no. 8 (April 3, 1983): pp. 101–3.

Currie, J., S. Trejo, and C. Goldin. *Gran Fury: Read My Lips.* New York: NYU Steinhardt, 2011.

Cvetkovich, Ann. "Legacies of Trauma, Legacies of Activism." In *Loss: The Politics of Mourning*, edited by David L. Eng, David Kazanjian, and Judith Butler, pp. 427–57. Berkeley: University of California Press, 2003.

Daston, Lorraine. "Cloud Physiognomy." *Representations* 135, no. 1 (2016): 45–71. doi:10.1525/rep.2016.135.1.45.

Daston, Lorraine, and Peter Galison. *Objectivity.* Cambridge, MA: Zone Books, 2007.

———. "The Image of Objectivity." *Representations*, no. 40 (1992): 81–128.

Delaney, Martin. "History of HAART – the True Story of How Effective Multi-Drug Therapy Was Developed for Treatment of HIV Disease." *Retrovirology* 3, Suppl 1 (December 21, 2006): 6. doi:10.1186/1742-4690-3-S1-S6.

Delaporte, François. *The History of Yellow Fever: An Essay on the Birth of Tropical Medicine.* Cambridge, MA: MIT Press, 1991.

Deleuze, Gilles. *Cinema 1: The Movement-Image.* New York: Bloomsbury Publishing, 2005.

Denkler, K., and J. Johnson. "A Lost Piece of Melanoma History." *Plastic and Reconstructive Surgery* 104, no. 7 (1999): 2149–53.

Derrida, Jacques. *Athens, Still Remains: The Photographs of Jean-François Bonhomme.* New York: Fordham University Press, 2010.

Of Grammatology. Baltimore: Johns Hopkins University Press, 1998.

De Saint-Maur, P. P. "The Birth of the Clinicopathological Method in France: The Rise of Morbid Anatomy in France during the First Half of the Nineteenth Century." *Virchows Archiv* 460, no. 1 (2012): 109–17. doi:10 .1007/s00428-011-1162-2.

Deschamps, M. "AIDS in the Caribbean." *Archives of AIDS Research* 2 (1988): 51–6.

Didi-Huberman, Georges. *Invention of Hysteria: Charcot and the Photographic Iconography of the Salpetriere.* Cambridge, MA: MIT Press, 2003.

Dijck, Jose Van. *The Transparent Body: A Cultural Analysis of Medical Imaging.* Seattle: University of Washington Press, 2015.

Dionisio, Daniele, ed. *Textbook-Atlas of Intestinal Infections in AIDS.* Milano: Springer, 2003.

Dolphijn, Rick, and Iris van der Tuin, eds. *New Materialism: Interviews and Cartographies.* Ann Arbor, MI: Open Humanities Press, 2012.

Dover, Jeffrey S. "Review: Color Atlas of AIDS." *Archives of Dermatology* 125, no. 6 (1989): 857–8.

Dubos, René, and Jean Dubos. *The White Plague: Tuberculosis, Man, and Society.* 3rd ed. New Brunswick, NJ: Rutgers University Press, 1996.

Dutt, Ashok K., Charles B. Monroe, Hiran M. Dutta, and Barbara Prince. "Geographical Patterns of AIDS in the United States." *Geographical Review* 77, no. 4 (1987): 456–71.

Echenberg, Myron J. *Plague Ports: The Global Urban Impact of Bubonic Plague, 1894–1901.* New York: New York University Press, 2007.

Eckholm, Erik. "AIDS in Africa: A Killer Rages On." *New York Times,* September 16, 1990.

Eckstein, Nicholas A. "Florence on Foot: An Eye-Level Mapping of the Early Modern City in Time of Plague." *Renaissance Studies* 30, no. 2 (2016): 273–97. doi:10.1111/rest.12144.

Edwards, Elizabeth. "Photographic Uncertainties: Between Evidence and Reassurance." *History and Anthropology* 25, no. 2 (March 15, 2014): 171–88. doi:10.1080/02757206.2014.882834.

Raw Histories: Photographs, Anthropology and Museums. London: Bloomsbury Academic, 2001.

Ehring, Franz. *Hautkrankheiten. 5 Jahrhunderte wissenschaftlicher Illustration – Skin diseases.* Stuttgart: Fischer, 1989.

Engelmann, Lukas. "What Are Medical Photographs of Plague?," *REMEDIA,* January 31, 2017. https://remedianetwork.net/2017/01/31/what-are-medical-photographs-of-plague/.

"Photographing AIDS:. Capturing AIDS in Pictures of People with AIDS." *Bulletin of the History of Medicine* 90, no. 2 (2016): 250–78.

"Eine analytische Bildpraxis. Die pathologisch-anatomischen Zeichnungen Jean Cruveilhiers in ihrem Verhältnis zu klinischen Beobachtungen." *Berichte zur Wissenschaftsgeschichte* 35 (2012): 7–24.

Engelmann, Lukas, and Janina Kehr. "Double Trouble? Towards an Epistemology of Co-Infection." *Medicine Anthropology Theory* 2 (2015): 1–31.

Epstein, Helen. *The Invisible Cure: Why We Are Losing the Fight against AIDS in Africa.* New York: Picador, 2008.

232   Bibliography

Epstein, Steven. "Activism, Drug Regulation, and the Politics of Therapeutic Evaluation in the AIDS Era: A Case Study of DdC and the 'Surrogate Markers' Debate." *Social Studies of Science* 27, no. 5 (1997): 691–726.

Impure Science: AIDS, Activism, and the Politics of Knowledge. Berkeley: University of California Press, 1996.

Fanon, Frantz. *A Dying Colonialism.* New York: Grove/Atlantic, 1994.

Farmer, Paul. *AIDS and Accusation: Haiti and the Geography of Blame.* Berkeley: University of California Press, 2006.

Farmer, Paul, Arthur Kleinman, Jim Kim, and Matthew Basilico, eds. *Reimagining Global Health.* Berkeley: University of California Press, 2013.

Farthing, Charles F., カラーアトラスAIDS. Tokyo: Igaku Shoin, 1987.

Farthing, Charles F., ed. *A Color Atlas of AIDS.* Chicago: Year Book Medical Publishers, 1988.

AIDS. Erworbenes Immundefekt-Syndrom. Ein Farbatlas. Stuttgart: Schwer, 1986.

Farthing, Charles F., Simon E. Brown, Richard C. D. Staughton, Jeffrey J. Cream, and Mark Mühlemann eds. *A Colour Atlas of AIDS (Acquired Immunodeficiency Syndrome).* London: Wolfe Medical Publications, 1986.

Fassin, Didier. *When Bodies Remember: Experiences and Politics of AIDS in South Africa.* Berkeley: University of California Press, 2007.

Fauci, Anthony S. "25 Years of HIV." *Nature* 453, no. 7193 (2008): 289–90. doi:10.1038/453289a.

Fee, Elizabeth, and Daniel M. Fox, eds. *AIDS: The Making of a Chronic Disease.* Berkeley: University of California Press, 1992.

AIDS: The Burdens of History. Berkeley: University of California Press, 1988.

Fee, Elizabeth, and Manon Parry. "Jonathan Mann, HIV/AIDS, and Human Rights." *Journal of Public Health Policy* 29, no. 1 (2008): 54–71.

Fend, Mechthild. *Fleshing Out Surfaces: Skin in French Art and Medicine, 1650–1850.* Oxford: Oxford University Press, 2016.

Fleck, Ludwik. *Genesis and Development of a Scientific Fact.* Chicago: University of Chicago Press, 1981.

Foucault, Michel. *Psychiatric Power: Lectures at the Collège de France, 1973–1974.* New York: St. Martin's Press, 2008.

"Polemics, Politics and Problematizations." In *Ethics: Subjectivity and Truth,* edited by Paul Rabinow and Robert Hurley, pp. 111–19. New York: New Press, 1997.

"Nietzsche, Genealogy, History." In *The Foucault Reader,* edited by Paul Rabinow, pp. 76–100. New York: Pantheon Books, 1984.

The Birth of the Clinic: An Archaeology of Medical Perception. New York: Pantheon Books, 1973.

Fox, Daniel M., and Christopher Lawrence. *Photographing Medicine: Images and Power in Britain and America since 1840.* New York: Greenwood Press, 1988.

France, David. *How to Survive a Plague: The Story of How Activists and Scientists Tamed AIDS.* London: Pan Macmillan, 2016.

Frey, Christiane. "Am Beispiel der Fallgeschichte. Zu Pinels 'Traité médico-philosophique sur l'aliénation.'" In *Das Beispiel. Epistemologie des Exemplarischen,* edited by Jens Ruchatz, Stefan Willer, and Nicolas Pethes, pp. 263–78. Berlin: Kulturverlag Kadmos, 2007.

Friedman-Kien, Alvin E., ed. *Color Atlas of AIDS*. Philadelphia: Saunders, 1989. "Disseminated Kaposi's Sarcoma Syndrome in Young Homosexual Men." *Journal of the American Academy of Dermatology* 5, no. 4 (1981): 468–71.

Friedman-Kien, Alvin E., and Clay J. Cockerell, eds. *Color Atlas of AIDS*. Philadelphia: W. B. Saunders, 1996.

Galison, Peter. "Images Scatter into Data: Data Gather into Images." In *Iconoclash: Beyond the Image Wars in Science, Religion and Art*, edited by Bruno Latour and Peter Weibel, pp. 300–23. Karlsruhe: Center for Arts and Media, 2002.

Gallo, R. C., P. S. Sarin, E. P. Gelmann, M. Robert-Guroff, E. Richardson, V. S. Kalyanaraman, D. Mann et al. "Isolation of Human T-Cell Leukemia Virus in Acquired Immune Deficiency Syndrome (AIDS)." *Science* 220, no. 4599 (May 20, 1983): 865–7. doi:10.1126/science.6601823.

Gallo, Robert. *Virus Hunting: AIDS, Cancer, and the Human Retrovirus*. New York: BasicBooks, 1991.

"HIV-The Cause of AIDS: An Overview on Its Biology, Mechanisms of Disease Induction, and Our Attempts to Control It." *Journal of Acquired Immune Deficiency Syndromes* 1, no. 6 (1988): 521–35.

"The AIDS Virus." *Scientific American* 256, no. 1 (January (1987): 46–57.

"The First Human Retrovirus." *Scientific American* 255, no. 6 (December 1986): 88–99.

Gallo, Robert, Syed Z. Salahuddin, Mikulas Popovic, Gene M. Shearer et al. "Frequent Detection and Isolation of Cytopathic Retroviruses (HTLV-III) from Patients with AIDS and at Risk for AIDS." *Science* 224, no. 4648 (1984): 500–3.

Galton, Francis, and F. A. Mahomed. "An Inquiry into the Physiognomy of Phthisis by the Method of 'Composite Portraiture.'" *Guy's Hospital Reports* 25 (1882): 475–93.

Gazzard, Brian. "Charles Farthing Obituary." *The Guardian*, May 11, 2014.

Gelfand, Toby. "A Clinical Ideal: Paris 1789." *Bulletin of the History of Medicine* 51 (1977): 397–411.

Geroulanos, Stefanos. *Transparency in Postwar France: A Critical History of the Present*. Stanford, CA: Stanford University Press, 2017.

Geroulanos, Stefanos, and Todd Meyers. "Introduction: Canguilhem's Critique of Medical Reason." In Georges Canguilhem, *Writings on Medicine*, pp. 1–25. New York: Fordham University Press, 2011.

Giles-Vernick, Tamara, and James L. A. Webb. *Global Health in Africa: Historical Perspectives on Disease Control*. Athens, Ohio: Ohio University Press, 2013.

Giles-Vernick, Tamara, Ch. Didier Gondola, Guillaume Lachenal, and William H. Schneider. "Social History, Biology, and the Emergence of HIV in Colonial Africa." *The Journal of African History* 54, no. 1 (2013): 11–30. doi:10.1017/S0021853713000029.

Gilman, Sander L. *Illness and Image: Case Studies in the Medical Humanities*. Piscataway, NJ: Transaction Publishers, 2014.

"The Beautiful Body and AIDS: The Image of the Body at Risk at the Close of the Twentieth Century." In *Picturing Health and Illness: Images of Identity and Difference*, edited by Sander L. Gilman, pp. 115–83. Baltimore: Johns Hopkins University Press, 1995.

"AIDS and Syphilis: The Iconography of Disease." In *AIDS, Cultural Analysis, Cultural Activism*, edited by Douglas Crimp, pp. 87–107. Cambridge, MA: MIT Press, 1988.

Disease and Representation: Images of Illness from Madness to AIDS. Ithaca, NY: Cornell University Press, 1988.

Giroux, Henry A. "Consuming Social Change: The 'United Colors of Benetton.'" *Cultural Critique*, no. 26 (1993): 5–32.

Goldstein, Richard. "The Implicated and the Immune: Cultural Responses to AIDS." *The Milbank Quarterly* 68 (1990): 295–319. doi:10.2307/3350055.

Golub, Andrew, Wilpen L. Gorr, and Peter R. Gould. "Spatial Diffusion of the HIV/AIDS Epidemic: Modeling Implications and Case Study of AIDS Incidence in Ohio." *Geographical Analysis* 25, no. 2 (1993): 85–100. doi:10.1111/j.1538-4632.1993.tb00282.x.

Gomes do Espirito Santo, M. E., and G. D. Etheredge. "Male Clients of Brothel Prostitutes as a Bridge for HIV Infection between High Risk and Low Risk Groups of Women in Senegal." *Sexually Transmitted Infections* 81, no. 4 (2005): 342–4. doi:10.1136/sti.2004.011940.

Gould, Deborah B. *Moving Politics: Emotion and ACT UP's Fight against AIDS*. Chicago: University of Chicago Press, 2009.

Gould, Peter. *The Slow Plague: A Geography of the AIDS Pandemic*. Oxford: Blackwell Publishers, 1993.

Gould, Peter, J. Kabel, W. Gorr, and A. Golub. "AIDS: Predicting the Next Map." *Interfaces* 21, no. 3 (1991): 80–92.

Gradmann, Christoph. "A Spirit of Scientific Rigour: Koch's Postulates in Twentieth-Century Medicine." *Microbes and Infection* 16, no. 11 (November 2014): 885–92. doi:10.1016/j.micinf.2014.08.012.

Grant, Alison D., and Kevin M. De Cock. "HIV Infection and AIDS in the Developing World." *British Medical Journal* 322, no. 7300 (June 16, 2001): 1475–8. doi:10.1136/bmj.322.7300.1475.

Grassi, Anita. "Review: A Color Atlas of AIDS." *Archives of Dermatology* 124, no. 1 (1988): 145.

Greco, Stephen. "Strong Bodies Gay Ways." *The Advocate*, July 7, 1983, pp. 20–3.

Greene, Jeremy A. *Generic: The Unbranding of Modern Medicine*. Baltimore: Johns Hopkins University Press, 2014.

Griesemer, John R., and Susan Leigh Star. "Institutional Ecology, 'Translations' and Boundary Objects: Amateurs and Professionals in Berkeley's Museum of Vertebrate Zoology, 1907–39." *Social Studies of Science* 19, no. 3 (1989): 387–420.

Grmek, Mirko D. *History of AIDS: Emergence and Origin of a Modern Pandemic*. Translated by Russell C. Maulitz and Jacalyn Duffin. Princeton, NJ: Princeton University Press, 1993.

Grover, Jan Zita. "OI: Opportunistic Identification, Open Identification in PWA Portraiture." In *Over Exposed : Essays on Contemporary Photography*, edited by Carol Squiers, pp. 105–22. New York: New Press, 1999.

"Visible Lesions: Images of PWA in America." In *Fluid Exchanges: Artists and Critics in the AIDS Crisis*, edited by James L. Miller, pp. 23–52. Toronto: University of Toronto Press, 1992.

Hacking, Ian. *The Social Construction of What?* Cambridge, MA: Harvard University Press, 1999.

The Taming of Chance. Cambridge: Cambridge University Press, 1990.

Haffner, Jeanne. *The View from Above: The Science of Social Space*. Cambridge, MA: MIT Press, 2013.

Hanley, Anne R. *Medicine, Knowledge and Venereal Diseases in England, 1886–1916*. Basingstoke, UK: Palgrave Macmillan, 2016.

Hansell, Peter. "Medical Photography: A Review." *The Lancet* 248, no. 6418 (August 31, 1946): 296–9. doi:10.1016/S0140-6736(46)90799-4.

Hansell, Peter, and Robert G. W. Ollerenshaw. "Applied Photography: Relation of the Photographic Department to the Teaching Hospital." *The Lancet* 250, no. 6479 (November 1, 1947): 663–6. doi:10.1016/S0140-6736(47)90689-2.

Hanson, Marta. *Speaking of Epidemics in Chinese Medicine: Disease and the Geographic Imagination in Late Imperial China*. New York: Routledge, 2012.

Haraway, Donna. *Primate Visions: Gender, Race and Nature in the World of Modern Science*. New York: Routledge, 1989.

Harden, Victoria A. *AIDS at 30: A History*. Washington, DC: Potomac Books, 2012.

Hardy, Anne. *The Epidemic Streets: Infectious Disease and the Rise of Preventive Medicine, 1856–1900*. Oxford: Clarendon Press, 1993.

Harley, John Brian. *The New Nature of Maps: Essays in the History of Cartography*. Baltimore: Johns Hopkins University Press, 2002.

"Deconstructing the Map." *Cartographica: The International Journal for Geographic Information and Geovisualization* 26, no. 2 (1989): 1–20.

Heinrich, Ari Larissa. *The Afterlife of Images: Translating the Pathological Body between China and the West*. Durham, NC: Duke University Press, 2008.

Helleringer, Stéphane, and Hans-Peter Kohler. "Sexual Network Structure and the Spread of HIV in Africa: Evidence from Likoma Island, Malawi." *AIDS* 21, no. 17 (November 2007): 2323–32. doi:10.1097/QAD .0b013e328285df98.

Herzberg, Joachim J. "Edmund Lesser und seine (vergessene) Schule." *Der Hautarzt* 39 (1988): 598–601.

Herzberg, Kurt. *Virus-Atlas*. Berlin: Transmare-Photo, 1951.

Hess, Volker. *Von der semiotischen zur diagnostischen Medizin. Die Entstehung der klinischen Methode zwischen 1750 und 1850*. Husum, Germany: Matthiesen, 1993.

Hess, Volker, and Andrew Mendelsohn. "'Sauvages' Paperwork: How Disease Classification Arose from Scholarly Note-Taking." *Early Science and Medicine* 19, no. 5 (2014): 471–503.

Hess, Volker, and J. Andrew Mendelsohn. "Case and Series: Medical Knowledge and Paper Technology, 1600–1900." *History of Science* 48, no. 161 (2010): 287–314.

Hirsch, August. *Handbook of Geographical and Historical Pathology*. London: New Sydenham Society, 1883.

HIV Plus. Los Angeles: Here Media, 2008.

Holcomb, R. C. *Who Gave the World Syphilis? The Haitian Myth*. New York: Froben Press, 1937.

Honigsbaum, Mark. "'Tipping the Balance': Karl Friedrich Meyer, Latent Infections, and the Birth of Modern Ideas of Disease Ecology." *Journal of the History of Biology* 49, no. 2 (2016): 261–309.

Hubbard, Jim. "Fever in the Archive." *GLQ: A Journal of Lesbian and Gay Studies* 7, no. 1 (2001): 183–92.

United in Anger: A History of ACT UP. Documentary, New York, 2012.

Hughes, Alun D. "Commentary: 'On the Cards': Collective Investigation of Disease and Medical Life Histories in the Nineteenth Century." *International Journal of Epidemiology* 42, no. 3 (June 1, 2013): 683–8. doi:10.1093/ije/dyt062.

Hüppauf, Bernd, and Peter Weingart. "Images in and of Science." In *Science Images and Popular Images of the Sciences.* Vol. 8, edited by Bernd Hüppauf and Peter Weingart, 3–31. New York: Routledge, 2008.

eds. *Science Images and Popular Images of Sciences.* New York: Routledge, 2008.

Jacobi, Eduard. *Atlas der Hautkrankheiten. Mit Einschluß der wichtigsten venerischen Erkrankungen für praktische Aerzte und Studierende.* Berlin, Vienna: Urban & Schwarzenberg, 1903.

Jarcho, Saul. "Yellow Fever, Cholera, and the Beginnings of Medical Cartography." *Journal of the History of Medicine and Allied Sciences* 25, no. 2 (1970): 131–42.

Jinxin, Liu, and Tang Xiaoping. *Atlas of AIDS Co-Infection.* Berlin and Boston: De Gruyter, 2015. doi:10.1515/9783110353945.

Jones, Caroline A., and Peter Galison. "Introduction." In *Picturing Science, Producing Art,* edited by Caroline A. Jones and Peter Galison, pp. 1–26. London: Psychology Press, 1998.

Jones, Rodney H. "Marketing the Damaged Self: The Construction of Identity in Advertisements Directed towards People with HIV/AIDS." *Journal of Sociolinguistics* 1, no. 3 (1997): 393–418. doi:10.1111/1467-9481.00022.

Jordanova, Ludmilla. *The Look of the Past: Visual and Material Evidence in Historical Practice.* Cambridge: Cambridge University Press, 2012.

Junge, Sophie. *Art about AIDS, Nan Goldin's Exhibition Witnesses: Against Our Vanishing.* Berlin: De Gruyter, 2016. doi:10.1515/9783110453072.

Kalichman, Seth C. *Denying AIDS: Conspiracy Theories, Pseudoscience, and Human Tragedy.* New York: Springer Science, 2009.

Kaposi, Moritz. *Handatlas der Hautkrankheiten für Studierende und Ärzte.* Vienna: Braumüller, 1898.

Kaslow, Richard A., and Donald P. Francis, eds. *The Epidemiology of AIDS: Expression, Occurrence, and Control of Human Immunodeficiency Virus Type 1 Infection.* New York: Oxford University Press, 1989.

Kassell, Lauren. "Casebooks in Early Modern England: Medicine, Astrology, and Written Records." *Bulletin of the History of Medicine* 88, no. 4 (2014): 595–625. doi:10.1353/bhm.2014.0066.

Kehr, Janina. "Blind Spots and Adverse Conditions of Care: Screening Migrants for Tuberculosis in France and Germany." *Sociology of Health and Illness* 34, no. 2 (2012): 251–65. doi:10.1111/j.1467-9566.2011.01415.x.

Keiller, William. "The Craze for Photography in Medical Illustration." *New York Medical Journal* 59 (1894): 788–9.

Kevles, Bettyann. *Naked to the Bone: Medical Imaging in the Twentieth Century.* Boston: Addison-Wesley, 1998.

King, Nicholas B. "The Scale Politics of Emerging Disease." *Osiris* 19 (2004): 62–76.

Knorr-Cetina, Karin. *Epistemic Cultures: How the Sciences Make Knowledge.* Cambridge, MA: Harvard University Press, 1999.

Koch, Robert. "Zur Untersuchung von pathogenen Organismen." *Mittheilungen aus dem Kaiserlichen Gesundheitsamte* 1 (1881): 112–63.

"Die Ätiologie der Milzbrand-Krankheit, begründet auf die Entwicklungsgeschichte des Bacillus anthracis." *Cohns Beiträge zur Biologie der Pflanzen* 2, no. 2 (1876): 277–310.

Koch, Tom. *Disease Maps: Epidemics on the Ground.* Chicago: University of Chicago Press, 2011.

Cartographies of Disease: Maps, Mapping, and Medicine. Redlands, CA: ESRI Press, 2005.

Koch, Tom, and Ken Denike. "Essential, Illustrative, or ... Just Propaganda? Rethinking John Snow's Broad Street Map." *Cartographica: The International Journal for Geographic Information and Geovisualization* 45, no. 1 (March 2010): 19–31. doi:10.3138/carto.45.1.19.

Koch, Tom, and Kenneth Denike. "Crediting His Critics' Concerns: Remaking John Snow's Map of Broad Street Cholera, 1854." *Social Science and Medicine* 69 (2009): 1246–51.

Koop, C. Everett. *Surgeon General's Report on Acquired Immune Deficiency Syndrome.* Washington, DC: US Public Health Service, 1986.

Kosoy, Michael, and Roman Kosoy. "Complexity and Biosemiotics in Evolutionary Ecology of Zoonotic Infectious Agents." *Evolutionary Applications*, June 29, 2017. doi:10.1111/eva.12503.

Krause, Richard M. "Koch's Postulates and the Search for the AIDS Agent." *Public Health Reports* 99, no. 3 (1984): 291–9.

Lam, Nina Siu-Ngan, Ming Fan, and Kam-biu Liu. "Spatial-Temporal Spread of the AIDS Epidemic, 1982–1990: A Correlogram Analysis of Four Regions of the United States." *Geographical Analysis* 28, no. 2 (1996): 93–107. doi:10.1111/j.1538-4632.1996.tb00923.x.

Langer, Erich. *Atlas der Syphilis.* Berlin: Berliner Medizinische Verlagsanstalt, 1949.

Latour, Bruno. *We Have Never Been Modern.* Cambridge, MA: Harvard University Press, 2012.

Pandora's Hope: Essays on the Reality of Science Studies. Cambridge, MA: Harvard University Press, 1999.

Latour, Bruno, and Steve Woolgar. *Laboratory Life: The Social Construction of Scientific Facts.* Princeton, NJ: Princeton University Press, 1979.

Lesser, Edmund. *Lehrbuch der Haut- und Geschlechtskrankheiten für Studierende und Ärzte.* Leipzig: F. C. W. Vogel, 1888.

Levy, Jay A., A. D. Hoffman, S. M. Kramer, J. A. Landis, J. M. Shimabukuro, and L. S. Oshiro. "Isolation of Lymphocytopathic Retroviruses from San Francisco Patients with AIDS." *Science* 225, no. 4664 (1984): 840–2.

Livingston, Julie. "Figuring the Tumor in Botswana." *Raritan* 34, no. 1 (2014): 10–24.

Improvising Medicine: An African Oncology Ward in an Emerging Cancer Epidemic. Durham, NC: Duke University Press, 2012.

"AIDS as Chronic Illness: Epidemiological Transition and Health Care in South-Eastern Botswana." *African Journal of AIDS Research* 3, no. 1 (2004): 15–22.

Ljungberg, Christina. "The Diagrammatic Nature of Maps." In *Thinking with Diagrams: The Semiotic Basis of Human Cognition*, edited by Christina Ljungberg and Sybille Krämer, pp. 139–59, Berlin: De Gruyter, 2016.

Löwy, Ilana. "Ways of Seeing: Ludwig Fleck and Polish Debates on the Perception of Reality." *Studies in History and Philosophy of Science* 39 (2008): 375–83.

Lüdtke, Karlheinz. *Zur Geschichte der Frühen Virusforschung*. Berlin: Max-Planck-Inst. für Wissenschaftsgeschichte, 1999.

Lwoff, André. "The Concept of Virus." *Journal of General Microbiology* 17 (1957): 239–53.

Lynteris, Christos. "Zoonotic Diagrams: Mastering and Unsettling Human-Animal Relations." *Journal of the Royal Anthropological Institute* 23, no. 3 (2017): 463–85. doi:10.1111/1467-9655.12649.

Ethnographic Plague: Configuring Disease on the Chinese-Russian Frontier. Basingstoke, UK: Palgrave Macmillan, 2016.

Lynteris, Christos, and Ruth J. Prince. "Anthropology and Medical Photography: Ethnographic, Critical and Comparative Perspectives." *Visual Anthropology* 29, no. 2 (March 14, 2016): 101–17. doi:10.1080/08949468.2016.1131104.

Lyons, Maryinez. *The Colonial Disease: A Social History of Sleeping Sickness in Northern Zaire, 1900–1940*. Cambridge: Cambridge University Press, 2002.

Macher, Abe M., ed. *AIDS: An Atlas of Cases for Diagnosis*. Baltimore: Williams & Wilkins, 1988.

Mandell, Gerald L., and Donna Mildvan, eds. *Atlas of AIDS*. 3rd ed. Philadelphia: Springer, 2001.

Mann, Jonathan M. *"The Global AIDS Situation."* Geneva: World Health Organization, 1987. www.who.int/iris/handle/10665/53236.

Mann, Jonathan M., H. Francis, T. Quinn et al. "Surveillance for AIDS in a Central African City: Kinshasa, Zaire." *JAMA* 255, no. 23 (1986): 3255–9. doi:10.1001/jama.1986.03370230061031.

Mann, Jonathan M., Daniel J. M. Tarantola, and Thomas W. Netter. *AIDS in the World*. Cambridge, MA: Harvard University Press, 1992.

Marcus, Sharon, Heather Love, and Stephen Best. "Building a Better Description." *Representations* 135, no. 1 (2016): 1–21. doi:10.1525/rep.2016.135.1.1.

Marsh, Ronald J. "Review: A Colour Atlas of AIDS and HIV Disease." *British Jounral of Ophthalmology* 74, no. 1 (1990): 64.

Matthews, J. Rosser. *Quantification and the Quest for Medical Certainty*. Princeton, NJ: Princeton University Press, 1995.

May, Jacques Meyer. *The Ecology of Human Disease*. New York: MD Publications, 1958.

Mbali, Mandisa. *South African AIDS Activism and Global Health Politics*. Basingstoke, UK: Palgrave Macmillan, 2013.

McKay, Richard A. *Patient Zero and the Making of the AIDS Epidemic*. Chicago: University of Chicago Press, 2017.

"Before HIV: Venereal Disease among Homosexually Active Men in England and North America." In *The Routledge History of Disease*, edited by Mark Jackson, pp. 439–57. Abingdon, UK: Routledge Handbooks Online, 2016. doi:10.4324/9781315543420.ch24.

"'Patient Zero': The Absence of a Patient's View of the Early North American AIDS Epidemic." *Bulletin of the History of Medicine* 88, no. 1 (2014): 161–94. doi:10.1353/bhm.2014.0005.

McLeod, Kari S. "Our Sense of Snow: The Myth of John Snow in Medical Geography." *Social Science and Medicine* 50, no. 7 (2000): 923–35.

Meade, Melinda S. *Medical Geography*. New York: Guilford Press, 2010.

Meli, Domenico Bertoloni. "The Rise of Pathological Illustrations: Baillie, Bleuland, and Their Collections." *Bulletin of the History of Medicine* 89, no. 2 (2015): 209–42. doi:10.1353/bhm.2015.0034.

Mersch, Dieter. "Visuelle Argumente. Zur Rolle der Bilder in den Naturwissenschaften." In *Bilder als Diskurse, Bilddiskurse*, edited by Sabine Maasen, Torsten Mayerhauser, and Cornelia Renggli, pp. 95–116. Weilerswist, Germany: Velbrück, 2006.

Mifflin, Jeffrey. "Visual Archives in Perspective: Enlarging on Historical Medical Photographs." *The American Archivist* 70, no. 1 (2007): 32–69.

Mildvan, Donna, ed. *International Atlas of AIDS*. 4th ed. Philadelphia: Springer, 2008.

AIDS. 2nd ed. Vol. 1. Atlas of Infectious Diseases. Philadelphia: Current Medicine, 1996.

AIDS. Vol. 1. Atlas of Infectious Diseases. Philadelphia: Current Medicine, 1995.

Mildvan, Donna, U. Mathur, R. W. Enlow, P. L. Romain, R. J. Winchester, C. Colp, H. Singman, B. R. Adelsberg, and I. Spigland. "Opportunistic Infections and Immune Deficiency in Homosexual Men." *Annals of Internal Medicine* 96, no. 6 (1982): 700–4.

Mindock, Clark. "'Critical Milestones' Reached for HIV Vaccine." *International Business Times*, September 9, 2016. www.ibtimes.com/cure-aids-hiv-vaccine-eyed-broadly-neutralizing-antibodies-human-mice-2413719.

Mirzoeff, Nicholas. *An Introduction to Visual Culture*. Hove, UK: Psychology Press, 1999.

Mitchell, W. J. T. "Image Science." In *Science Images and Popular Images of the Sciences*, edited by Bernd Hueppauf and Peter Weingart, pp. 55–68. New York: Routledge, 2008.

What Do Pictures Want? The Lives and Loves of Images. Chicago: University of Chicago Press, 2005.

"Showing Seeing: A Critique of Visual Culture." *Journal of Visual Culture* 1 (2002): 165–81.

Moffett, Alexander. "Generic Images of Disease: The Uses of Collective Investigation, 1880–1900." Presentation at AAHM 2015, New Haven, CT, 2015.

Monmonier, Mark. "Maps as Graphic Propaganda for Public Health." In *Imagining Illness: Public Health and Visual Culture*, edited by David Harley Serlin, 108–25. Minneapolis: University of Minnesota Press, 2010.

Monson, Thomas. "Review: International Atlas of AIDS." *JAMA: The Journal of the American Medical Association* 300, no. 5 (2008): 585–6.

Morimoto, Ryo. "Message without a Coda: On the Rhetoric of Photographic Records." *Signs and Society* 2, no. 2 (September 1, 2014): 284–313. doi:10.1086/677923.

Morris, C. N., and A. G. Ferguson. "Estimation of the Sexual Transmission of HIV in Kenya and Uganda on the Trans-Africa Highway: The Continuing Role for Prevention in High Risk Groups." *Sexually Transmitted Infections* 82, no. 5 (October 2006): 368–71. doi:10.1136/sti.2006.020933.

Morrison, Joel L. "The Science of Cartography and Its Essential Processes." *Cartographica: The International Journal for Geographic Information and Geovisualization* 14, no. 1 (1977): 58–71.

Moss, Andrew R., Peter Bacchetti, Michael Gorman, Selma Dritz, Marcus Conant, Donald Abrams, Paul Volberding, and John Ziegler. "AIDS in the 'Gay' Areas of San Francisco." *The Lancet* 321, no. 8330 (1983): 923–4. doi:10.1016/S0140-6736(83)91346-6.

Mracek, Franz. *Atlas der Syphilis und der venerischen Krankheiten mit einem Grundriss der Pathologie und Therapie derselben. Lehmann's Medicin. Handatlanten.* München: J. F. Lehmann, 1898.

Murphy, Michelle. *Sick Building Syndrome and the Problem of Uncertainty. Environmental Politics, Technoscience, and Women Workers.* Durham, NC: Duke University Press, 2006.

Nattrass, Nicoli. *The AIDS Conspiracy: Science Fights Back.* New York: Columbia University Press, 2013.

Nayler, J. R. "Clinical Photography: A Guide for the Clinician." *Journal of Postgraduate Medicine* 49, no. 3 (September 2003): 256–62.

Neuse, W. H., N. J. Neumann, P. Lehmann, T. Jansen, and G. Plewig. "The History of Photography in Dermatology: Milestones from the Roots to the 20th Century." *Archives of Dermatology* 132, no. 12 (December 1996): 1492–8.

Nguyen, Vinh-Kim. "Antiretroviral Globalism, Biopolitics, and Therapeutic Citizenship." In *Global Assemblages*, edited by Aihwa Ong and Stephen J. Collier, pp. 124–44. London: Blackwell Publishing, 2007.

Nguyen, Vinh-Kim, Pierre-Marie David, and Gabriel Girard. "AIDS and Biocapitalisation: The Ambiguities of a 'World without AIDS." *Books and Ideas*, December 11, 2015. www.booksandideas.net/AIDS-Biocapitalisation.html.

Nixon, Nicholas, and Peter Galassi, Museum of Fine Arts Boston, Detroit Institute of Arts, and San Francisco Museum of Modern Art. *Nicholas Nixon: Pictures of People.* New York: Museum of Modern Art, 1988.

Noble, Gary R. "International Conference on Acquired Immunodeficiency Syndrome: 14–17 April 1985, Atlanta, Georgia." *Annals of Internal Medicine* 103, no. 5 (November 1, 1985): 653. http://doi:10.7326/0003-4819-103-5-653.

"NOVA Online/Odyssey of Life/Behind the Lens: Interview with Lennart Nilsson." Accessed September 21, 2016. www.pbs.org/wgbh/nova/odyssey/nilsson.html.

O'Connor, Erin. "Camera Medica." *History of Photography* 23, no. 3 (September 1, 1999): 232–44. doi:10.1080/03087298.1999.10443326.

Ogdon, Bethany. "Through the Image: Nicholas Nixon's 'People with AIDS.'" *Discourse* 23, no. 3 (2001): 75–105.

Oppenheimer, Gerald M. "In the Eye of the Storm: The Epidemiological Construction of AIDS." In *AIDS: The Burdens of History*, edited by Elizabeth Fee and Daniel M. Fox, pp. 267–300. Berkeley: University of California Press, 1988.

Oppenheimer, Gerald, and Ronald Bayer. "An Epidemic of Unknown Proportions: The First Decade of HIV/AIDS." In *HIV/AIDS in the Post-HAART Era: Manifestations, Treatment, and Epidemiology*, edited by John C. Hall, Clay J. Cockerell, and Brian J. Hall, pp. 3–19. Sheldon, IA: PMPH-USA, 2011.

Orland, Barbara. "Repräsentation von Leben. Visualisierung, Embryonenmanagement und Qualitätskontrolle im reproduktionsmedizinischen Labor." In *The Picture's Image: Wissenschaftliche Visualisierung als Komposit.*, edited by Inge Hinterwaldner and Markus Buschhaus, pp. 222–42. München: Wilhelm Fink Verlag, 2006.

Ostherr, Kirsten. *Medical Visions: Producing the Patient through Film, Television and Imaging Technologies*. Oxford: Oxford University Press, 2013.

Patton, Cindy. *Globalizing AIDS*. Minneapolis: University of Minnesota Press, 2002.

"From Nation to Family: Containing African AIDS." In *The Lesbian and Gay Studies Reader*, edited by Michèle Aina Barale, David M. Halperin, and Henry Abelove, pp. 127–41. Hove, UK: Psychology Press, 1993.

Paul, Diane B., and Jeffrey P. Brosco. *The PKU Paradox: A Short History of a Genetic Disease*. Baltimore: Johns Hopkins University Press, 2013.

Paul, Gerhard, ed. *Visual History: Ein Studienbuch*. Göttingen: Vandenhoeck & Ruprecht, 2006.

Peirce, Charles Sanders. *Peirce on Signs: Writings on Semiotic*. Chapel Hill: University of North Carolina Press, 1991.

Pepin, Jacques. *The Origins of AIDS*. Cambridge: Cambridge University Press, 2011.

Pichel, Beatriz. "From Facial Expressions to Bodily Gestures: Passions, Photography and Movement in French 19th-Century Sciences." *History of the Human Sciences* 29, no. 1 (February 1, 2016): 27–48. doi:10.1177/0952695115618592.

Pinel, Philippe. *Nosographie philosophique; ou La méthode de l'analyse appliquée a la médecine*. Paris: J. A. Brosson, 1818.

Piot, P., T. C. Quinn, H. Taelman, F. M. Feinsod, K. B. Minlangu, O. Wobin, N. Mbendi, P. Mazebo, K. Ndangi, and W. Stevens. "Acquired Immunodeficiency Syndrome in a Heterosexual Population in Zaire." *Lancet* 2, no. 8394 (1984): 65–9.

Pisani, Elizabeth. *The Wisdom of Whores: Bureaucrats, Brothels and the Business of AIDS*. London: Granta Books, 2010.

Preda, Alex. *AIDS, Rhetoric, and Medical Knowledge*. Cambridge: Cambridge University Press, 2005.

Prince, Ruth J. "The Diseased Body and the Global Subject: The Circulation and Consumption of an Iconic AIDS Photograph in East Africa."

Visual Anthropology 29, no. 2 (2016): 159–86. doi:10.1080/08949468.2016 .1131517.

Quétel, Claude. *History of Syphilis.* Cambridge: Polity Press, 1990.

Rasmussen, Nicolas. *Picture Control: The Electron Microscope and the Transformation of Biology in America, 1940–1960.* Stanford, CA: Stanford University Press, 1999.

Rawling, Katherine. "'She Sits All Day in the Attitude Depicted in the Photo': Photography and the Psychiatric Patient in the Late Nineteenth Century." *Medical Humanities* 43, no. 2 (June 1, 2017): 99–100. doi:10.1136/medhum-2016-011092.

"Repercussion, N." *OED Online.* Oxford University Press, June 2018. www.oed .com/view/Entry/162762 (accessed 19/06/2018).

"Review: Color Atlas of AIDS." *The Ulster Medical Journal* 58, no. 1 (1989): 118.

Rheinberger, Hans-Jörg. "Difference Machines: Time in Experimental Systems." *Configurations* 23, no. 2 (2015): 165–76. doi:10.1353/con.2015.0013.

"Preparations, Models, and Simulations." *History and Philosophy of the Life Sciences* 36, no. 3 (January 2015): 321–34. doi:10.1007/s40656-014-0049-3.

"Experimental Systems. Historiality, Narration, and Deconstruction." In *The Science Studies Reader,* edited by Mario Biagioli, pp. 417–29. New York: Routledge, 1999.

Toward a History of Epistemic Things: Synthesizing Proteins in the Test Tube. Stanford, CA: Stanford University Press, 1997.

Roberts, Bill D. "HIV Antibody Testing Methods: 1985–1988." *Journal of Insurance Medicine* 26 (1994): 13–14.

Rodenwaldt, Ernst, ed. *Welt-Seuchen-Atlas. Weltatlas der Seuchenverbreitung und Seuchenbewegung; in drei Teilen – World-Atlas of Epidemic Diseases.* Hamburg: Falk, 1952.

Roitman, Janet. *Anti-Crisis.* Durham, NC: Duke University Press, 2013.

Rondanelli, Elio Guido, ed. *Atlante Di Clinica e Laboratorio, AIDS, Clinical and Laboratory Atlas.* Pavia, Italy: Edizioni Medico-Scientifiche, 1989.

Rosario, Vernon A. *Homosexuality and Science: A Guide to the Debates. Controversies in Science.* Santa Barbara, CA: ABC-CLIO, 2002.

Rosenberg, Charles E. "What Is an Epidemic? AIDS in Historical Perspective." In *Living with AIDS,* edited by Stephen R. Graubard, pp. 1–17. Cambridge, MA: MIT Press, 1989.

"Disease and Social Order in America: Perceptions and Expectations." *The Milbank Quarterly* 64, no. 1 (1986): 34–55.

Rosenbrock, Rolf, F. Dubois-Arber, M. Moers, P. Pinell, D. Schaeffer, and M. Setbon. "The Normalization of AIDS in Western European Countries." *Social Science and Medicine* 50, no. 11 (June 2000): 1607–29.

Rosengarten, Marsha. *HIV Interventions: Biomedicine and the Traffic between Information and Flesh.* Seattle: University of Washington Press, 2009.

Rubin, Gayle S. "Thinking Sex: Notes for a Radical Theory of the Politics of Sexuality." In *The Lesbian and Gay Studies Reader,* edited by Henry Abelove, Michele Aina Barale, and David M. Halperin, pp. 143–78. New York: Routledge, 1993.

Rupke, Nicolaas A., ed. *Medical Geography in Historical Perspective*. London: Wellcome Trust Centre for the History of Medicine at UCL, 2000.

Sauerteig, Lutz. *Krankheit, Sexualität, Gesellschaft. Geschlechtskrankheiten und Gesundheitspolitik in Deutschland im 19. und frühen 20. Jahrhundert*. Stuttgart: Steiner, 1999.

Schappach, Beate. *AIDS in Literatur, Theater und Film. Zur kulturellen Dramaturgie eines Störfalls*. Zürich: Chronos, 2012.

"AIDS-Bilder – Zur Bedeutung des Kaposi Sarkoms im AIDS-Diskurs." In *Bild und Gestalt. Wie formen Medienpraktiken das Wissen in Medizin und Humanwissenschaft?*, edited by Frank Stahnisch and Heiko Bauer, pp. 199–210. Hamburg: Wilhelm Fink Verlag, 2007.

Schlich, Thomas. "Repräsentationen von Krankheitserregern. Wie Robert Koch Bakterien als Krankheitsursache dargestellt hat." In *Räume des Wissens – Repräsentation, Codierung, Spur*, edited by Hans-Jörg Rheinberger, Michael Hagner, and Bettina Wahrig-Schmidt, pp. 165–90. Berlin: Akademie Verlag, 1997.

"'Wichtiger als der Gegenstand selbst' – Die Bedeutung des fotografischen Bildes in der Begründung der bakteriologischen Krankheitsauffassung durch Robert Koch." In *Neue Wege in der Seuchengeschichte*, edited by Martin Dinges and Thomas Schlich, pp. 143–52. Medizin, Gesellschaft und Geschichte. Stuttgart: Franz Steiner Verlag, 1995.

Schmidt, Gunnar. *Anamorphotische Körper. Medizinische Bilder vom Menschen im 19. Jahrhundert*. Köln: Böhlau, 2001.

"Todeszeichen. Zu literarischen und medizinischen Bildern im 19. Jahrhundert." In *Bildkörper. Verwandlungen des Menschen zwischen Medium und Medizin*, edited by Marianne Schuller, Claudia Reiche, and Gunnar Schmidt, pp. 47–75. Hamburg: Lit Verlag, 1998.

Schnalke, Thomas. *Diseases in Wax: The History of the Medical Moulage*. Chicago: Quintessence Publications, 1995.

"Moulagen und Photografie." *Photomed* 2 (1989): 21–4.

Schnurrer, Friedrich. "Die geographische Verteilung der Krankheiten, vorgelesen in der Versammlung der deutschen Aerzte und Naturforscher zu München den 22. Sept. 1827." *Das Ausland* 1, no. März (1828): 357–9.

Schulze, Elke. "Zeichnung und Fotografie – Statusfragen. Universitäres Zeichnen und Naturwissenschaftliche Bildfindung." *Berichte zur Wissenschaftsgeschichte* 28 (2005): 151–9.

Seckinelgin, Hakan. "The Global Governance of Success in HIV/AIDS Policy: Emergency Action, Everyday Lives and Sen's Capabilities." *Health and Place* 18, no. 3 (May 2012): 453–60. doi:10.1016/j.healthplace.2011.09.014.

Sendziuk, Paul. "Philadelphia or Death." *GLQ* 16, no. 3 (2010): 444–9.

Learning to Trust: Australian Responses to AIDS. Sydney: University of New South Wales Press, 2003.

Serlin, David Harley, ed. *Imagining Illness. Public Health and Visual Culture*. Minneapolis: University of Minnesota Press, 2010.

Serwadda, David, N. K. Sewankambo, J. W. Carswell, A. C. Bayley, R. S. Tedder, R. A. Weiss, R. D. Mugerwa et al. "Slim Disease: A New Disease in Uganda and Its Association with HTLV-III Infection." *The Lancet* 326, no. 8460 (1985): 849–52.

Shah, Nayan. *Contagious Divides: Epidemics and Race in San Francisco's Chinatown*. Berkeley: University of California Press, 2001.

Shannon, Gary W., and Gerald F. Pyle. "The Origin and Diffusion of AIDS: A View from Medical Geography." *Annals of the Association of American Geographers* 79, no. 1 (1989): 1–24.

Sheehan, Tanya. *Doctored: The Medicine of Photography in Nineteenth-Century America*. University Park: Pennsylvania State University Press, 2011.

Sick, Andrea. "Viren 'bilden.' Visualisierungen des Tabakmosaikvirus (TMV) und anderer infektiöser Agenten." In *Sichtbarkeit und Medium. Austausch, Verknüpfung und Differenz naturwissenschaftlicher und ästhetischer Bildstrategien*, edited by Anja Zimmermann, pp. 257–87. Hamburg: Hamburg University Press, 2005.

Siddique, Haroon. "Scientists Testing HIV Cure Report 'Remarkable' Progress after Patient Breakthrough." *The Guardian*, October 2, 2016. www.theguardian.com/society/2016/oct/02/scientists-testing-cure-for-hiv-report-progress.

Silverman, Sol. *Color Atlas of Oral Manifestations of AIDS*. Toronto and Philadelphia: Mosby, 1989.

Smallman-Raynor, Matthew, Andrew Cliff, and Peter Haggett, eds. *London International Atlas of AIDS*. Oxford and Cambridge: Blackwell Publishers, 1992.

Snow, John. *On the Mode of Communication of Cholera*. London: John Churchill, 1855.

Solomon, Rosalind. *Portraits in the Time of AIDS*. Edited by Grey Art Gallery & Study Center. New York.: Grey Art Gallery & Study Center, New York University, 1988.

Sonnabend, J., S. S. Witkin, and D. T. Purtilo. "Acquired Immunodeficiency Syndrome, Opportunistic Infections, and Malignancies in Male Homosexuals: A Hypothesis of Etiologic Factors in Pathogenesis." *JAMA* 249, no. 17 (1983): 2370–4. doi:10.1001/jama.1983.03330410056028.

Sontag, Susan. *Regarding the Pain of Others*. New York: Farrar, Straus and Giroux, 2003.

AIDS and Its Metaphors. New York: Farrar, Straus and Giroux, 1989.

Stahnisch, Frank, and Heiko Bauer. *Bild und Gestalt. Wie formen Medienpraktiken das Wissen in Medizin und Humanwissenschaft?* Hamburg: Lit Verlag, 2007.

Stanford, Brian. "The Hospital Photographic Department." *The Lancet* 248, no. 6418 (August 31, 1946): 299–301. doi:10.1016/S0140-6736(46)90800-8.

Stein, Claudia, and Roger Cooter. "Visual Objects and Universal Meanings: AIDS Posters and the Politics of Globalisation and History." *Medical History* 55 (2011): 85–108.

Sturdy, Steven, and Roger Cooter. "Science, Scientific Management, and the Transformation of Medicine in Britain c. 1870–1950." *History of Science* 36, no. 114 (1998): 421–66.

Stüttgen, Günter. "Edmund Lesser and the International Congress on Dermatology." *International Journal on Dermatology* 27 (1988): 269–73.

Tan, W. Y. *Stochastic Modeling of AIDS Epidemiology and HIV Pathogenesis.* London: World Scientific, 2000.

Tanne, Janice Hopkins. "Fighting AIDS: On the Front Lines against the Plague," *New York Magazine,* no. 12. February (1987).

Taussig, Michael T. "Reification and the Consciousness of the Patient." *Social Science and Medicine* 14B, no. 1 (1980): 3–13.

Tedjasukmana, Chris. *Mechanische Verlebendigung. Ästhetische Erfahrung im Kino.* Paderborn: Wilhelm Fink Verlag, 2014.

Temkin, Owsei. *The Double Face of Janus.* Baltimore and London: Johns Hopkins University Press, 1977.

Thomas, Ann, and Marta Braun, eds. *Beauty of Another Order: Photography in Science.* New Haven, CT: Yale University Press, 1997.

Thornton, Robert. *Unimagined Community: Sex, Networks, and AIDS in Uganda and South Africa.* Berkeley: University of California Press, 2008.

Tobler, Waldo R. "Analytical Cartography." *The American Cartographer* 3, no. 1 (1976): 21–31.

Treichler, Paula A. *How to Have Theory in an Epidemic: Cultural Chronicles of AIDS.* Durham, NC: Duke University Press, 1999.

"AIDS, Africa, and Cultural Theory." *Transition,* no. 51 (1991): 86–103. doi:10.2307/2935080.

"AIDS, Homophobia, and Biomedical Discourse: An Epidemic of Signification." In *AIDS, Cultural Analysis, Cultural Activism,* edited by Douglas Crimp, pp. 31–70. Cambridge, MA: MIT Press, 1988.

Tucker, Jennifer. *Nature Exposed: Photography as Eyewitness in Victorian Science.* Baltimore: Johns Hopkins University Press, 2005.

"Photography as Witness, Detective, and Impostor: Visual Representation in Victorian Science." In *Victorian Science in Context,* edited by Bernard Lightman, pp. 378–408. Chicago: University of Chicago Press, 1997.

Vaughan, Megan. *Curing Their Ills, Colonial Power and African Illness.* Cambridge: Polity Press, 1991.

Verghese, Abraham. *My Own Country: A Doctor's Story.* New York: Vintage Books, 1994.

Verghese, Abraham, Steven L. Berk, and Felix Sarubbi. "Urbs in Rure: Human Immunodeficiency Virus Infection in Rural Tennessee." *Journal of Infectious Diseases* 160, no. 6 (1989): 1051–5.

Vidler, Anthony. "Diagrams of Diagrams: Architectural Abstraction and Modern Representation." *Representations* 72 (2000): 1–20. doi:10.2307/2902906.

Virchow, Rudolf. "Ueber die Standpunkte in der Wissenschaftlichen Medicin." *Archiv für Pathologische Anatomie und Physiologie* 1 (1847): 3–19.

Von Zumbusch, Leo. *Atlas der Syphilis.* Leipzig, Germany: F. C. W. Vogel, 1922.

Wailoo, Keith. *Dying in the City of the Blues: Sickle Cell Anemia and the Politics of Race and Health.* Chapel Hill: University of North Carolina Press, 2014.

Wainer, Howard. *Picturing the Uncertain World: How to Understand, Communicate, and Control Uncertainty Through Graphical Display.* Princeton, NJ: Princeton University Press, 2011.

Waldby, Catherine. *AIDS and the Body Politic: Biomedicine and Sexual Difference.* London: Routledge, 1996.

Walsh, Fergus. "Why Talk of a Cure for HIV Is Premature." *BBC News*, October 3, 2016. www.bbc.co.uk/news/health-37545953.

Warner, John Harley. *Dissection: Photographs of a Rite of Passage in American Medicine, 1880–1930.* New York: Blast Books, 2009.

"The History of Science and the Sciences of Medicine." *Osiris* 10 (1995): 164–93.

Watney, Simon. "Photography and AIDS." In *The Critical Image: Essays on Contemporary Photography*, edited by Carol Squiers, pp. 173–92. Seattle, WA: Bay Press, 1990.

Weingart, Brigitte. "Viren visualisieren: Bildgebung und Popularisierung." In *Virus! Mutationen einer Metapher*, edited by Ruth Mayer and Brigitte Weingart, pp. 97–130. Bielefeld, Germany: Transcript Verlag, 2004.

Ansteckende Wörter, Repräsentationen von AIDS. Frankfurt am Main: Suhrkamp, 2002.

Whooley, Owen. *Knowledge in the Time of Cholera: The Struggle over American Medicine in the Nineteenth Century.* Chicago: University of Chicago Press, 2013.

Wilder, Kelley E. *Photography and Science.* Exposures. London: Reaktion, 2009.

Witkin, Joel-Peter, and Stanley Burns, eds. *Masterpieces of Medical Photography: Selection from the Burns Archive.* Pasadena, CA: Twelvetrees Press, 1987.

Worboys, Michael. *Spreading Germs: Disease Theories and Medical Practice in Britain, 1865–1900.* Cambridge: Cambridge University Press, 2000.

World Health Organization. *AIDS: Images of the Epidemic.* Geneva: World Health Organization, 1994.

"Workshop on AIDS in Central Africa." *Bangui, Central African Republic: World Health Organization*, October 22, 1985. www.who.int/hiv/strategic/en/bangui1985report.pdf?ua=1.

"Geographical Reconnaissance for Malaria Eradication Programmes." Geneva: World Health Organization, 1965. www.who.int/iris/handle/10665/70045.

Yingling, Thomas. *AIDS and the National Body.* Durham, NC: Duke University Press, 1997.

"AIDS in America: Postmodern Governance, Identity and Experience." In *Inside/out: Lesbian Theories, Gay Theories*, edited by Diana Fuss, pp. 292–310. New York: Routledge, 1991.

Ziegler, John L. "Review: Color Atlas of AIDS and HIV Diesaese." *JAMA: The Journal of the American Medical Association* 261, no. 24 (1989): 3621–2.

Index

Printed in the United States
By Bookmasters